EMERGENCY MEDICINE

PEARLS OF WISDOM

Third Edition

Jonathan Adler, M.D.

Scott H. Plantz, M.D.

Copyright © 1994 by Jonathan Adler, M.D. and Scott H. Plantz, M.D.

Printed with support from the Office of the Publisher, Harvard Medical School by Mount Auburn Press, Watertown, MA.

Distributed by Mosby-Year Book, Inc., St. Louis, MO and by Gallagher and Forsythe Ltd., Yarmouth Port, MA.

ISBN 0-8151-6798-9
987654321

Cover design by Sharon Plantz, Jonathan Adler and Scott H. Plantz. Figures by Jonathan Adler. Cover line drawing by Sharon Plantz.

This book was produced with word processing software and computer based graphics using a Macintosh® Quadra 700.

For my father, Alan Huntly Plantz, whose love, support and brilliance has always been my guiding light.

Scott

For my brothers, David and Peter, for your fellowship, love, and your wonderful extended families!

Jonathan

AUTHOR/EDITORS

Jonathan Adler, M.D.
Assistant in Emergency Medicine,
Massachusetts General Hospital
Instructor in Medicine,
Harvard Medical School
Boston, MA

Scott H. Plantz, M.D.
Assistant Director, Department of
Emergency Medicine,
Mt. Sinai Medical Center
Instructor in Medicine,
Chicago Medical School
Chicago, IL

CONTRIBUTING AUTHORS

Felix Ankel, M.D.
Assistant Professor, Emergency Medicine
University of Wisconsin Medical Center
Madison, WI

Chuck McCart, M.D.
University of Illinois
St. Francis Medical Center
Peoria, IL

Stephen Emond, M.D.
Assistant in Emergency Medicine,
Massachusetts General Hospital
Instructor in Medicine,
Harvard Medical School
Boston, MA

Tony Russo, M.D.
University of Illinois
St. Francis Medical Center
Peoria, IL

Gordon Larsen, M.D.
University of Illinois
St. Francis Medical Center
Peoria, IL

Dana Stearns, M.D.
Assistant in Emergency Medicine,
Massachusetts General Hospital
Instructor in Medicine,
Harvard Medical School
Boston, MA

Nicholas Y. Lorenzo, M.D.
Department of Neurology
Cellular Neurobiology Laboratory
Mayo Clinic
Rochester, MN

Jack "Lester" Stump, M.D.
Attending Physician, Rogue Valley
Medical Center
Medford, OR

Grant Mansell, M.D.
University of Illinois
St. Francis Medical Center
Peoria, IL

Greg Tudor, M.D.
University of Illinois
St. Francis Medical Center
Peoria, IL

CONTRIBUTING EDITORS

Timothy J. Schaefer, M.D.
Clinical Assistant Professor
University of Illinois College of Medicine
Assistant Program Director,
Emergency Medicine Residency
St. Francis Medical Center
Peoria, IL

Marc D. Squillante, D.O., FACEP
Program Director,
Emergency Medicine Residency
University of Illinois College of Medicine
St. Francis Medical Center
Peoria, IL

José M. Vega, M.D.
Assistant in Emergency Medicine,
Massachusetts General Hospital
Instructor in Medicine,
Harvard Medical School
Boston, MA

Therese M. Whitt, M.D.
Clinical Instructor of Emergency
Medicine
University of Illinois College of Medicine
St. Francis Medical Center
Peoria, IL

Joseph P. Wood, M.D., J.D.
Chairman, Department of Emergency
Medicine
Edward Hospital
Naperville, IL
Staff Physician, Department of
Emergency Medicine
EHS Christ Hospital and Medical Center
Oak Lawn, IL

Table of Contents

Introduction

Congratulations! Emergency Medicine *Pearls of Wisdom*, Third Edition, will help you learn some emergency medicine. Originally designed as a study aid to improve performance on the EM Written Boards/Recertification or EM Inservice exam, "Pearls" is full of useful information. First intended for EM specialists, we have learned that "Pearls" unique format has also been found to be useful by house officers and medical students rotating in the ED. A few words are appropriate discussing intent, format, limitations and use.

The primary intent of "Pearls" is to serve as a study aid to improve performance on the EM Written Boards/Recertification or EM Inservice Exam. To achieve this goal the text is written in rapid-fire question/answer format. Questions receive immediate gratification with a correct answer. Misleading or confusing "foils" are <u>not</u> provided. This eliminates the risk of erroneously assimilating an incorrect piece of information that made a big impression. Questions themselves often contain a pearl intended to be reinforced in association with the question/answer. Additional hooks are often attached to the answer in various forms including mnemonics, evoked visual imagery, repetition and humor. Additional information not requested in the question may be included in the answer. The same information is often sought in several different questions. Emphasis has been placed on distilling true trivia and key facts that are easily overlooked, are quickly forgotten and that somehow seem to be needed on Board exams.

Many questions have answers without explanations. This is done to enhance ease of reading and rate of learning. Explanations often occur in a later question/answer. It may happen that upon reading an answer the reader may think - "Hmm, why is <u>that</u>?!" or, "Are you sure...?!" If this happens to you, GO CHECK! Truly assimilating these disparate facts into a framework of knowledge <u>absolutely requires</u> further reading of the surrounding concepts. Information learned in response to seeking an answer to a particular question is retained much better than that passively observed. Take advantage of this! Use "Pearls" with your preferred source texts handy and open!

The short question/answer format of the First Edition has been retained. The structure of "Pearls" was enhanced significantly in the Second Edition. The most important addition was that of eighteen new Pearls Topics sections. These sections are presented in descending order of relative importance on the EM board exam. Information presented in the Pearls Topics sections is mostly limited to straightforward and more basic facts. The second section of the book consists of random pearls - questions grouped into small clusters by topic presented in no particular order. The random pearls section repeats much of the factual information contained in the Pearls Topics and builds on this foundation with greater emphasis on linking information and filling in gaps from the Pearls Topics.

A second significant format change in the Second Edition was the incorporation of questions produced by Contributing Authors. The book has also been improved by the input of Contributing Editors whose assistance will be appreciated by you, the reader. We extend heartfelt thanks on behalf of ourselves and the readers for the contributions of these individuals. The Third Edition contains several hundred additional improvements to questions.

"Pearls" has limitations (directly proportional to those of the senior editor/authors!). We have found *many* conflicts between sources of information. Variation between the definition of "apneustic" breathing provided in Tintinalli vs. Stedman's causes little consternation. Variations between half-life of paralyzing agents and of naloxone, or between rankings of stability of cervical spine fractures, provided in Tintinalli vs. Rosen are more concerning. We have tried to verify in other references the most accurate information. Some texts have internal discrepancies further confounding clarification of information.

"Pearls" risks accuracy by aggressively pruning complex concepts down to the simplest kernel - the dynamic knowledge base and clinical practice of emergency medicine is not like that! For the most part, the information taken as "correct" is that indicated in the text, Emergency Medicine A Comprehensive Study Guide, Third Edition, edited by Tintinalli, Krome and Ruiz and published in association with the American College of Emergency Physicians.

Further, new research and practice occasionally deviates from that which likely represents the "right" answer for test purposes. In such cases we have selected the information that we believe is most likely "correct" for test purposes. This text is designed to maximize your score on a test. Refer to your most current sources of information and mentors for direction for practice.

"Pearls" is designed to be used, not just read. It is an *interactive* text. Use a 3x5 card and cover the answers; attempt <u>all</u> questions.

A study method we strongly recommend is oral, group study, preferably over an extended meal or pitchers. The mechanics of this method are simple and no one ever appears stupid.

One person holds "Pearls", with answers covered, and reads the question. Each person, including the reader, says "Check!" when he or she has <u>an</u> answer in mind. After everyone has "checked" in, someone states their answer. If this answer is correct, on to the next one, if not, another person says their answer or the answer can be read. Usually the person who "checks" in first gets the first shot at stating the answer. If this person is being a smarty-pants answer-hog, then others can take turns. Try it, its almost fun!

"Pearls" is also designed to be re-used several times to allow, dare we use the word, memorization. One co-author (Plantz), a pessimist, suggests putting a check mark ✔ in each box ❐ provided every time a question is missed. Thus, three boxes have been arbitrarily provided. If you fill all three boxes on three re-uses of "Pearls", forget this question! You will get it wrong on the exam!

Another suggestion is to place a check mark when the question is answered correctly once; skip all questions with check marks thereafter. Utilize whatever scheme of using the check boxes you prefer.

We welcome your comments, suggestions and criticism. Great effort has been made to verify these questions and answers. There will be answers we have provided that are at variance with the answer you would prefer. Most often this is attributable to the variance between original sources (previously discussed). <u>Please</u> make us aware of any errata you find. We hope to make continuous improvements in a fourth edition and would greatly appreciate any input with regard to format, organization, content, presentation, or about specific questions. Leave a message with Betsy at Gallagher and Forsythe Ltd. at 508-362-7005 or fax a note to 508-362-4220. We look forward to hearing from you.

Study hard and good luck!

J.N.A & S.H.P.

CARDIOVASCULAR PEARLS

☑ ❏ ❏ ➣ **What is the most common symptom of aortic dissection?**

Interscapular back pain.

☑ ❏ ❏ ➣ **What is the most common side effect of esmolol, labetalol, and bretylium?**

Hypotension.

☑ ❏ ❏ ➣ **What side effect is expected with too rapid an infusion of procainamide?**

Hypotension. Other side effects include: myocardial depression, QRS/QT prolongation, V-fib, and torsade de pointes.

☑ ❏ ❏ ➣ **Adverse drug effects of lidocaine?**

Drowsiness, nausea, vertigo, confusion, ataxia, tinnitus, muscle twitching, respiratory depression, and psychosis.

☑ ❏ ❏ ➣ **What are the three stages of CXR findings in CHF?**

1st -   PAWP 12-18 mmHg. Blood flow increases in upper lung fields.
2nd -   PAWP 18 -25 mmHg. Interstitial edema with blurred edges of blood vessels and Kerley A and B lines.
3rd -   PAWP > 25. Fluid exudes into alveoli with generation of the classic butterfly pattern of perihilar infiltrates.

☑ ❏ ❏ ➣ **Do nitrates affect preload or afterload?**

Mostly preload.

☑ ❏ ❏ ➣ **Does hydralazine affect preload or afterload?**

Afterload.

☑ ❏ ❏ ➣ **Do prazosin, captopril, and nifedipine affect preload or afterload?**

Both.

☑ ❏ ❏ ➣ **When is dobutamine used in CHF?**

Inotrope with little vasoconstrictor action, as a result, used when heart failure is <u>not</u> accompanied by severe hypotension.

☑ ❏ ❏ ➣ **When is dopamine selected in CHF?**

Vasoconstrictor and positive inotrope, used if shock is present.

☑ ❏ ❏ ➤ **Causes of MAT?**

COPD is a common cause. CHF, sepsis, and methylxanthine toxicity are other causes, particularly among the elderly. Treat the underlying disorder. Magnesium, verapamil, and ß-adrenergic agents are thought to be helpful.

☑ ❏ ❏ ➤ **How is atrial flutter treated?**

Initiate A-V nodal blockade with ß-adrenergic or calcium channel blockers or with digoxin. If necessary, in a stable patient, attempt chemical cardioversion with a class IA agent such as procainamide or quinidine. If such treatment fails, or if patient is unstable and requires immediate electrocardioversion, do so with 25-50 J.

☑ ❏ ❏ ➤ **What are the causes of atrial fibrillation?**

Hypertension, rheumatic heart disease, thyrotoxicosis and ischemic heart disease are reasonably common causes. Pericarditis, EtOH intoxication, PE, CHF and COPD are other causes.

☑ ❏ ❏ ➤ **How is atrial fibrillation treated?**

Control rate with digitalis or verapamil then convert with procainamide, quinidine, or verapamil. Synchronized cardioversion at 100 to 200 J in an unstable patient requiring cardioversion. In a stable patient with a-fib of unclear duration anticoagulation for 2-3 wk should be considered prior to chemical or electrical cardioversion.

☑ ❏ ❏ ➤ **Causes of SVT?**

Ectopic SVT may be due to digitalis toxicity (25% of digitalis induced arrhythmias), pericarditis, MI, COPD, preexcitation syndromes, mitral valve prolapse, rheumatic heart disease, pneumonia, and EtOH.

☑ ❏ ❏ ➤ **How is SVT caused by digitalis toxicity treated?**

Stop digitalis, treat hypokalemia. Give Mg, phenytoin, or lidocaine. Provide digoxin specific antibodies in the unstable patient. Avoid cardioversion.

☑ ❏ ❏ ➤ **Treatment of SVT not caused by dig toxicity?**

Adenosine, verapamil, ß-blockers, vagal maneuvers, Mg.

☑ ❏ ❏ ➤ **Describe the key features of Mobitz I (Wenckebach) 2° AV block.**

Progressive prolongation of the PR interval until atrial impulse is not conducted. If symptomatic, atropine and transcutaneous/transvenous pacing.

☑ ❏ ❏ ➤ **Describe the features and treatment of Mobitz II 2° AV block.**

Constant PR interval. One or more beats fail to conduct. Treat with atropine and transcutaneous/transvenous pacing.

☑ ❑ ❑ ➢ **What artery is most commonly associated with embolism in mesenteric ischemia?**

Superior mesenteric artery.

☑ ❑ ❑ ➢ **Name 5 causes of mesenteric ischemia.**

Arterial thrombosis at sites of atherosclerotic plaques, emboli from left atrium in patients with a-fib or rheumatic heart disease who are not anticoagulated, arterial embolism most commonly to the superior mesenteric artery, insufficient arterial flow, and venous thrombosis.

☑ ❑ ❑ ➢ **What is the most common source for acute mesenteric ischemia.**

Arterial embolism 40-50%. Source is usually the heart, most often from a mural thrombus. Most common point of obstruction is the superior mesenteric artery.

☑ ❑ ❑ ➢ **What lab abnormalities are expected in a patient with mesenteric ischemia?**

Leukocytosis >15,000, metabolic acidosis, hemoconcentration, and elevation of phosphate and amylase.

☑ ❑ ❑ ➢ **For how long do ST and T changes persist after an episode of pain in unstable angina?**

Several hours.

☑ ❑ ❑ ➢ **What is the cause of Prinzmetal's variant angina?**

Spasm of epicardial coronary arteries.

☑ ❑ ❑ ➢ **Contraindications to ß-blockers?**

CHF, variant angina, AV block, COPD, asthma (relative), bradycardia, hypotension and IDDM.

☑ ❑ ❑ ➢ **What percentage of LV myocardium must be damaged to cause cardiogenic shock?**

40%. 25% results in heart failure.

☑ ❑ ❑ ➢ **What percentage of MI's are clinically unrecognized?**

About 5 - 10%.

☑ ❑ ❑ ➢ **What may a new systolic murmur indicate in a patient with an AMI?**

Ventriculoseptal rupture or mitral regurgitation as a result of papillary muscle rupture or dysfunction.

☑ ☐ ☐ ➤ **A non-Q-wave infarction is associated with:**

Non-Q-wave infarctions are more commonly associated with subsequent angina or recurrent infarction. They also have a lower in-hospital mortality than Q-wave MIs.

☑ ☐ ☐ ➤ **Why do T waves invert in an AMI?**

Infarction or ischemia causes a reversal of the sequence of repolarization (endocardial-to-epicardial as opposed to normal epicardial-to-endocardial).

☑ ☐ ☐ ➤ **What ECG changes are seen in a true posterior infarction?**

Large R-wave and ST depression in V1 and V2.

☑ ☐ ☐ ➤ **What conduction defects are commonly seen in an AWMI?**

The dangerous kind. Damage to the conducting system results in a Mobitz II 2° or in a 3° AVB.

☑ ☐ ☐ ➤ **What conduction defects are commonly seen in an IWMI?**

IWMI affects the autonomic fibers in the atrial septum which increases vagal tone and impairs AV nodal conduction; 1° AV block and Mobitz type I 2° (Wenckebach) AV block are common.

☑ ☐ ☐ ➤ **How quickly will a Technetium - 99 pyrophosphate scan show infarcted myocardial tissue?**

A "hot spot" will show up in 10 to 12 h. Sensitivity is higher with Q-wave infarctions.

☑ ☐ ☐ ➤ **How should PSVT be treated during an AMI?**

Vagal maneuvers, adenosine, or cardioversion. Stable patients may be able to tolerate verapamil or even ß-adrenergic blockers which are negative inotropes.

☑ ☐ ☐ ➤ **A patient presents 1 day after discharge for an AMI with a new harsh systolic murmur along the left sternal border and pulmonary edema. Diagnosis?**

Ventricular septal rupture. Diagnosis is confirmed with Swanz-Ganz catheterization or echo. Treatment includes nitroprusside for afterload reduction and possible intra-aortic balloon pump.

☑ ☐ ☐ ➤ **In a patient who has suffered an AMI, when would cardiac rupture be expected?**

50% in the 1st 5 d and 90% within the 1st 14 d post MI.

☑ ❑ ❑ ➤ **What type of infarct commonly leads to papillary muscle dysfunction?**

IWMI. Signs and symptoms include a mild transient systolic murmur and pulmonary edema.

☑ ❑ ❑ ➤ **A patient presents 2 wk post AMI with chest pain, fever, and pleuropericarditis. A pleural effusion is seen on CXR. Diagnosis?**

Dressler's (postmyocardial infarction) syndrome which is caused by an immunologic reaction to myocardial antigens.

☑ ❑ ❑ ➤ **Can patients be retreated with streptokinase or APSAC?**

Antibodies persist for 6 mo. Retreatment is not recommended.

☑ ❑ ❑ ➤ **What type of thrombolytic agent is fibrin specific?** *TPA*

Tissue plasminogen activator. It is a human protein with no antigenic properties.

☑ ❑ ❑ ➤ **What side effects are seen with urokinase?**

Shaking chills which respond to meperidine and Benadryl. Allergic reactions and hypotension are not commonly seen.

☑ ❑ ❑ ➤ **What maneuvers will increase hypertrophic cardiomyopathy murmurs?**

↓VR

Valsalva, standing, and amyl nitrate.

☑ ❑ ❑ ➤ **What maneuvers will decrease hypertrophic cardiomyopathic murmurs?**

Handgrip, squatting and leg elevation in the supine patient. *↑VR*

☑ ❑ ❑ ➤ **What is the most common symptom of acute pericarditis?**

Sharp or stabbing retrosternal or precordial chest pain. Pain increases when supine and decreases when sitting-up and leaning forward. Pain may be increased with movement and deep breaths. Other symptoms include fever, dyspnea described as pain with inspiration, and dysphagia.

☑ ❑ ❑ ➤ **What physical findings are associated with acute pericarditis?**

Pericardial friction rub is the most common. Rub is best heard at the left sternal border or apex in a sitting leaning forward position. Other findings include fever and tachycardia.

☑ ❑ ❑ ➤ **What ECG changes are seen in acute pericarditis?**

ST segment elevation in the precordial leads, especially V5 and V6 and in lead I. PR depression is seen in leads II, aVF, V4-V6.

☑ ❑ ❑ ➢ **What percentage patients with angiogram proven pulmonary embolism have an initial ventilation-perfusion scan reported as low probability.**

12%!

☑ ❑ ❑ ➢ **What are the most common symptoms and signs of PE?**

CP (90%).
Tachypnea (90%).
Dyspnea (80%).
Anxiety (60%).
Fever (30%).
Tachycardia (30%).
DVT (30%).
Hypotension (25%).
Syncope (10-20%).

☑ ❑ ❑ ➢ **Can a patient with a PE have a PaO_2 greater than 90 mmHg?**

About 5% have a PaO_2 > 90 mmHg.

☑ ❑ ❑ ➢ **What is the most common CXR finding in PE?**

Elevated dome of one hemidiaphragm as a result of decreased lung volume observed in 50% of PEs. Other common findings include pleural effusions, atelectasis, and pulmonary infiltrates.

☑ ❑ ❑ ➢ **What are two relatively specific findings in PE on CXR?**

Hampton's Hump - Area of lung consolidation with a rounded border facing the hilus. Westermark's sign - Dilated pulmonary outflow tract ipsilateral to the emboli with decreased perfusion distal to the lesion.

☑ ❑ ❑ ➢ **What does a normal perfusion scan rule out?**

Rules out a PE. An abnormal scan can be caused by PE, asthma, emphysema, bronchitis, pneumonia, pleural effusion, carcinoma, CHF, and atelectasis.

☑ ❑ ❑ ➢ **What does normal ventilation with decreased perfusion suggest?**

PE.

☑ ❑ ❑ ➢ **What are some of the indications for pulmonary angiography in a patient thought to have a PE?**

1. Patients at high risk for bleeding complications with anticoagulation.
2. Negative test for DVT and low or medium probability lung scans.
3. Unstable patients for whom fibrinolytic therapy is being considered.

☑ ❑ ❑ ➢ **What is the most common cause of mitral stenosis?**

Rheumatic heart disease. The most common initial symptom is dyspnea.

❑ ❑ ❑ ➣ **What is the earliest chest x-ray finding seen with mitral stenosis?**

Straightening of the left heart border as a result of left atrial enlargement.

❑ ❑ ❑ ➣ **What physical findings may be found with mitral stenosis?**

Prominent a-wave, early-systolic left parasternal lift, 1st heart sound is loud and snapping, and early-diastolic opening snap with a low-pitched, mid-diastolic rumble that crescendos into S1.

❑ ❑ ❑ ➣ **What are the most common causes of acute mitral regurgitation?**

Rupture of the chordae tendineae, rupture of the papillary muscles, or perforation of the valve leaflets. Common causes include AMI and infectious endocarditis.

❑ ❑ ❑ ➣ **What are the two most common causes of valvular aortic stenosis?**

Rheumatic heart disease or congenital bicuspid valve.

❑ ❑ ❑ ➣ **What triad of symptoms is characteristic of aortic stenosis?**

Syncope, angina, and left heart failure. As the disease progresses, systolic BP decreases and pulse pressure narrows.

❑ ❑ ❑ ➣ **What are the signs and symptoms of acute aortic regurgitation?**

Dyspnea, tachycardia, tachypnea, and chest pain. Causes include: infectious endocarditis, acute rheumatic fever, trauma, spontaneous rupture of valve leaflets, or aortic dissection.

❑ ❑ ❑ ➣ **What physical findings are characteristic of chronic aortic regurgitation?**

Bobbing of the head with systole, bounding carotid pulse (water-hammer), pistol shot sound, the to-and-fro murmur of Duroziez's sign over the femoral arteries, and capillary pulsation of the nailbeds (Quincke's sign).

❑ ❑ ❑ ➣ **What is the most common cause of tricuspid stenosis?**

Rheumatic heart disease.

❑ ❑ ❑ ➣ **A patient presents to the ED 10 d after placement of a mechanical prosthetic valve with fever, chills, and a leukocytosis. Endocarditis is suspected. What type of bacterium is most common?**

Staphylococci or Gram-negative rods. Delayed endocarditis is most commonly caused by Strep. viridans or Staphylococcus epidermidis.

❑ ❑ ❑ ➣ **Define a hypertensive emergency.**

8

Increased BP with associated end-organ dysfunction or damage. A controlled drop in BP over one h should be attempted.

☑ ❑ ❑ ➤ **Define a hypertensive urgency.**

BP elevated to dangerous level, typically a diastolic greater than 115 mmHg. Gradually reduce BP over 24 to 48 h.

☑ ❑ ❑ ➤ **Define uncomplicated hypertension.**

Diastolic BP less than 115 mmHg with no symptoms of end-organ damage. Does not require acute treatment.

❑ ❑ ❑ ➤ **What lab findings would suggest a hypertensive emergency?**

UA - RBCs, red cell casts, and proteinuria.
BUN and CR - elevated.
X-ray - Aortic dissection, pulmonary edema, or coarctation of the aorta.
ECG - LVH and cardiac ischemia.

❑ ❑ ❑ ➤ **What are the signs and symptoms of hypertensive encephalopathy?**

Nausea, vomiting, headache, lethargy, coma, blindness, nerve palsies, hemiparesis, aphasia, retinal hemorrhage, cotton wool spots, exudates, sausage linking, and papilledema. Treat with labetalol or sodium nitroprusside, lower the mean arterial pressure to approximately 120 mmHg.

❑ ❑ ❑ ➤ **In general, how quickly should severe elevations in BP (>210/130) be treated?**

Initial diastolic decrease of 20 - 30% over 30 to 60 min.

❑ ❑ ❑ ➤ **At what point does magnesium sulfate become toxic?**

Loss of reflexes occurs at levels >8 mEq/l and respiratory arrest at levels >12 mEq/l.

☑ ❑ ❑ ➤ **Can eclampsia occur post-partum?**

YES. Up to 2 weeks.

☑ ❑ ❑ ➤ **What two drugs are used to treat eclampsia?**

Magnesium sulfate 4 to 6 g bolus IV followed by a 2 g/h infusion as well as hydralazine 10 to 20 mg IV. Labetalol may also be used.

☑ ❑ ❑ ➤ **What antihypertensives should be avoided in patients with a history of CHF?**

Hydralazine, diazoxide, and labetalol.

☑ ❑ ❑ ➤ **What drugs should be used to lower BP in a patient with thoracic aortic dissection?**

Sodium nitroprusside, propranolol, and trimethaphan.

☑ ❏ ❏ ➤ **A patient presents with a history of episodic elevations in BP. She complains of headache, diarrhea, and skin flushing. Diagnosis.**

Pheochromocytoma.

☑ ❏ ❏ ➤ **A patient with a psychiatric history taking a MAO inhibitor, has ingested a 12 pack of beer with a meal of pickled herring and a nice aged cheese. He complains of severe headache. On exam, BP is elevated. A diagnosis of acute hypertension is made secondary to hyperstimulation of the adrenergic receptors. Treatment?**

An α- and ß-adrenergic antagonist such as labetalol.

☑ ❏ ❏ ➤ **What drug can be used for all hypertensive emergencies?**

Sodium nitroprusside (not DOC for eclampsia). Sodium nitroprusside works through production of cGMP which relaxes smooth muscle. This results in decreased preload and afterload, decreased oxygen demand, slight increased heart rate with no change in myocardial blood flow, cardiac output, or renal blood flow. Duration of action is 1 to 2 min. Sometimes, ß-blockade is required to treat rebound tachycardia.

☑ ❏ ❏ ➤ **What is the most common complication of nitroprusside?**

Hypotension. Thiocyanate toxicity with blurred vision, tinnitus, change in mental status, muscle weakness, and seizures is seen more often in patients with renal failure and after prolonged infusions. Cyanide toxicity is uncommon, it may occur with hepatic dysfunction, after prolonged infusions, and in rates greater than 10 μg/kg per minute.

☑ ❏ ❏ ➤ **A patient presents with sudden onset chest pain and back pain. Further work-up reveals an ischemic right leg. Diagnosis?**

Suspect an acute aortic dissection when chest or back pain is associated with ischemic or neurologic defects.

☑ ❏ ❏ ➤ **What physical findings are suspicious for acute aortic dissection?**

BP differences between arms, cardiac tamponade, and aortic insufficiency murmur. An abnormal ECG may also be present.

☑ ❏ ❏ ➤ **What CXR findings occur with a thoracic aortic aneurysm?**

Change in appearance of aorta, mediastinal widening, hump in the aortic arch, pleural effusion (most common on the left), and extension of the aortic shadow.

☑ ❏ ❏ ➤ **How are Stanford type A and B aortic dissections defined and treated?**

Type A - Ascending, proximal to left subclavian (Debakey I & II) - surgery.
Type B - Descending, distal to left subclavian (Debakey III) - usually medical treatment.

☑ ❏ ❏ ➤ A 74 y old male presents with acute onset testicular pain. Ecchymosis is present in the groin and scrotal sac. Diagnosis?

Ruptured aortic or iliac artery aneurysm.

☑ ❏ ❏ ➤ In a patient with an abdominal mass and a suspected ruptured AAA, what x-ray study should be ordered?

None. They should go to the OR ASAP. About 60% of AAA's will have calcification and appear on lateral abdominal x-ray.

☑ ❏ ❏ ➤ What percentage of patients beyond the age of 80 experience CP with a AMI?

50% experience CP. 20% experience diaphoresis, stroke, syncope, and/or acute confusion.

☑ ❏ ❏ ➤ In a patient with substantial aortic stenosis, what murmur would be expected?

Prolonged, harsh, loud (IV, V, or VI) systolic murmur.

❏ ❏ ❏ ➤ What historical findings suggest an embolus vs. a thrombosis in a lower extremity?

Embolus - arrhythmia, valvular disease, MI, no skin changes of chronic arterial insufficiency, and no symptoms in the opposite extremity.
Thrombosis - opposite extremity shows evidence of chronic arterial occlusive disease with history of rest pain claudication, etc.

☑ ❏ ❏ ➤ How is thrombus vs. embolus distinguished on arteriogram?

Thrombus - tapering lumen. Embolus - sharp cutoff.

☑ ❏ ❏ ➤ What is the risk of PE in a patient with an axillary or subclavian vein thrombus?

The risk of PE is about 15%.

❏ ❏ ❏ ➤ Rheumatic heart disease is the most common cause of stenosis of what 3 heart valves?

Mitral, aortic (along with congenital bicuspid valve) and tricuspid.

TRAUMA PEARLS

"The only missing clotting factor is silk."

Donald Trunkey, M.D.

☑ ☐ ☐ ➤ **A radial pulse on exam indicates a BP of at least ____.**

80 mmHg.

☑ ☐ ☐ ➤ **A femoral pulse on exam indicates a BP of at least____.**

70 mm Hg.

☑ ☐ ☐ ➤ **A carotid pulse indicates a BP of at least____.**

60 mm Hg.

☑ ☐ ☐ ➤ **What is the most common long bone fractured?**

The tibia.

☑ ☐ ☐ ➤ **A trauma patient presents with decreasing level of consciousness and an enlarging right pupil. Diagnosis?**

Probable uncal herniation with oculomotor nerve compression.

☑ ☐ ☐ ➤ **The corneal reflex tests?**

Ophthalmic branch (V_1) of the trigeminal (5th) nerve afferent and the facial (7th) nerve efferent.

☑ ☐ ☐ ➤ **Name five clinical signs of basilar skull fracture.**

Periorbital ecchymosis (raccoon's eyes), retroauricular ecchymosis (Battle's sign), otorrhea or rhinorrhea, hemotympanum or bloody ear discharge, and 1st, 2nd, 7th, and 8th CN deficits.

☑ ☐ ☐ ➤ **A trauma patient presents with anisocoria, neurological deterioration, and/or lateralizing motor findings. Treatment?**

Mannitol 1 g/kg infused rapidly. (Avoid if hypovolemic). Elevate head of bed 30°. Some authors recommend dexamethasone 1 mg/kg, and phenytoin 18 mg/kg at 20 mg/min.

☑ ☐ ☐ ➤ **How is posterior column function tested and why is it significant?**

Position and vibration sensation are carried in the posterior columns and are usually spared in anterior cord syndrome. Light touch sensation may also be spared. Pain and temperature sensation cross near the level of entry and are carried in the more posterior spinothalamic tract.

❑ ❑ ❑ ➤ **What is the most common cause of upper airway obstruction in a comatose patient?**

Tongue prolapse into the pharynx.

❑ ❑ ❑ ➤ **At what point of airway obstruction will inspiratory stridor become evident?**

70% occlusion.

❑ ❑ ❑ ➤ **What is the most common cause of shock in patients with blunt chest trauma?**

Pelvic or extremity fractures.

❑ ❑ ❑ ➤ **What nerve should be avoided during pericardiotomy?**

Open the pericardium vertically, anterior (medial) to the phrenic nerve. The nerve runs along the superolateral aspect of the pericardium.

❑ ❑ ❑ ➤ **Differential diagnosis of distended neck veins in a trauma patient?**

Tension pneumothorax, pericardial tamponade, air embolism, and cardiac failure. Neck vein distention may not be present until hypovolemia has been treated.

❑ ❑ ❑ ➤ **A trauma patient presents with a "rocking-horse" type of ventilation. Diagnosis?**

Probable high spinal cord injury with intercostal muscle paralysis.

❑ ❑ ❑ ➤ **What should be checked prior to inserting a chest tube in an intubated patient with respiratory distress and decreased breath sounds on one side?**

Position of the ET tube.

❑ ❑ ❑ ➤ **Should a chest tube be placed into a bullet hole apparent in the 4th lateral interspace?**

No. The tube might follow the bullet track into the diaphragm or lung.

❑ ❑ ❑ ➤ **A trauma patient presents with subcutaneous emphysema. Diagnosis?**

Pneumothorax or pneumomediastinum; if emphysema is severe, consider a major bronchial injury.

❑ ❑ ❑ ➤ **A pneumothorax is suspected but does not show up on PA and Lat CXR. What**

other x-rays should be considered?

Expiratory films.   A pneumothorax is usually best seen on expiratory films.

❑ ❑ ❑ ➢ **What rib fracture has the worst prognosis?**

First rib. First and second rib fractures are associated with bronchial tears, vascular injury, and myocardial contusions.

❑ ❑ ❑ ➢ **What cardiovascular injury is commonly associated with sternal fractures?**

Myocardial contusions (blunt myocardial injury).

❑ ❑ ❑ ➢ **How much fluid needs to collect in the chest to be seen on decubitus or upright chest x-rays?**

200 to 300 ml; if supine, greater than 1 liter may be necessary to be seen on AP CXR.

❑ ❑ ❑ ➢ **Describe Beck's triad.**

Muffled heart tones, hypotension, and distended neck veins.   Causes include: myocardial contusion, AMI, pericardial tamponade, and tension pneumothorax. Tamponade may also cause pulsus paradoxus and distention of neck veins during inspiration. Total electrical alternans is highly specific for pericardial tamponade.

❑ ❑ ❑ ➢ **Which valve is most commonly injured with blunt trauma?**

Aortic valve.

❑ ❑ ❑ ➢ **What is the most likely cause of a new systolic murmur and ECG infarct pattern observed in a patient with chest trauma?**

Ventricular septal defect.

❑ ❑ ❑ ➢ **With a myocardial contusion (blunt myocardial injury), when should the CPK-MB peak?**

About 18 to 24 h.

❑ ❑ ❑ ➢ **What is the most accurate plain film x-ray finding indicating traumatic rupture of the aorta?**

Deviation of the esophagus > 2 cm right of the spinous process of T4.

❑ ❑ ❑ ➢ **What is the basic disorder contributing to the pathophysiology of compartment syndrome ?**

Increased pressure within closed tissue spaces compromising blood flow to muscle & nerve tissue. There are three prerequisites to the development of compartment syndrome:

1) Limiting space.
2) Increased tissue pressure.
3) Decreased tissue perfusion.

☐ ☐ ☐ ➤ **What are the two basic mechanisms for elevated compartment pressure?**

1) External compression -- by burn eschar, dressings, splints, or casts.
2) Volume increase within the compartment -- hemorrhage into the compartment, IV infiltration, or post-ischemic swelling.

☐ ☐ ☐ ➤ **Which long bone fracture is most commonly associated with compartment syndrome?**

The tibia, resulting most often in anterior compartment involvement.

☐ ☐ ☐ ➤ **What are the general signs & symptoms of compartment syndrome?**

Pain, paralysis (or weakness), paresthesia, pallor, then pulselessness. The compartment is tense too.

☐ ☐ ☐ ➤ **What are the four compartments of the leg?**

Anterior, lateral, deep posterior, and superficial posterior compartments.

☐ ☐ ☐ ➤ **What signs & symptoms would be noted for a compartment syndrome involving the superficial posterior compartment of the leg?**

Pain on foot dorsi/plantar - flexion and hypesthesia of the lateral foot (sural nerve).

☐ ☐ ☐ ➤ **What signs & symptoms would be noted for a compartment syndrome involving the deep posterior compartment of the leg?**

Pain on foot eversion or toe dorsiflexion and hypesthesia of plantar surface of foot.

☑ ☐ ☐ ➤ **What intracompartmental pressure raises concern?**

It is generally agreed that > 30 mm Hg mandates fasciotomy, however in patients who are unreliable (i. e. with altered level of consciousness) > 20 mm Hg requires surgical consultation.

☐ ☐ ☐ ➤ **What are the two major wounding mechanisms of ballistic injuries?**

Tissue crush and tissue stretch. Crush creates a permanent cavity; the degree of crush is largely determined by the missile. Stretch is primarily determined by the tissue itself.

☐ ☐ ☐ ➤ **What bullet characteristics determine the degree of tissue crushing?**

Yaw, deformation, & fragmentation (of missile and bone). These three factors determine the surface area of the missile(s) and subsequent tissue damage.

☑ ☐ ☐ ➢ **Why are civilian bullets usually more damaging than military bullets?**

Military bullets are usually jacketed and are less prone to fragmentation/"mushrooming" than hollow/soft point civilian bullets.

☑ ☐ ☐ ➢ **Which tissues are more prone to significant wounding due to temporary cavitation?**

Less elastic tissues such as brain, spleen & liver; fluid-filled organs such as bladder, bowel, and heart; and dense tissue such as bone.

☑ ☐ ☐ ➢ **Why do simple through-and-through wounds of the extremities fare well regardless of velocity of bullet?**

The short path in the tissue results in:
1) little or no deformation of slower bullets,
2) less time for higher velocity bullet to yaw, thereby resulting in a lesser degree of tissue damage.

☑ ☐ ☐ ➢ **Is the heat of firing significant enough to sterilize a bullet and its wound?**

No, contaminants from body surface & from viscera can be carried along the bullet's path.

☑ ☐ ☐ ➢ **What features of the brain/skull result in higher severity of head wounds?**

The brain is highly sensitive to cavitation due to poor elasticity & cohesiveness, enclosure of calvarium contains the cavitation forces.
Also, the brain is really important in most people and causes a lot of problems when it is shot.

☑ ☐ ☐ ➢ **What anatomic locations of bullets/pellets are associated with lead intoxication?**

Within bursa, joints, or disc spaces.

☑ ☐ ☐ ➢ **Other than lead intoxication, why should intraarticular bullets be removed?**

Potential for lead synovitis leading to severe damage of articular cartilage.

☑ ☐ ☐ ➢ **What causes a boutonnière deformity?**

A disruption of the extensor hood at the PIP joint in the hand.

☑ ☐ ☐ ➢ **Describe a Gamekeeper's thumb.**

Disruption of the ulnar collateral ligament of the MP joint of the thumb (stress testing showing > 20° opening indicates need for surgical repair).

☑ ☐ ☐ ➢ **For which condition does Finkelstein's test test?**

Tenosynovitis of the extensor pollicis brevis & abductor pollicis (DeQuervan's stenosing tenosynovitis).

✓☐☐ ➤ **What is the treatment of a felon?**

10 - 12 with time-off for good behavior.
A felon is a subcutaneous infection of the pulp space of the fingertip, usually S. aureus; treat by incising the pulp space.

✓☐☐ ➤ **What is a paronychia?**

An infection of the lateral nail fold. Usually from S. aureus or Streptococcus. Treat with I&D followed by warm soaks.

✓☐☐ ➤ **Describe Tinel's and Phalen's tests.**

Tinel's - Tapping the volar aspect of the wrist over the median nerve produces paresthesia's that extend along the index & long finger.
Phalen's - Full flexion at the wrist for one minute leads to paresthesia along distribution of median nerve. Both test for carpal tunnel syndrome.

✓☐☐ ➤ **What are the three most common carpal fractures?**

The scaphoid, dorsal chip (triquetrum), and the lunate. All may be 2° falls on an outstretched hand. The scaphoid is the most common.

✓☐☐ ➤ **What is Keinbach's disease?**

Avascular necrosis of the lunate with collapse of the lunate secondary to fracture. As with a navicular (scaphoid) fracture, initial wrist x-rays may not demonstrate the fracture. Therefore, tenderness over the lunate warrants immobilization.

✓☐☐ ➤ **Which bone is most commonly fractured at birth?**

The clavicle.

✓☐☐ ➤ **Most common shoulder dislocation?**

Anterior (95%).

✓☐☐ ➤ **A patient cannot actively abduct her shoulder. What injury does this suggest?**

Rotator cuff tear. The cuff is comprised of the supraspinatus, infraspinatus, subscapularis, and the teres minor muscles and tendons.

✓☐☐ ➤ **Why is the displaced supracondylar fracture (of distal humerus) in a child considered a true emergency?**

The injury often results in injury to brachial artery or median nerve.

☑ ☐ ☐ ➤ **What is the significance of the fat pad sign with an elbow injury?**

Fat pad sign or radiolucency just anterior to the distal humerus is indicative of effusion or hemarthrosis of the elbow joint; this suggests an occult fracture of the radial head.

☑ ☐ ☐ ➤ **Define increased intracranial pressure.**

ICP > than 15 mmHg.

☑ ☐ ☐ ➤ **What is the most common site of a basilar skull fracture?**

Petrous portion of the temporal bone.

☑ ☐ ☐ ➤ **What is the most common artery involved with an epidural hematoma?**

Meningeal artery, specifically the middle.

☑ ☐ ☐ ➤ **Where are epidural hematomas located?**

Between the dura and inner table of the skull.

☑ ☐ ☐ ➤ **Where are subdural hematomas located?**

Beneath the dura and over the brain and arachnoid. Caused by tears of pial arteries or of bridging veins. Subdurals typically become symptomatic within 24 h to 2 wk after injury.

☑ ☐ ☐ ➤ **For a trauma victim, which test is most helpful for evaluating retroperitoneal organs?**

CT.

☑ ☐ ☐ ➤ **How should a DPL be performed in a trauma victim with a fractured pelvis?**

Supraumbilical incision to avoid pelvic hematoma.

☑ ☐ ☐ ➤ **Absolute contraindication to DPL?**

None.
Relative contraindications: clear indication for laparotomy, previous abdominal surgery and gravid uterus (use open technique).

☑ ☐ ☐ ➤ **What findings represent a positive DPL in blunt trauma?**

RBC > 100,000 cells/mm^3, WBC > 500 cells/mm^3, bile, bacteria, or vegetable material.

☑ ☐ ☐ ➤ **What clues are evident with duodenal injury?**

Increased serum amylase and retroperitoneal free air.

❑ ❑ ❑ ➢ **What is the most frequently injured organ with blunt trauma?**

Spleen.

❑ ❑ ❑ ➢ **What is Kehr's sign?**

Left shoulder pain with splenic rupture.

❑ ❑ ❑ ➢ **What type of injury most commonly damages the pancreas?**

Penetrating.

❑ ❑ ❑ ➢ **Inability to pass a nasogastric tube in a trauma victim suggests damage to what organ?**

Diaphragm, usually on the left.

❑ ❑ ❑ ➢ **What type of contrast medium should be used to evaluate the esophagus if traumatic injury is suspected?**

Gastrograffin.

❑ ❑ ❑ ➢ **Describe the 3 zones of the neck and their evaluation?**

I -   Below the cricoid cartilage - Arteriogram.

II-   Between the cricoid and the mandible - Surgery. "2 surgery!"

III -   Above the angle of the mandible - Arteriogram.

❑ ❑ ❑ ➢ **A stress fracture is suspected, but none is found on initial x-rays. How long before a 2nd set of x-rays will likely be positive?**

10 - 14 d.

❑ ❑ ❑ ➢ **The three steps of bone healing after a fracture are:**

Union - consolidation - remodeling.

❑ ❑ ❑ ➢ **How long after a fracture does callus start to form?**

5 - 7 d.

❑ ❑ ❑ ➢ **The most common Salter-Harris class fracture?**

Type II. A triangular fracture involving the metaphysis and an epiphyseal separation.

❑ ❑ ❑ ➢ **What tarsal bone is most commonly fractured?**

Calcaneus (60%). Calcaneal fractures are commonly associated with lumbar compression injuries (10%).

□ □ □ ➢ **The tarsal-metatarsal joint is also called:**

Lisfranc's joint.

□ □ □ ➢ **The second metatarsal is the locking mechanism of the mid-part of the foot. A fracture at the base of the second metatarsal should raise suspicion of:**

A disrupted joint - treatment may require ORIF.

□ □ □ ➢ **What is a ballet fracture?**

An avulsion fracture at the base of the 5th metatarsal usually secondary to plantar flexion and inversion.

□ □ □ ➢ **What is the 2nd most common foot fracture?**

Talus.

□ □ □ ➢ **What is the most common metatarsal fracture?**

5th.

□ □ □ ➢ **What is the most common foot fracture?**

Calcaneus.

□ □ □ ➢ **Which patellar fracture requires orthopedic consultation?**

Displaced transverse fracture, comminuted fractures, and open fractures.

□ □ □ ➢ **What is the most common mechanism for fractures of the femoral condyles?**

Direct trauma, fall or blow to the distal femur.

□ □ □ ➢ **Of tibial plateau fractures, where is the most common site?**

Lateral, more common in the older population, usually presenting with swollen painful knee and limited range of motion.

□ □ □ ➢ **With complete rupture of medial or collateral ligaments, how much laxity is expected on exam?**

>1 cm without endpoint as compared to uninjured knee.

□ □ □ ➢ **What is the most common ligamentous injury to the knee?**

Anterior cruciate ligament, usually from non-contact injury.

➤ **Why 'tap' a knee with an acute hemarthrosis?**

Relieve pressure and pain and see if fat globules are present indicating a fracture.

➤ **How would you 'un-lock' a 'locked' knee?**

Hang leg over table at 90 degree flexion, allow relaxation and apply longitudinal traction with internal and external rotation.

➤ **Where is the most common site of compartment syndrome?**

Anterior compartment of the leg - contains tibialis anteriorus, extensor digitorum longus, extensor hallucis longus, and peroneus muscles, as well as anterior tibial artery and deep peroneal nerve.

➤ **Who gets Achilles' tendon rupture?**

Middle aged men most commonly on the left side.

➤ **Where is the most common site for a palpable defect of Achilles' tendon?**

2 - 6 cm proximal to its insertion.

➤ **What are the most common lower extremity injuries to bone in children?**

Tibial and fibular shaft fractures, usually secondary to twist forces.

➤ **What radiograph would one order with suspected patellar fracture in a child?**

Standard radiographs including patellar or "sunrise" views, plus comparison radiographs of uninvolved knee.

➤ **What are the differences between Osgood-Schlatter disease and avulsion of tibial tubercle?**

Both occur at tibial tubercle, avulsion presents with acute inability to walk, lateral view of the knee is most diagnostic, treatment is surgical.
Osgood-Schlatter's has vague history of intermittent pain, is bilateral in 25% of cases, has pain with range of motion but not with rest; treatment is symptomatic and not surgical.

➤ **What is a toddler fracture?**

Common cause of limp or refusal to walk in this age group is a spiral fracture of the tibia without fibular involvement.

➤ **What is the most common cause of a painful hip joint in infants?**

Septic arthritis. Staphylococcus is the most common cause in infancy. Hip usually abducted, flexed, and externally rotated.

☑ ☐ ☐ ➢ **Most common cause of painful hip in older children?**

Transient synovitis.

☐ ☐ ☐ ➢ **8 y old male presents with a limp. On exam, hip range of motion is decreased. What rare disease should be considered?**

Children 5 - 9 y may get idiopathic avascular necrosis of the femoral heal (Legg-Calvé-Perthes Disease).

☑ ☐ ☐ ➢ **Describe a common patient with a slipped capital femoral epiphysis?**

Obese boy, age 10 to 16 y. Groin or knee discomfort increases with activity; may have a limp. Often bilateral. The slip is best seen on a lateral view.

☑ ☐ ☐ ➢ **What is the most important complication of a proximal tibial metaphyseal fracture?**

Arterial involvement, especially when there is a valgus deformity.

☑ ☐ ☐ ➢ **What is the most common ankle injury?**

75% of ankle injuries are sprains with 90% of these involving the lateral complex. 90% of lateral ligament injuries are anterior talofibular.

☑ ☐ ☐ ➢ **What is the most helpful physical exam test for anterior talofibular ligament injury?**

Anterior drawer test, >3 mm of excursion might be significant (compare sides), >1 cm is always significant.

☐ ☐ ☐ ➢ **How are sprains classified?**

1st° - stretching of ligament, normal x-ray.
2nd° - severe stretching with partial tear, marked tenderness swelling and pain with weight bearing, normal x-ray (now stressed).
3rd° - complete tendon rupture, no weight bearing possible, marked tenderness, swelling and obviously deformed joint. X-ray shows abnormal talus-mortise relationship.

☑ ☐ ☐ ➢ **What is unique about avulsion fractures at the base of the fifth metatarsal?**

It is one of the most commonly missed fractures, history is of ankle injury from plantar flexion and inversion.

☐ ☐ ☐ ➢ **A 21 y old female complains of pain and 'clicking' sound located at the posterior lateral malleolus. You sense a 'fullness' beneath the lateral malleolus. Dx?**

Peroneal tendon subluxation, with associated tenosynovitis.

❑ ❑ ❑ ➢ **What percentage of distal tibial (medial malleolus) fractures treated closed result in non-union?**

10 - 15%.

❑ ❑ ❑ ➢ **Traumatic arthritis occurs in what percentage of ankle fractures?**

20 - 40%.

❑ ❑ ❑ ➢ **Name the function of, and spinal level innervating, the biceps, triceps, flexor digitorum, interossei, quadriceps, extensor hallucis, biceps femoris, soleus and gastrocnemius, and rectal sphincter.**

Muscle	Action	Spinal Level
Biceps	Forearm flexion	C 5,6
Triceps	Forearm extensors	C7
Flexor digitorum	Finger flexion	C8
Interossei	Finger Add/Abd	T1
Quadriceps	Knee extension	L3,4
Extensor hallucis	Great toe dorsiflexion	L5
Biceps femoris	Knee Flexion	S1
Soleus and gastrocnemius	Foot plantar flexion	S1,2
Rectal sphincter	Sphincter tone	S2-4

❑ ❑ ❑ ➢ **What is the dose of methylprednisolone used to treat acute spinal cord injury?**

30 mg/kg load over 15 min in the 1st h followed by 5.4 mg/kg per h over the next 23 h.

❑ ❑ ❑ ➢ **Sensory innervation to the nipple, umbilicus, and perianal region?**

Nipple   - T4
Umbilicus - T10.
Perianal   - S2-4.

❑ ❑ ❑ ➢ **What percent of fractures are seen on lateral, odontoid, AP films of the neck?**

Lateral 90%
Odontoid 10%.
AP just a few.

❑ ❑ ❑ ➢ **On lateral Csp, how much soft tissue prevertebral swelling is normal from C1-4?**

Up to 4 mm is normal; >5 mm suggests fracture.

❑ ❑ ❑ ➢ **How much anterior subluxation is normal on an adult lateral Csp?**

3.5 mm.

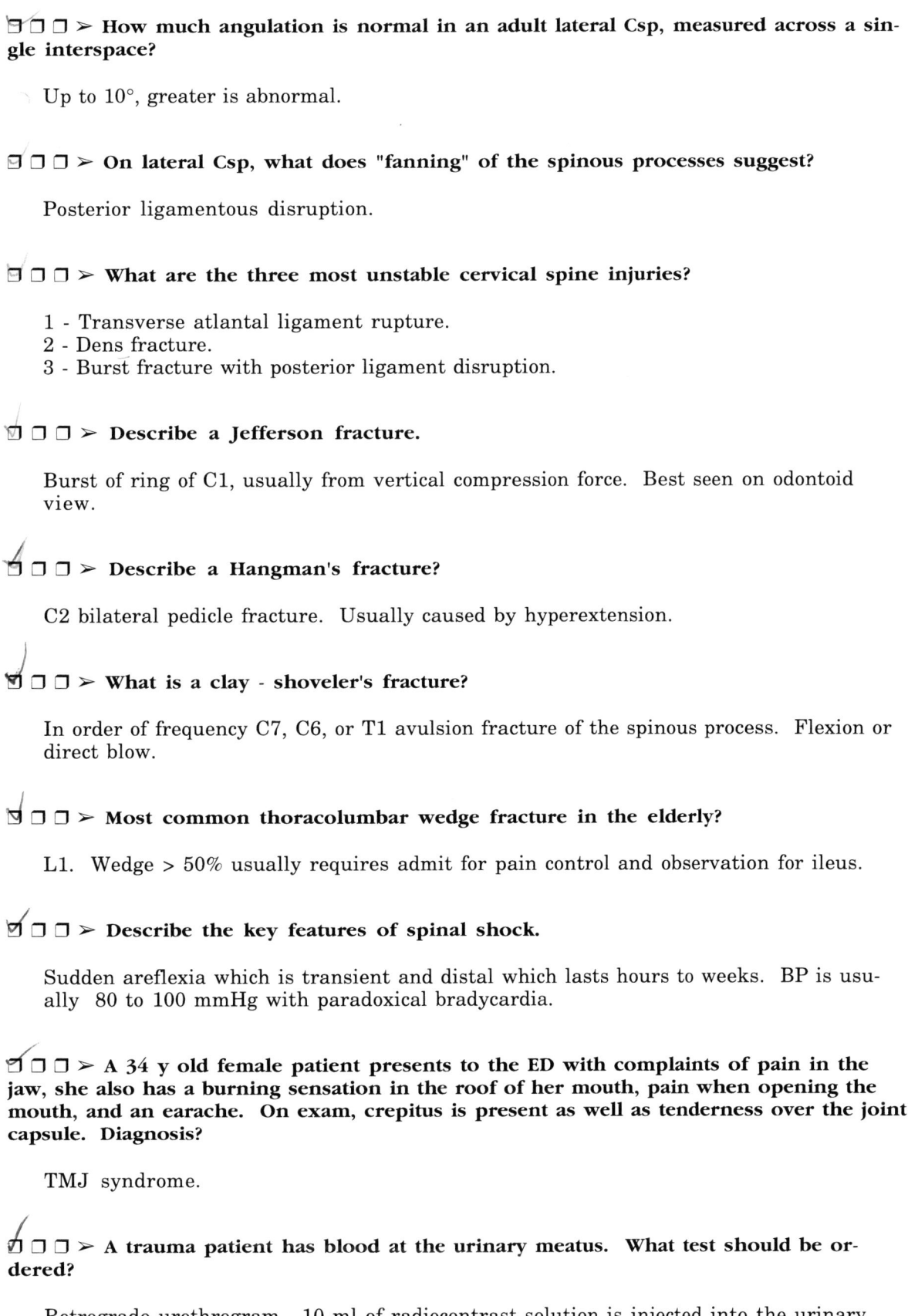

❏ ❏ ❏ ➢ **How much angulation is normal in an adult lateral Csp, measured across a single interspace?**

Up to 10°, greater is abnormal.

❏ ❏ ❏ ➢ **On lateral Csp, what does "fanning" of the spinous processes suggest?**

Posterior ligamentous disruption.

❏ ❏ ❏ ➢ **What are the three most unstable cervical spine injuries?**

1 - Transverse atlantal ligament rupture.
2 - Dens fracture.
3 - Burst fracture with posterior ligament disruption.

❏ ❏ ❏ ➢ **Describe a Jefferson fracture.**

Burst of ring of C1, usually from vertical compression force. Best seen on odontoid view.

❏ ❏ ❏ ➢ **Describe a Hangman's fracture?**

C2 bilateral pedicle fracture. Usually caused by hyperextension.

❏ ❏ ❏ ➢ **What is a clay - shoveler's fracture?**

In order of frequency C7, C6, or T1 avulsion fracture of the spinous process. Flexion or direct blow.

❏ ❏ ❏ ➢ **Most common thoracolumbar wedge fracture in the elderly?**

L1. Wedge > 50% usually requires admit for pain control and observation for ileus.

❏ ❏ ❏ ➢ **Describe the key features of spinal shock.**

Sudden areflexia which is transient and distal which lasts hours to weeks. BP is usually 80 to 100 mmHg with paradoxical bradycardia.

❏ ❏ ❏ ➢ **A 34 y old female patient presents to the ED with complaints of pain in the jaw, she also has a burning sensation in the roof of her mouth, pain when opening the mouth, and an earache. On exam, crepitus is present as well as tenderness over the joint capsule. Diagnosis?**

TMJ syndrome.

❏ ❏ ❏ ➢ **A trauma patient has blood at the urinary meatus. What test should be ordered?**

Retrograde urethrogram. 10 ml of radiocontrast solution is injected into the urinary meatus.

24

☑☐☐ ➤ **What are the 2 most commonly injured genitourinary organs?**

1.) - Kidney.
2.) - Bladder (associated with pelvic fracture).

☑☐☐ ➤ **In blunt trauma, what is the most common renal pedicle injury?**

Renal artery thrombosis.

☑☐☐ ➤ **Describe a type I pelvic fracture.**

Fracture of a single bone without a break in the pelvic ring structure. Stable - treat with bedrest.

☑☐☐ ➤ **Describe a type II pelvic fracture.**

Fracture with a single break in the pelvic ring. Stable - treat with bedrest.

☑☐☐ ➤ **Describe a type III pelvic fracture.**

Double break in the pelvic ring. Unstable - Associated with hemorrhage, visceral, and soft tissue injuries.

☑☐☐ ➤ **Describe a type IV pelvic fracture.**

Fracture of the acetabulum. Associated with dislocation of the hip.

☑☐☐ ➤ **Describe the leg position in a patient with a femoral neck fracture.**

Shortened, abducted, and slightly externally rotated.

☑☐☐ ➤ **Describe the leg position in a patient with an anterior dislocation.**

Abducted and externally rotated. 10% of hip dislocations. Mechanism is forced abduction.

☑☐☐ ➤ **Describe the leg position in a patient with a posterior hip dislocation.**

Shortened, adducted, and internally rotated. 90% of hip dislocations. Force applied to a flexed knee directed posteriorly. Associated with sciatic nerve injury.

☑☐☐ ➤ **A pneumatic tourniquet can be inflated on an extremity to more than a patient's systolic blood pressure for how long?**

2 h without damage to underlying vessels or nerves.

☑☐☐ ➤ **For how long can wound care be delayed before proliferation of bacteria that may result in infection?**

3 h.

☑ ❏ ❏ ➢ **What mechanisms of injury create wounds that are most susceptible to infection?**

Compression or tension injuries. They are 100 times more susceptible to infection.

☑ ❏ ❏ ➢ **What are the 3 anatomic subdivisions of the body created by composition of skin microflora?**

Moist areas: axilla & peritoneum - 10^4 to 10^6/cm^2.
Dry areas: trunk, upper arms & legs - 10^1 to 10^3/cm^2.
Exposed areas: head, face, hands, feet - 10^4 to 10^6/cm^2.

☑ ❏ ❏ ➢ **What is the dose of bacteria necessary to cause wound infection without a foreign body & with a foreign body?**

Without foreign body - > 10^6 bacteria/gm of tissue.
With foreign body - 100 bacteria.

☑ ❏ ❏ ➢ **What 2 factors determine the ultimate appearance of a scar?**

Static & dynamic skin tension on surrounding skin.

☑ ❏ ❏ ➢ **What has been proven to decrease the pain of local anesthetic administration?**

Buffering the solution with sodium bicarbonate, decreasing the speed of injection and use of a subdermal injection instead of superficial or intradermal injections.

☑ ❏ ❏ ➢ **Why is epinephrine added to local anesthesia?**

To increase the duration of the anesthesia. Epinephrine also causes vasoconstriction & decreased bleeding, which weakens tissue defenses and increases the incidence of wound infection.

☑ ❏ ❏ ➢ **Where does one inject local anesthesia for an ulnar nerve block?**

On the anterior wrist, proximal volar skin crease, between the ulnar artery & the flexor carpi ulnaris.

☑ ❏ ❏ ➢ **Where does one inject local anesthesia for a median nerve block?**

On the anterior wrist, proximal volar skin crease, between the tendon of the palmaris longus & the flexor carpi radialis.

☑ ❏ ❏ ➢ **What nerve block is used for anesthesia of the sole of the foot?**

Tibial nerve block. Tibial nerve block does not provide anesthesia to the lateral aspect of the heel and foot.

☑ ☐ ☐ ➤ **What is the preferred route for anesthesia for deep lacerations of the anterior tongue?**

Lingual nerve block.

☑ ☐ ☐ ➤ **What local anesthetic, ester or amide, is responsible for most allergic reactions?**

Esters - procaine.

☑ ☐ ☐ ➤ **How should hair be removed prior to wound repair?**

By clipping the hair around the wound, not by using razor preparation which increases infection rates.

☑ ☐ ☐ ➤ **What are the 4 C's in determining muscle viability?**

Color, Consistency, Contraction, and Circulation.

☑ ☐ ☐ ➤ **How long should one wait before delayed primary closure?**

4 d. This will decrease the infection rate and is used for severely contaminated wounds.

☑ ☐ ☐ ➤ **Bacterial endocarditis secondary to soft tissue infections may be caused by which two organisms?**

Staphylococcus aureus & Staphylococcus epidermidis.

☑ ☐ ☐ ➤ **What factors increase the likelihood of wound infection?**

Dirty or contaminated wounds, stellate or crushing wounds, wounds longer than 5 cm, wounds older than 6 h, and infection prone anatomic sites.

☑ ☐ ☐ ➤ **Gabriella Sabatini, the famous tennis star, presents to your "fast-track" after stepping on a nail that went right through her favorite, oldest pair of tennis shoes. What organism might infect her puncture wound?**

Pseudomonas aeruginosa.

☑ ☐ ☐ ➤ **What is the common bacteria seen in cat bite wounds which can also occur with dog bites?**

Pasteurella multocida.

☑ ☐ ☐ ➤ **Which has greater resistance to infection, sutures or staples?**

Staples.

☑ ❑ ❑ ➢ **What types of wounds result in the majority of tetanus cases?**

Lacerations, punctures, & crush injuries.

☑ ❑ ❑ ➢ **Characterize tetanus prone wounds.**

Age of wound:	> 6 h.
Configuration:	Stellate wound.
Depth:	> 1 cm.
Mechanism of injury:	Missile, crush, burn, frostbite.
Signs of infection:	Present.
Devitalized tissue:	Present.
Contaminants:	Present.
Denervated &/or ischemic tissue:	Present.

☑ ❑ ❑ ➢ **T/F- It is acceptable to clip or shave an eyebrow if needed to repair the skin.**

False. Eyebrows are valuable landmarks. 15% will not regrow.

☑ ❑ ❑ ➢ **When is a scar considered mature so that scar revision can be performed?**

6 - 12 mo.

☑ ❑ ❑ ➢ **What is the risk associated with not treating a septal hematoma of the nose?**

Absorption of the septal cartilage resulting in septal perforation.

☑ ❑ ❑ ➢ **What are the important structures to be considered when repairing lacerations of the cheek?**

Facial nerve, and parotid duct & gland.

☑ ❑ ❑ ➢ **What is the resultant deformity if an auricular hematoma is not properly treated?**

Cauliflower ear.

☑ ❑ ❑ ➢ **What percent of nailbed injuries have associated fracture of the distal phalanx?**

50%.

☑ ❑ ❑ ➢ **How are tattoos and teeth related to trama frequency?**

The frequency of trauma is directly proportional to the tattoo/tooth ratio. In addition, the more distal the tattoos, the worse the injury.

EENT PEARLS

☑ ☐ ☐ ➢ **Define Ellis Class I, II, and III.**

I   - Enamel.
II   - Enamel plus dentin exposure (pink). Complain of sensitivity to heat and cold.
III - Enamel, dentin, and pulp. Complain of pain or no pain depending on nerve involvement. Treat by application of tinfoil, analgesics, and immediate referral. Avoid topical analgesics which may cause sterile abscesses.

☑ ☐ ☐ ➢ **How is a Schiotz tonometer interpreted?**

Low scale readings suggest high pressure and high scale readings suggest low pressure. A scale of 4 or greater is equal to 20 mmHg or less (normal).

☑ ☐ ☐ ➢ **A patient is seen with herpetic lesions on the tip of the nose. Why is this a problem?**

The tip of the nose and the cornea are both supplied by the nasociliary nerve. Thus, the cornea may also be involved.

☑ ☐ ☐ ➢ **A patient presents with an itching, tearing, right eye. On exam huge cobblestone papillae are found under the upper lid. Diagnosis?**

Allergic conjunctivitis.

☑ ☐ ☐ ➢ **A patient presents with inflammation of the conjunctiva and lid margins. Slit-lamp exam reveals a "greasy" appearance of lid margins with scaling, especially around the base of the lashes. Diagnosis?**

Blepharitis. Often caused by staphylococcal infection of the oil glands and skin next to the lash follicles. Treatment consists of scrubbing with baby shampoo and, in consultation with an ophthalmologist, sulfacetamide drops and steroid.

☑ ☐ ☐ ➢ **A patient presents with a painful red eye. On slit-lamp exam, a localized white flocculent infiltrate is seen in the anterior chamber. Diagnosis?**

Hypopyon is an accumulation of white inflammatory exudate in the anterior chamber. Obtain cultures, consult an ophthalmologist immediately, and admit the patient.

☑ ☐ ☐ ➢ **A welder presents with severe eye pain. What would be the expected finding on slit-lamp exam?**

Diffuse punctate keratopathy. Multiple pinpoint areas of fluorescein uptake representing ruptured corneal epithelial cells.

☑ ☐ ☐ ➢ **A patient presents with a pustular vesicle at the lid margin. Diagnosis and treatment?**

Hordeolum (Stye). Acute inflammation of the meibomian gland most commonly of the upper lid. Treat with topical antibiotics and warm compresses. Surgical drainage may be necessary.

❑ ❑ ❑ ➢ **A patient presents with a chronic nontender uninflamed nodule of the upper lid. Diagnosis?**

Chalazion. Treat with surgical curettage.

❑ ❑ ❑ ➢ **A patient presents with blurred vision, photophobia, and dull pain in the temporal area. Exam reveals a red eye, constricted pupil, ciliary flush, and red sclera at the limbus. Visual acuity is decreased and intraocular pressure is decreased in the affected eye. What would be expected on slit-lamp exam?**

Flare and cells are expected with uveitis. Treatment consists of cycloplegics (cyclopentolate or homatropine) and topical steroids in consultation with an ophthalmologist.

❑ ❑ ❑ ➢ **A patient presents with a history of dull eye pain which developed shortly after entering a dark, sleezy bar. They also have nausea and vomiting, blurred vision, and see "halos" around lights. Exam reveals a red congested eye with decreased visual acuity. The cornea is hazy and pupil is mid-dilated and fixed to light. What reading is expected on the Schiotz tonometer?**

Usually 50 mmHg or greater. Treatment of acute angle closure glaucoma consists of acetazolamide (Diamox) 500 mg and topical timolol 0.5% (Timoptic) 1 drop repeated in 10 min. Avoid timolol in patients with COPD or heart disease. Give oral glycerol or IV mannitol. Pilocarpine 1% q 15 min for 1st h followed by one drop every 30 to 60 min.

❑ ❑ ❑ ➢ **A patient presents with the sensation of a foreign body in the eye. Slit-lamp exam reveals a dendritic figure which has a Christmas tree pattern. Treatment?**

Herpes simplex keratitis is treated with antiviral agents and cycloplegics. Steroids spell disaster!

❑ ❑ ❑ ➢ **A patient presents with sudden, painless, loss of vision in one eye. What physical findings would be expected?**

Central retinal artery occlusion typically results in a pale retina and a small pink dot near the fovea. Digital massage and immediate ophthalmic consultation with anterior chamber paracentesis is the treatment of choice.

❑ ❑ ❑ ➢ **A patient presents with a physical finding of a chaotically blood-streaked retina with congested and dilated veins. Diagnosis?**

Central retinal vein occlusion. Patients often complain of painless decrease in vision in one eye.

❑ ❑ ❑ ➢ **A patient presents with loss of vision in one eye. Physical exam demonstrates a loss of central vision, peripheral vision is preserved. Diagnosis?**

Retrobulbar neuritis. Twenty-five percent of cases of retrobulbar neuritis are associated with MS.

☑ ❏ ❏ ➢ **A patient presents with sudden loss of vision is one eye which returned quickly. Diagnosis?**

Amaurosis fugax. Usually caused by central retinal artery emboli from extracranial atherosclerosis.

☑ ❏ ❏ ➢ **A patient presents with the sensation of painless loss of vision in one eye described as a wall slowly developing in the visual field. Findings expected on exam?**

Gray detached retina. Patient may also complain of flashing lights in the peripheral visual field or "spider webs" in the visual field. Inferior detachment is treated with the patient sitting up. Superior detachment is treated with the patient lying flat.

☑ ❏ ❏ ➢ **What five lid lacerations should be referred to an ophthalmologist?**

1. Near the lacrimal canaliculi (between the medial canthus and the punctum).
2. Near the levator (transverse lacerations of the upper lid).
3. Near the orbital septum (upper lid deep wounds, between the tarsus and the superior orbital rim).
4. Canthal tendons (wounds penetrating the lateral and medial canthi).
5. Lid Margins (wounds through the tarsal plate and lid margins).

☑ ❏ ❏ ➢ **A patient presents with a history of being struck in the eye with a tennis ball. On exam, no abnormalities are evident. What should the discharge instructions state?**

Return to ED if ocular pain or blurred vision develop. Repeat exam within 24 h. Hyphemas caused by blunt eye trauma may not be present on initial exam.

☑ ❏ ❏ ➢ **A patient presents to the ED with a history of blunt trauma to the orbit. On exam, the patient is found to have diplopia and pain on upward gaze. What x-ray should be ordered?**

Modified stereo (Water's view) will show a blowout fracture of the orbit.
Some clinicians prefer the "Caldwell" view - the orbital floor is projected <u>above</u> petrous ridges.

☑ ❏ ❏ ➢ **A patient presents with a history of trauma to the orbit with a dull ocular pain, decreased visual acuity, and photophobia. Exam reveals a constricted pupil and ciliary flush. What will be found on slit-lamp exam?**

Flare and cells in the anterior chamber are present with traumatic iritis.

☑ ❏ ❏ ➢ **An anxious 24 y old female presents with a complaint of blurred vision made worse when looking at objects far away. On exam, the eyes are convergent, the pupils are constricted, and accommodation is at a maximum. Diagnosis?**

Spasm of accommodation. Treat anxiety. A short-acting cycloplegic may stop the cycle.

☑ ❏ ❏ ➢ **A very anxious 16 y old male presents stating that his vision is like "looking down a gun barrel". How should physiologic versus hysterical scotoma be differentiated?**

Physiologic -double the distance between the patient and tangent screen (visual screen test) results in a doubling of the size of the central visual field.
Hysterical - Visual field size remains the same.

☑ ☐ ☐ ➤ **Which anesthetic works the fastest and which lasts the longest: proparacaine or tetracaine?**

Proparacaine - Rapid onset, duration 20 min.
Tetracaine - Delayed onset, duration 1 h.

☑ ☐ ☐ ➤ **Place the following mydriatic-cycloplegic medications in order of duration of activity: tropicamide, homatropine, atropine, and cyclopentolate?**

Tropicamide - Onset 15-20 min, brief duration.
Cyclopentolate - Onset 30-60 min, duration < 24 h.
Homatropine - Long lasting, 2-3 d.
Atropine - Very long lasting, 2 wk.

☑ ☐ ☐ ➤ **What are miotics used to treat?**

Glaucoma. Pilocarpine is the most common, instilled 4 times daily.

☑ ☐ ☐ ➤ **Function of acetazolamide and glycerol?**

Acetazolamide - carbonic anhydrase inhibitor. Decreases ciliary body aqueous output.
Glycerol - hyperosmotic agent. Decreases intraocular pressure by making plasma hypertonic to aqueous humor.

☑ ☐ ☐ ➤ **A 48 y old diabetic male presents with pain, itching, and discharge from the right ear. On exam, the drum is intact. Diagnosis?**

Otitis externa. Treat by suctioning ear and treating for one week with an antibiotic-steroid otic solution. May use an earwick to improve delivery of antibiotic. Suspect malignant external otitis in the diabetic patient.

☑ ☐ ☐ ➤ **A patient presents with ear pain. On exam, the tympanic membrane has blisters which appear to contain fluid. Diagnosis?**

Bullous myringitis, commonly caused by Mycoplasma or viruses.
Treat with erythromycin.

☑ ☐ ☐ ➤ **A 16 y old former "Golden Gloves" champ presents with right ear pain and swelling after receiving a blow to the ear. Treatment?**

If the ear is not treated appropriately, cauliflower deformity may result. As such, the ear should be aseptically drained by incision or aspiration and a mastoid-conforming dressing should be applied. ENT follow-up is mandatory.

☑ ☐ ☐ ➤ **A patient presents with a swollen, tender, red left auricle. Diagnosis?**

Perichondritis caused by Pseudomonas.

❏ ❏ ❏ ➤ **A lower airway foreign body is suspected. What will plain films show?**

Plain films may show air trapping on the affected side. Inspiration and expiration views demonstrate mediastinal shift away from the affected side.

❏ ❏ ❏ ➤ **A patient presents with trismus, painful swallowing, a stiff neck, altered voice, and fever. On exam, pharyngeal swelling and tonsillar displacement is present as well as external swelling in the parotid regions. Diagnosis?**

Parapharyngeal abscess. Usually treated by a lateral approach I & D through the neck.

❏ ❏ ❏ ➤ **What potential complication of a nasal fracture should always be considered on physical exam?**

Septal hematoma. If not drained, aseptic necrosis of the septal cartilage or septal abscess may develop.

❏ ❏ ❏ ➤ **In what age group is retropharyngeal abscess most common?**

Children less than four. Symptoms may include difficulty breathing, fever, enlarged cervical nodes, difficulty swallowing, and a stiff neck. Exam may reveal a mass or fullness in the posterior pharyngeal area.

❏ ❏ ❏ ➤ **In what age group are peritonsillar abscesses most common?**

Adolescents and young adults. Symptoms may include ear pain, trismus, drooling, and alteration of voice.

❏ ❏ ❏ ➤ **A 5 y old child presents with a history of sinus infection. On exam, the child's eyelid is red and swollen, the globe is displaced laterally and inferiorly, and proptosis is present. Diagnosis?**

The child may have orbital cellulitis and an abscess associated with ethmoid sinusitis.

❏ ❏ ❏ ➤ **A patient with a history of frontal sinusitis presents with a large forehead abscess. Diagnosis?**

Pott's puffy tumor.

❏ ❏ ❏ ➤ **A patient presents 3 d after tooth extraction with severe pain and a foul mouth odor and taste. Diagnosis?**

Alveolar osteitis (dry socket). Treat by irrigation of the socket, medicated dental packing, or iodoform with Campho-Phenique or eugenol.

❏ ❏ ❏ ➤ **A patient presents with gingival pain and foul odor and taste in the mouth. On exam, fever and lymphadenopathy are present. The gingiva is bright red and the papillae are ulcerated and covered with a gray membrane. Diagnosis?**

Acute necrotizing ulcerative gingivitis.

❏ ❏ ❏ ➤ **A 47 y old female presents to the ED with a complaint of excruciating sudden waxing and waning pain in the right cheek. She says it feels like an electric shock. Diagnosis and treatment?**

Tic douloureux. Carbamazepine (100 mg bid starting dose and increase to 1200 mg daily if needed). Referral to neurologist and dentist. Rule out cerebellopontine angle tumor, MS, nasopharyngeal carcinoma, cluster headache, polymyalgia rheumatica, temporal arteritis, and oral pathology.

❏ ❏ ❏ ➤ **What are the signs and symptoms of a mandibular fracture?**

Malocclusion, pain, decreased range of motion, bony deformity, swelling, ecchymosis, and mental nerve anesthesia.

❏ ❏ ❏ ➤ **What is the most common type of mandibular fracture?**

Alveolar (tooth-bearing segment of the mandible). Numbness of the lower lip suggests a mandibular fracture.

❏ ❏ ❏ ➤ **Signs and symptoms of fracture of the zygomaticomaxillary complex?**

Emphysema of the tissue, edema, ecchymosis, facial flattening, unilateral epistaxis, anesthesia, step deformity, decreased mandibular movement and diplopia.

❏ ❏ ❏ ➤ **What are the two most common findings with an orbital floor injury?**

Diplopia and globe lowering.

❏ ❏ ❏ ➤ **Describe a Le Fort I fracture.**

Fracture line starting at the nasal apertures to the wall of the maxillary sinuses bilaterally, across the pterygomaxillary tissue, and involving the lateral pterygoid plates. X-rays often miss this fracture.

❏ ❏ ❏ ➤ **Describe the physical findings of a Le Fort II fracture.**

Swelling of the nose, lips, eyes, and midface. Sub-conjunctival hemorrhage may be present with blood in the nares. Suspect cerebrospinal involvement and check for rhinorrhea. Water's view and bilateral tomograms should be ordered. Fracture involves facial aspects of the maxillae extending to the nasal and ethmoid bones. Fracture also involves the maxillary sinuses and infraorbital rims bilaterally across the bridge of the nose.

❏ ❏ ❏ ➤ **Describe the fracture line in a Le Fort III fracture.**

Runs through the frontozygomatic suture lines bilaterally, through the orbits, and through the base of the nose and ethmoid region. Also called a "Dishface" fracture. Movement of the zygoma and midface is suggestive. Water's view and bilateral orbital tomograms confirm the diagnosis.

❏ ❏ ❏ ➤ **Is cerebrospinal rhinorrhea most common with Le Fort I, II, or III?**

III.

❏ ❏ ❏ ➢ **A 42 y old female presents with dull jaw and ear pain and a burning sensation in the roof of her mouth. The pain is worse in the evening. She also hears a "popping" sound when she opens and closes her mouth. Exam reveals tenderness of the joint capsule. Diagnosis?**

TMJ syndrome. Treat with physiotherapy, analgesics, soft diet, muscle relaxants, and occlusive therapy. Apply warm moist compresses 4 to 5 times daily for 15 min for 7 to 10 d.

❏ ❏ ❏ ➢ **A 48 y old male presents with a history of high fever and swelling of the inferior borders of the mandible and lateral neck. Pain is severe. The patient has increased pain with swallowing and trismus. Diagnosis?**

Parapharyngeal space infection.

❏ ❏ ❏ ➢ **What is the most common site associated with Ludwig's angina?**

Lower 2nd and 3rd molars. It is a boardlike swelling in the region of the submandibular, sublingual, and submental spaces. The most common organisms are hemolytic Streptococci, Staphylococcus, and mixed anaerobes and aerobes.

PULMONARY PEARLS

"We rarely gain a higher or larger view except when it is forced upon us through struggles which we would avoid if we could."

Charles Cooney

❏ ❏ ❏ ➢ **What is the <u>most</u> <u>common</u> cause of bacterial pneumonia?**

Pneumococcus.

❏ ❏ ❏ ➢ **What percentage of upper respiratory infectious agents are non-bacterial?**

Non-bacterial agents account for over 90% of pharyngitis, laryngitis, tracheal bronchitis, and bronchitis.

❏ ❏ ❏ ➢ **Name two anti-viral medications that are useful for viral pneumonia.**

Amantadine for influenza A and aerosolized Ribavirin for RSV.

❏ ❏ ❏ ➢ **If a patient has a patchy infiltrate on a chest x-ray and bullous myringitis, what antibiotic should be given.**

Erythromycin for Mycoplasma.

❏ ❏ ❏ ➢ **What kind of pneumonia occurs in alcoholics and other persons who develop aspiration pneumonia?**

Anaerobe and gram-negative pneumonia.

❏ ❏ ❏ ➢ **What bacterial pneumonia often occurs following a viral pneumonia?**

Staph. aureus pneumonia.

❏ ❏ ❏ ➢ **What are the number of PMNs and squamous cells necessary for an adequate sputum sample?**

Greater than 25 PMNs and less than 10 squamous epithelial cells per low powered field.

❏ ❏ ❏ ➢ **A 40 y old alcoholic presents with rigors and shortness of breath. Currant jelly sputum shows short, plump gram-negative bacilli. Chest x-ray shows a necrotizing lobar pneumonia in the right upper lobe. What is the etiologic agent?**

Klebsiella pneumonia.

❐ ❐ ❐ ➢ **Legionella pneumoniae occurs in summer or winter?**

Predominantly in the summer.
Staph pneumonia also occurs more frequently in summer.

❐ ❐ ❐ ➢ **An older patient with GI symptoms and relative bradycardia usually has what kind of pneumonia?**

Legionella.

❐ ❐ ❐ ➢ **What is the treatment for Legionella pneumonia?**

IV erythromycin.

❐ ❐ ❐ ➢ **Should steroids be used in aspiration pneumonia?**

No.

❐ ❐ ❐ ➢ **Who will benefit from pentamidine prophylactic therapy for PCP?**

People with previous history of PCP and those with CD4 counts less than 200.
Criteria for pentamidine prophylaxis are becoming more relaxed.

❐ ❐ ❐ ➢ **Are aspirated foreign bodies more likely to be found in the right or left bronchus?**

Right.

❐ ❐ ❐ ➢ **T/F - Flora of lung abscesses are usually polymicrobial.**

True.

❐ ❐ ❐ ➢ **What are some common organisms of empyema?**

Staph, gram negatives, and anaerobes.

❐ ❐ ❐ ➢ **Describe the chest x-ray of Mycoplasma pneumonia.**

Patchy densities involving the entire lobe are most common. Pneumatoceles, cavities, abscesses and pleural effusions can occur, but are uncommon. Erythromycin.

❐ ❐ ❐ ➢ **Describe the chest x-ray findings in Legionella pneumonia.**

Dense consolidation and bulging fissures. Expect elevated liver enzymes and hypophosphatemia.

❐ ❐ ❐ ➢ **What are the classic signs and symptoms of TB?**

Night sweats, fever, weight loss, malaise, cough, and a green/yellow sputum most commonly seen in the mornings.

❐ ❐ ❐ ➤ **Why are the lung zones of initial tubercle bacillus infection in the apical and posterior segments of the upper lobe and the superior segments of the lower lobe?**

The tubercle bacillus requires a relatively high oxygen tension for survival.

❐ ❐ ❐ ➤ **What are some common extrapulmonary TB sites?**

Pleura, lymph node, bone, GI tract, GU tract, meninges, liver and the pericardium.

❐ ❐ ❐ ➤ **Right upper lobe cavitation with parenchymal involvement is classic for:**

TB.
Lower lung infiltrates, hilar adenopathy, atelectasis, and pleural effusion are common.

❐ ❐ ❐ ➤ **T/F - People under 35 y of age with positive TB skin tests should have at least six months of isoniazid chemoprophylaxis.**

True.

❐ ❐ ❐ ➤ **Is there a higher incidence of spontaneous pneumothorax among males or females?**

Males.

❐ ❐ ❐ ➤ **Is a pneumothorax more evident on an inspiratory or expiratory film?**

Expiratory.

❐ ❐ ❐ ➤ **What kind of pneumonias may be associated with pneumothorax?**

Staph, TB, Klebsiella, and PCP.

❐ ❐ ❐ ➤ **What diagnostic test is helpful in sub-clinical PCP infection?**

Exertional pulse oximetry is helpful in making the diagnosis of PCP, if clinically suspicious.

❐ ❐ ❐ ➤ **Elevated LDH may be an indicator of what opportunistic infection?**

PCP.

❐ ❐ ❐ ➤ **Most common radiographic finding of PCP?**

A reticulonodular pattern.

❐ ❐ ❐ ➤ **The initial therapy for PCP includes what antibiotics?**

TMP-SMZ or pentamidine.

❏ ❏ ❏ ➤ **Are corticosteroids recommended for severe PCP?**

Yes.

❏ ❏ ❏ ➤ **List two drugs that can cause ARDS.**

Heroin and aspirin.

❏ ❏ ❏ ➤ **How long after an initial insult does ARDS usually occur?**

12 to 72 h.

❏ ❏ ❏ ➤ **Are sedatives beneficial in acutely asthmatic patients?**

No. They may be dangerous.

❏ ❏ ❏ ➤ **Discuss some agents that may be used to induce unconsciousness.**

Agent	aka	Class	Onset	Duration	Dose
Thiopental	Pentothal	Barbiturate	≈ 30 s	2 - 30 min. dep. on source	2.0-5.0 mg/kg @ 40 mg/min
Methohexital	Brevital	Barbiturate	Fast	Very short	5-12 ml of 1% solution @ 1 ml/5 sec
Fentanyl	Sublimaze	Opiate	2 min	≈ 20 min	20 - 150 μg/kg
Midazolam	Versed	Benzodiazepine	≈ 5 min	≈ 30 min	0.1 mg/kg
Etomidate	Amidate	Benzoderiv.	1 min	3-12 min	0.2-0.4 mg/kg

❏ ❏ ❏ ➤ **How is the A-a gradient calculated for a patient breathing room air?**

$$A - a = 150 - Pa_{O_2} - (Pa_{CO_2} \times 1.25) \quad \text{Normal} \approx 2\text{-}10.$$

❏ ❏ ❏ ➤ **The summit of Mt. Everest is at 8,848 m (29,029 ft). What is the PaO_2 for a climber at this altitude?**

PaO_2 = 26 - 33 mm Hg. Measured $PaCO_2$ = 9.5 - 13.8 mm Hg with a corresponding SaO_2 of 58%. Whoa!

❏ ❏ ❏ ➤ **T/F- Pulse oximetry provides a reliable means of estimating oxyhemoglobin saturation in a patient suffering CO poisoning.**

False. COHb has light absorbance that can lead to a falsely elevated pulse oximiter transduced saturation level. The <u>calculated</u> value from a standard ABG may also be falsely elevated. The oxygen saturation should be <u>measured</u> using a co-oximiter that <u>measures</u> the amounts of unsaturated O_2Hb, of COHb and of MetHb.

❐ ❐ ❐ ➤ **What is the half-life of COHb for a patient breathing room air, breathing 100% oxygen and breathing 100% oxygen @ 3 atm pressure?**

Source	$FIO_2 = 0.21$	$FIO_2 = 1.0$	$FIO_2 = 1.0$ @ 3 atm
Tintinalli, 3rd Ed., pg 59.	2 - 3 h	20 - 30 min	
Tintinalli, 3rd Ed., pg 706.	8.67 h	80 min	23 min
Rosen, 3rd Ed., pg 2675	4 - 6 h	90 min	30 min
Bryson, 2nd Ed., pg 234.	4 - 5.3 h	80 - 100 min	20 - 30 min

Using weighted averages and throwing out the outlying values it seems safe to try to remember these values as ≈ 6 h, 1.5 h and 0.5 h.

GI PEARLS

❐ ❐ ❐ ➢ **A patient has trouble swallowing cold liquids because they "end up in my nose." The likely condition(s)?**

Motor disorders such as CVA, bulbar palsies, polio and myositis.

❐ ❐ ❐ ➢ **After a week, an ill-appearing patient says her sore throat got worse and she complains of spiking fevers and central chest burning. What is your concern?**

Retro- or parapharyngeal abscess with extension to superior mediastinitis.

❐ ❐ ❐ ➢ **A child presents with odynophagia and drooling. What should you expect on examination of the oropharynx?**

Trouble, if you look with a tongue blade! A patient with suspected epiglottitis is at high risk for upper airway compromise; intubation with direct visualization, typically in the OR, is best. This dogma may be evolving.

❐ ❐ ❐ ➢ **A patient says food gets stuck in his mid-chest, then is regurgitated as a putrid, undigested mess. A barium study shows a dilated esophagus with a distal "beak." Diagnosis?**

Achalasia.

❐ ❐ ❐ ➢ **A woman with telangiectasias, "tight knuckles," and "acid indigestion" might have what findings on an upper GI series?**

Aperistalsis, characteristic of scleroderma.

❐ ❐ ❐ ➢ **A 40 y old smoker describes acute, crescendo substernal chest tightness going to his back, unrelieved by antacids. An ECG shows ST changes, and his pain resolves 7-10 minutes after a nitroglycerin tablet. Is this angina?**

Maybe, though the delayed response to nitrates characterizes "esophageal colic" caused by segmental esophageal spasm, often triggered by reflux.

❐ ❐ ❐ ➢ **Over a mo, an elderly woman has had progressive trouble swallowing first solids, then liquids. She presents with sudden drooling after dinner. Your concern?**

A peptic stricture or esophageal cancer complicated by bolus obstruction.

❐ ❐ ❐ ➢ **A patient with an "acid stomach" develops melena and vomits bright red blood. Is esophagitis a likely cause?**

No. Capillary bleeding rarely causes impressive acute blood loss. Arterial bleeding (from a complicated ulcer, foreign body, or Mallory-Weiss tear) or variceal bleeding are much more likely.

❒ ❒ ❒ ➤ **A cirrhotic vomits bright red blood. He is dizzy, and has a systolic blood pressure of 90 mm Hg. After an aggressive fluid resuscitation, 4 units of red cells, and gastric lavage, his pressure is 90 mm Hg. What next?**

Assume a coagulopathy and transfuse fresh frozen plasma; start a vasopressin drip; and arrange for emergent endoscopic intervention for sclerotherapy or banding.

❒ ❒ ❒ ➤ **Recurrent pneumonias, especially in the right middle lobe or the superior segments of the bilateral upper lobes, suggests what syndrome?**

Aspiration, associated with motor diseases and gastroesophageal reflux.

❒ ❒ ❒ ➤ **List 4 contraindications to introduction of a nasogastric tube.**

1.) Suspected esophageal laceration or perforation.
2.) Near obstruction due to stricture.
3.) Esophageal foreign body.
4.) Severe head trauma with rhinorrhea.

❒ ❒ ❒ ➤ **Repeated, violent bouts of vomiting can result in both Mallory-Weiss tears and Boerhaave's syndrome. Differentiate the two.**

Mallory-Weiss tears involve the submucosa and mucosa, typically in the right posterolateral wall of the GE junction.
Boerhaave's is from a full-thickness tear, usually in the unsupported left posterolateral wall of the abdominal esophagus.

❒ ❒ ❒ ➤ **After a high-speed MVA, an unrestrained driver develops abdominal and chest pain radiating to the neck. An upper chest film shows left pleural fluid. What gastroesophageal catastrophe might have occurred?**

Impact against a steering wheel, like repeated, violent Valsalva-ing, can result in Boerhaave's syndrome with esophageal perforation and mediastinitis.

❒ ❒ ❒ ➤ **You suspect a perforated esophagus; what's the next test to order?**

A water-soluble contrast study. In the mean time, start broad-spectrum antibiotics and call the surgeons ASAP.

❒ ❒ ❒ ➤ **In kids, foreign bodies stick at what esophageal levels?**

Typically at levels of the cricopharyngeus muscles (most usual), thoracic inlet, aortic arch, tracheal bifurcation, and lower esophageal sphincter.

❒ ❒ ❒ ➤ **When is removing a button battery lodged in the esophagus indicated?**

Always. If this corrosive foreign body was swallowed <u>less than 2 hours</u> ago, and endoscopy is <u>not</u> available, consider attempting Foley balloon removal. More wisely, find a scope doc for immediate endoscopic removal.

❒ ❒ ❒ ➤ **X-rays are crucial in the search for a suspected swallowed foreign body. In**

kids, what physical findings can tip you off?

Besides a child's distress, you may also find a red or scratched oropharynx, dysphagia, a high fever, or peritoneal signs. Subcutaneous air suggests perforation.

❏ ❏ ❏ ➢ **Most objects, even sharp ones, pass thorough the GI tract without incident. What objects should be removed?**

Any object that obstructs or perforates, that is > 5 cm long and >2 cm wide (won't make it past the GE junction), or is toxic (batteries) should be removed, either endoscopically or surgically. Sharp or pointed objects (sewing needles and razor blades) should be removed if they haven't passed the pylorus.

❏ ❏ ❏ ➢ **An obstructing meat bolus should be removed within 12 hours. What's the best approach?**

Endoscopy, through a trial of IV glucagon (given as 1 mg push after a small test dose, then repeated as a 2 mg dose at 20 min if no relief), or sublingual nifedipine, 10 mg, may work. Both relax esophageal smooth muscle. Meat tenderizer is best avoided, since perforation has occurred.

❏ ❏ ❏ ➢ **Which test is mandatory after the food bolus is cleared?**

A barium study to both confirm the passage/removal of the foreign body and to look for underlying pathology (present in virtually all adults with obstructing food boluses).

❏ ❏ ❏ ➢ **Are there clinical findings that reliably distinguish duodenal ulcer from gastric ulcer?**

No. Some findings are suggestive: A typical DU causes pain 2 h after a meal that may radiate to the back, and wake a patient from sleep, while GU often causes immediate postprandial pain and is more often due to ethanol or NSAID use.

❏ ❏ ❏ ➢ **Name two endocrine problems that cause peptic ulcer.**

Zollinger-Ellison syndrome and hyperparathyroidism (hypercalcemia).

❏ ❏ ❏ ➢ **Postprandial midabdominal pain might suggest what ectopic syndrome?**

Peptic ulcer in a Meckel's diverticulum.

❏ ❏ ❏ ➢ **T/F - H_2--blockers decrease the risk of perforation and rebleeding in peptic ulcer disease.**

False. However, cimetidine has reduced the need for surgery, improved rates of ulcer healing, and reduced the mortality from the initial bleeding episode.

❏ ❏ ❏ ➢ **Any worries in giving cimetidine to a wheezing, anticoagulated patient with a seizure disorder?**

Maybe. By decreasing blood flow to the liver and competing with the drug-eliminating cytochrome p450 system, cimetidine can increase the levels of theophylline, warfarin, and phenytoin, not to mention diazepam, propranolol, and lidocaine.

❐ ❐ ❐ ➢ **A patient with "half a stomach" after surgery for a bleeding ulcer presents with weight loss, epigastric burning, and diarrhea. Potential reasons?**

An obstructed afferent loop (Billroth II), bile reflux gastritis, dumping syndrome, malabsorption (poor mixing, of gastric/pancreatic juices, bacterial overgrowth), or gastric remnant carcinoma. Anemia (from B_{12}, iron, and folate malabsorption) and osteoporosis (from vitamin D and calcium malabsorption) are common.

❐ ❐ ❐ ➢ **Is a person with massive upper GI bleeding likely to have a perforated ulcer?**

No.

❐ ❐ ❐ ➢ **After fluid and blood resuscitation for a bleeding ulcer, the most useful diagnostic test?**

Endoscopy, which can also be therapeutic, with cryo- or electrocautery of an arterial bleeder.

❐ ❐ ❐ ➢ **In a patient with early satiety and ulcer symptoms, what clinical finding essentially rules out a gastric outlet obstruction?**

Bilious vomitus.

❐ ❐ ❐ ➢ **T/F - Upright abdominal, left lateral decubitus, or upright chest films show free air in most perforations.**

True, but just barely. Some 49% of cases show no free air (typically they are walled off). Insufflate 300-500 cc of air through a nasogastric tube, then clamp it, and have the patient sit up for 10 min to up the yield.

❐ ❐ ❐ ➢ **Are "stress ulcers" a surgical problem?**

Not usually. The diffuse gastric bleeding that results from CNS tumors, head trauma, burns, sepsis, shock, steroids, aspirin, or alcohol is usually mucosal, can be life-threatening, and can most often be managed medically. Endoscopic diagnosis is key.

❐ ❐ ❐ ➢ **Burning epigastric pain shooting to the back, hypovolemic shock, and a high amylase suggests . . .**

Posterior perforation of a duodenal ulcer.

❐ ❐ ❐ ➢ **Can non-gallstone cholecystitis perforate?**

Yes. Up to 40% of gall bladder perforations are associated with acalculous cholecystitis.

❐ ❐ ❐ ➢ **Who gets acalculous cholecystitis?**

Dehydrated post-op, post-trauma, and burn patients, as well as those with transfusion related hemolysis or narcotic use (illicit or prescribed).

❏ ❏ ❏ ➤ **Enteric coated potassium tablets, typhoid, tuberculosis, tumors, and strangulated hernia may cause what rare process?**

Non-traumatic small-bowel perforation.

❏ ❏ ❏ ➤ **The most common cause of lower GI perforation?**

Diverticulitis, followed by tumor, colitis, foreign bodies, and instrumentation.

❏ ❏ ❏ ➤ **A pregnant woman with right upper quadrant pain should be assumed to have what intraabdominal pathology until proven otherwise?**

Acute appendicitis.

❏ ❏ ❏ ➤ **Rovsing's, psoas, and obturator signs can all indicate an inflamed posterior appendix. Please describe these signs.**

Rovsing's sign - right lower quadrant pain on left lower quadrant palpation.
Psoas sign - right lower quadrant pain on right thigh extension.
Obturator sign - right lower quadrant pain on internal rotation of the flexed right thigh.

❏ ❏ ❏ ➤ **What does ultrasound show in acute appendicitis?**

A fixed, tender, non-compressible mass, but only in 75 to 90% of cases.

❏ ❏ ❏ ➤ **What does abdominal CT scanning show in acute appendicitis?**

Not much in early appendicitis; the study is useful to distinguish the causes of a right lower quadrant <u>mass</u> (late appendicitis, perforation/abscess, carcinoma, and pseudomyxoma).

❏ ❏ ❏ ➤ **What does laparoscopy show in acute appendicitis?**

Appendicitis, if you're lucky. Unfortunately, just seeing an inflamed appendix does not prove appendicitis; finding another cause of abdominal pain does not rule out appendicitis.

❏ ❏ ❏ ➤ **What about blood tests?**

An elevated WBC or a left shift are seen in 95 to 99% of cases; this is a sensitive test (helps rule out appendicitis), but nonspecific (can't rule it in).

❏ ❏ ❏ ➤ **So what's the point of the last four questions?**

Don't rely on diagnostic studies to diagnose acute abdominal pain. Rely instead on an exam by an experienced clinician, hospital admission, serial exams, and surgical consultation.

❏ ❏ ❏ ➤ **The most common cause of small bowel obstruction?**

Adhesions are the most common causes of <u>extra</u>luminal obstruction, followed by incarcerated hernia, while gallstones and bezoars are the most common causes of <u>intra</u>luminal obstruction.

❐ ❐ ❐ ➤ **Recurrent small bowel obstruction in an elderly woman associated with unilateral pain into one thigh suggests what occult process?**

Obturator hernia incarceration. May often present with pain down medial thigh to knee.

❐ ❐ ❐ ➤ **The most common causes of colonic obstruction?**

Cancer, then diverticulitis followed by volvulus.

❐ ❐ ❐ ➤ **An elderly man presents with new constipation without tenesmus, abdominal pain, nausea or vomiting. He has hard stool in the vault on rectal exam. A KUB shows a colon "full of stool." Is an enema all he needs?**

No. Fecal impaction with "obstipation" is both common and benign, but it is usually associated with tenesmus. He needs a workup for a colorectal tumor.

❐ ❐ ❐ ➤ **A KUB is suspicious for a large bowel obstruction. The next step(s) in evaluation?**

Unprepped sigmoidoscopy to confirm obstruction, then a barium study to determine the cause. If you suspect pseudo-obstruction (typically due to medications), **don't** order a barium study (for fear of concretion and obstruction). Colonoscopy can be diagnostic and therapeutic.

❐ ❐ ❐ ➤ **List three classes of drugs that cause pseudo-obstruction.**

Anticholinergics, antiparkinsonian drugs, and tricyclic antidepressants.

❐ ❐ ❐ ➤ **While you're at it, list three types of <u>internal</u> hernias.**

Diaphragmatic hernia, lesser sac hernia (through the foramen of Winslow), and omental or mesenteric hernia.

❐ ❐ ❐ ➤ **Which is more dangerous, a small hernia or a large one?**

Incarceration is more likely with small hernias.

❐ ❐ ❐ ➤ **Is a hernia in Hesselbach's triangle (between the inguinal ligament, inferior epigastric vessels, and lateral border of the rectus abdominis) likely to incarcerate some day?**

Direct hernias rarely incarcerate.

❐ ❐ ❐ ➤ **What about a hernia that is lateral to the epigastric vessels?**

Indirect hernias are much more likely to incarcerate.

❒ ❒ ❒ ➤ **Which is the most common hernia in women, inguinal or femoral?**

Inguinal, <u>not</u> femoral. While it's true that femoral hernias are more common in women than in men, inguinal hernias remain the most common hernia in women.

❒ ❒ ❒ ➤ **Distinguish between a groin hernia, a hydrocele and a lymph node.**

Hydroceles transilluminate and are non-tender. Lymph nodes tend to be freely moving, firm, and multiple. Hernias don't transilluminate and may have bowel sounds.

❒ ❒ ❒ ➤ **A patient tells you that 2 d ago his groin bulged and he developed severe pain with progressive nausea and vomiting. He has a tender mass in his groin. What shouldn't you do?**

Don't try to reduce a long-standing, tender incarcerated hernia! The abdomen is no place for dead bowel.

❒ ❒ ❒ ➤ **How does the pathology of Crohn's disease differ from that of ulcerative colitis?**

Crohn's is a through-and-through, segmental, granulomatous process, while ulcerative colitis is a mucosal, juxtapositional, ulcerative process.

❒ ❒ ❒ ➤ **A young man with atraumatic chronic back pain, eye trouble, and painful red lumps on his shins develops <u>bloody diarrhea</u>. What is the point of this question?**

To remind you of extraintestinal manifestations of inflammatory bowel disease, such as ankylosing spondylitis, uveitis, and erythema nodosum, not to mention <u>kidney stones</u>.

❒ ❒ ❒ ➤ **At least a third of patients with Crohn's disease have kidney stones. Why?**

Dietary oxalate is usually bound to calcium and excreted. When terminal ileal disease leads to decreased bile salt absorption, the resulting fattier intestinal contents bind calcium by saponification. Free oxalate is "hyper-absorbed" in the colon, resulting in hyperoxaluria and calcium oxalate nephrolithiasis.

❒ ❒ ❒ ➤ **Complications of Crohn's include perirectal abscesses, anal fissures, rectovaginal fistulas, and rectal prolapse. How often is perirectal disease present?**

In around 90 percent of patients.

❒ ❒ ❒ ➤ **Which drugs maintain remission in Crohn's disease?**

Steroids, sulfasalazine, Imuran and azathioprine (steroid-sparing agents) suppress inflammation, but <u>no drugs maintain remission</u>. This was a trick question! Sulfasalazine <u>does</u> maintain remission in ulcerative colitis.

❒ ❒ ❒ ➤ **A patient with chronic, occasionally bloody diarrhea develops severe diarrhea** and abdominal pain with marked distention. What "can't-miss" diagnosis does this suggest?

Toxic megacolon, a life-threatening complication of ulcerative colitis.

❑ ❑ ❑ ➣ **What are the odds that a patient with severe ileal disease will be cured by surgery?**

Virtually zero. Crohn's almost invariably recurs in the remaining GI tract. In contrast, total proctocolectomy with ileostomy is curative in ulcerative colitis.

❑ ❑ ❑ ➣ **A patient with new diarrhea and abdominal pain tells you she took antibiotics for sinusitis a month ago. Sigmoidoscopy might reveal what?**

Yellowish superficial plaques suggestive of pseudomembranous colitis. Stool studies would show C. difficile toxin.

❑ ❑ ❑ ➣ **What's the treatment?**

Oral vancomycin, 125 mg qid or oral metronidazole, 500 mg qid. Either regimen should be given for 7 to 10 d. Cholestyramine, which binds the toxin, can help limit the diarrhea. Follow-up stool studies should confirm clearance of the toxin.

❑ ❑ ❑ ➣ **Is diverticulitis the likely diagnosis in a patient with low abdominal pain and bright red blood per rectum?**

No. Typically diverticulosis bleeds, while diverticulitis doesn't. Diverticular bleeding is typically painless.

❑ ❑ ❑ ➣ **Is sigmoidoscopy or contrast x-ray study indicated in acute diverticulitis?**

A controversial topic. The conventional wisdom says wait until the acute inflammation resolves.

❑ ❑ ❑ ➣ **Crampy abdominal pain with mucus in the stool suggests what syndrome?**

The irritable bowel one. Patients are afebrile, and often improve after passing flatus.

❑ ❑ ❑ ➣ **What barium findings distinguish colonic obstruction due to acute diverticulitis from that due to colon cancer?**

Diverticulitis is extraluminal, so the mucosa appears intact and involved bowel segments are longer. Adenocarcinoma distorts the mucosa, involves a short segment of bowel, and has overhanging edges.

❑ ❑ ❑ ➣ **Abdominal pain in a gray-haired patient should always suggest _____ _____, until proven otherwise.**

Mesenteric ischemia.

❑ ❑ ❑ ➣ **Prescribe an outpatient antibiotic regimen for uncomplicated diverticulitis.**

Ampicillin, Keflex, or tetracycline, 500 mg qid to cover aerobes, plus metronidazole, 500 mg qid to cover anaerobes.

❏ ❏ ❏ ➤ **Which is more sensitive for locating the source of GI bleeding, a radioactive Tc-labeled red cell scan, or angiography?**

A bleeding scan can find a site bleeding at a rate as low as 0.12 ml/min, while angiography requires rapid bleeding (greater than 0.5 ml/min).

❏ ❏ ❏ ➤ **A patient known to have gallstones presents with acute, postprandial right upper quadrant pain. What's the KUB likely to show?**

Nothing specific. Only around 10% of gallstones are radiopaque. Complications of cholelithiasis - emphysematous cholecystitis, perforation, and pneumobilia - are uncommon but useful findings.

❏ ❏ ❏ ➤ **A child with sickle cell disease presents with fever, shaking chills, and jaundice. The likely diagnosis?**

Charcot's triad suggests ascending cholangitis. The precipitating cause is most likely pigment stones resulting from chronic hemolysis.

❏ ❏ ❏ ➤ **A post-surgical patient develops right upper quadrant pain, nausea, and low-grade fevers. According to his surgeon, the gallbladder was normal intraoperatively. What's a probable diagnosis?**

Acalculous cholecystitis.

❏ ❏ ❏ ➤ **Eight years after her cholecystectomy, a woman develops right upper quadrant pain and jaundice. What's the chance of developing recurrent biliary tract stones after cholecystectomy?**

At least 10%, due either to retained stones or *in-situ* formation by biliary epithelium.

❏ ❏ ❏ ➤ **List the ultrasound findings suggestive of acute cholecystitis.**

Presence of gall stones (or sludge, in acalculous cholecystitis), gall bladder wall thickening > 5 mm, and pericholecystic fluid. A dilated common bile duct (>10 mm) suggests common duct obstruction.

❏ ❏ ❏ ➤ **Name two findings in acute cholecystitis that mandate emergent laparotomy.**

Emphysematous cholecystitis and perforation. Otherwise, timing of surgery is somewhat institution- and surgeon-dependent.

❏ ❏ ❏ ➤ **What simple test can distinguish between conjugated and unconjugated hyperbilirubinemia?**

A dipstick test for urobilinogen, which reflects conjugated (water soluble) hyperbilirubinemia.

❒ ❒ ❒ ➢ **In addition to conjugated hyperbilirubinemia, what liver function abnormalities suggest biliary tract disease?**

Elevated alkaline phosphatase out of proportion to transaminases.

❒ ❒ ❒ ➢ **Which two LFT abnormalities reflect a poor prognosis in acute viral hepatitis?**

A total bilirubin > 20 mg/dl, and prolongation of the prothrombin time > 3 seconds. The extent of transaminase elevation is not a useful marker.

❒ ❒ ❒ ➢ **Match the following hepatitis serologies with the right clinical description:**

(1) HBsAg (-), antiHBs(+)   ___ongoing viral replication; highly infectious.
(2) IgM HBcAg (+), antiHBs(-)   ___remote infection; not infectious.
(3) IgG HBcAg (+), antiHBs(-)   ___recent or ongoing infection; a high titer means high infectivity, while a low titer suggests chronic, active infection.
(4) HBeAg (+)   ___ prior infection or vaccination; not infectious.

Answers: 4,3,2,1.

HBeAg (+):   "e" = "eeeek! I'm infectious!", for e ANTIGEN, anti-HBe implies decreased infectivity.
IgG HBcAg (+):   "G" = Gone.
IgM HBcAg (+):   "M" = Might be contagious still.
ANTIHBs (+):   "s" = Stopped, Pt. has antibodies to surface antigen.

WARNING! YOU <u>MUST</u> SPECIFY WHETHER THE <u>ANTIGEN</u> OR THE <u>ANTIBODY</u> IS PRESENT WHEN LEARNING THESE LETTER CODES, OTHERWISE YOU WILL LEARN THESE THINGS THE WRONG WAY AROUND!! Go over it ten times or so in the text of your choice, then it will make sense and remembering the letters won't be necessary.

❒ ❒ ❒ ➢ **T/F - The "delta agent" can cause hepatitis D in a patient without active hepatitis B.**

False. The d-agent is an incomplete, "defective," RNA virus responsible for hepatitis D. It is an obligate covirus and requires hepatitis B for replication.

❒ ❒ ❒ ➢ **You stick yourself with a needle from a chronic hepatitis B carrier. You've been vaccinated, but never had your antibody status checked. What would be the appropriate post-exposure prophylaxis?**

Have your anti-HBs titer measured. If it's adequate (>10 mIU), you need no treatment. If it's inadequate, you need a single dose of HBIG as soon as possible and a vaccine booster.

❒ ❒ ❒ ➢ **Match the following hepatotoxic drugs with the correct toxic syndrome:**

(1) Halothane, methyldopa, isoniazid.

(2) Anabolic steroids, oral contraceptives, oral hypoglycemics, erythromycin estolate.

(3) Carbon tetrachloride, phosphorus, acetaminophen, *Amanita* mushrooms.

(4) Vinyl chloride, arsenic.

(5) Ethanol.

___chronic active hepatitis and cirrhosis.

___massive hepatic necrosis.

___acute hepatitis.

___steatosis, hepatocellular necrosis.

___cholestatic jaundice.

(Answer: 4, 3, 1, 5, 2)

❏ ❏ ❏ ➤ **A known alcoholic presents with abdominal pain, jaundice, and tender hepatomegaly. Lab evaluation reveals acute hepatitis with the SGOT (AST) elevated more than the SGPT (ALT). In addition to electrolyte repletion, folate, thiamine, and abstinence, what treatment may be indicated?**

Methylprednisolone has been shown to improve the outcome in severe alcoholic hepatitis.

❏ ❏ ❏ ➤ **A high fever and leukocytosis accompanying acute alcoholic hepatitis is worrisome. Why?**

Alcohol is marrow toxic, so leukocytosis often reflects serious associated infection. Get a chest x-ray, and obtain blood cultures, a urinalysis, and ascitic fluid for cell count and culture.

❏ ❏ ❏ ➤ **A cirrhotic presents with weakness and edema. What electrolyte imbalances might be present?**

Hyponatremia (dilutional or diuretic-induced), hypokalemia (from GI losses, secondary hyperaldosteronism, or diuretics), and hypomagsemia.

❏ ❏ ❏ ➤ **The best diuretic choice for most cirrhotics with ascites?**

Potassium-sparing agents (treat the hyperaldosterone state specifically).

❏ ❏ ❏ ➤ **A confused cirrhotic presents to the ED. She is afebrile and has asterixis. What should your exam consist of as you look for the precipitant of hepatic encephalopathy?**

Give thiamine and folate. Assess her mental status and search for localizing neurologic signs (occult head injury); look for dry mucous membranes and a low jugular venous pressure (hypovolemia and azotemia); check a stool guaiac (GI bleeding). Focused lab testing can pinpoint other causes (diuretic overuse and hypokalemia, hypoglycemia, anemia, hypoxia, and infection).

❏ ❏ ❏ ➤ **Aside from fixing the above, what therapy is useful?**

Lactulose, which produces an acidic diarrhea that traps nitrogenous wastes in the gut.

❏ ❏ ❏ ➤ **Are there any useful therapies for the rapid renal failure that can complicate cirrhosis?**

Unfortunately not. The hepatorenal syndrome still has a mortality that approaches 100%.

❐ ❐ ❐ ➤ **An ascitic patient presents with fever but no localizing signs or symptoms of infection, and a normal WBC. Because you know that spontaneous bacterial peritonitis can be an occult disease, you perform an abdominal paracentesis. What WBC in ascitic fluid suggests SBP?**

Greater than 250/mm^3. You should also Gram stain the fluid and send at least 10 cc in blood culture bottles for aerobic and anaerobic culture.

❐ ❐ ❐ ➤ **The most common organism responsible for SBP?**

E. coli, followed by pneumococci.

❐ ❐ ❐ ➤ **So the best therapy is . . .?**

Intravenous penicillin G (10 million units daily) or ampicillin (12 g daily) **plus** an aminoglycoside is reasonable empiric therapy pending culture results.

❐ ❐ ❐ ➤ **What two therapies can reduce the risk of recurrent SBP?**

Diuretics decrease ascitic fluid, and nonabsorbable oral antibiotics decrease the gut bacterial load, limiting bacterial translocation. Both treatments have cut the risk of recurrence in compliant patients.

❐ ❐ ❐ ➤ **A non-drinker presents with acute pancreatitis. What conditions may underlie this acute process?**

Biliary tract disease, trauma (blunt or penetrating), ulcers (posterior penetrating duodenal ulcer), diabetes (ketoacidosis), and hypertriglyceridemia.

❐ ❐ ❐ ➤ **Which is a more sensitive test for pancreatitis, serum amylase or lipase?**

Amylase elevation is 70-90% sensitive for pancreatitis; lipase is 75-100% sensitive; the combination is up to 95-97% sensitive. Remember that up to 10% of patients with severe acute pancreatitis may have a normal amylase. In chronic pancreatitis, up to 30% may have a normal amylase.

❐ ❐ ❐ ➤ **What are Ranson's five predictors of complications from acute pancreatitis upon admission?**

Age over 55, blood glucose >200 mg/dl, WBC > 16,000/mm^3, SGOT (AST) >250 U/l, and LDH > 700 IU/l.

❐ ❐ ❐ ➤ **Forty-eight h after admission, what six findings predict poor outcome?**

Hematocrit drop > 10%, rise in BUN > 5 gm/dl, calcium lower than 8 mg/dl, PaO$_2$ < 60 mm Hg, large third-space fluid accumulation, and base deficit > 4 mEq/l.

❏ ❏ ❏ ➤ **Is a nasogastric tube always indicated in acute pancreatitis?**

Only if nausea and vomiting are severe. One trial showed a <u>worse</u> outcome with NG tubes because of complications, including aspiration.

❏ ❏ ❏ ➤ **When are antibiotics useful in acute pancreatitis?**

Pancreatitis is a chemical disease, and antibiotics are only useful for treating <u>complications</u> such as abscess or sepsis. The only exception is in pancreatitis associated with choledocholithiasis, when cefotetan or ampicillin plus gentamicin are indicated.

❏ ❏ ❏ ➤ **Symptoms that last longer than a week or the presence of an abdominal mass, hyperamylasemia, and leukocytosis suggest what potentially disastrous complications of pancreatitis?**

Pancreatic abscess or pseudocyst.

❏ ❏ ❏ ➤ **Are there any useful plain film findings in pancreatitis?**

Right upper quadrant calcifications suggests gallstone pancreatitis, air in the region of the pancreas suggests abscess, and calcific stippling in the epigastrium suggests chronic pancreatitis.

❏ ❏ ❏ ➤ **Portal hypertension produces internal hemorrhoids through which veins?**

Internal hemorrhoids are proximal to the fabled dentate line in the **2**-, **5**-, and **9**-o'clock position in the prone patient, and are typically not palpable on rectal exam. They occur in the superior rectal and inferior mesenteric veins.

❏ ❏ ❏ ➤ **Are painful hemorrhoids always external hemorrhoids?**

No. Though hemorrhoidal pain is more likely to be due to thrombosed external hemorrhoids, be on the lookout for prolapsed and/or incarcerated internal hemorrhoids.

❏ ❏ ❏ ➤ **Distinguish, by location, the following: anal cryptitis, anal fissure, anorectal abscess, and fistula in ano.**

Cryptitis, fissures and perianal abscess typically occur in the posterior midline; deep abscesses can point to areas far from the anus. Goodsall's rule on fistulas: those that open anteriorly go straight to the anal canal, while those that open posteriorly may follow a circuitous route.

❏ ❏ ❏ ➤ **T/F - Antibiotics are unnecessary after an uncomplicated perirectal abscess is incised and drained.**

True, assuming the patient has no underlying immunoincompetence (HIV, diabetes, malignancy). Sitz baths beginning the next day are the primary after-care.

❏ ❏ ❏ ➤ **Distinguish anal chancres and herpetic ulcers.**

Anal chancres of primary syphilis are <u>painful</u>, symmetric, indurated, and diagnosed by dark-field microscopy.

Herpes simplex produces perianal paresthesias and pruritus, followed by red-haloed vesicles and apthous ulcers (ruptured vesicles); a Tzanck smear is diagnostic. Both cause painful inguinal adenopathy.

❒ ❒ ❒ ➤ **A patient presents with proctitis, and a Gram stain of a rectal swab reveals neutrophils with Gram-negative intracellular diplococci. The treatment?**

Ceftriaxone, 250 mg IM, once, with tetracycline, 500 mg qid (or doxycycline 100 mg bid) for 10 days to cover possible Chlamydia co-infection (send a Chlamydia swab and a serologic test for syphilis to the lab, as well). Sexual partners should be notified, and follow-up cultures obtained after therapy. (Note: some authors suggest empiric treatment for Chlamydia in women only, since Chlamydial proctitis is less common in men).

❒ ❒ ❒ ➤ **Procidentia in adults mandates what intervention?**

Rectal prolapse can be manually reduced in children with good results; adults typically require proctosigmoidoscopy and surgical repair.

❒ ❒ ❒ ➤ **Is it better to have cancer of the anal margin or of the anal canal?**

Anal margin cancer is usually low-grade, and late to metastasize, while anal canal cancers are more aggressive and metastasize early.

❒ ❒ ❒ ➤ **Watery diarrhea with profuse rectal discharge and weakness might suggest what uncommon tumor?**

Villous adenoma, with watery diarrhea and hypokalemia.

❒ ❒ ❒ ➤ **Do pilonidal abscesses communicate with the anal canal?**

Nope. They are virtually always midline and overly the lower sacrum. Posterior-opening, horseshoe-type anorectal fistulas can find their way to the lower sacrum, but are rarely in the midline. Remember Goodsall's rule.

❒ ❒ ❒ ➤ **Should pilonidal cysts be excised in the emergency department?**

Probably not. Incision and drainage is OK, followed by a bulky dressing, analgesics, and hot sitz baths beginning the next day; antibiotics are not typically necessary. One study suggests that minimal excision, marsupialization, and packing amounts to incomplete surgery, and excision should be complete and definitive (in the OR), once the acute infection clears up.

❒ ❒ ❒ ➤ **In adults, pruritus ani is seen with dietary factors contributing to liquid stool (caffeine, mineral oil), sexually transmitted infections, fecal contamination, overzealous hygiene, and vitamin deficiencies. The most common cause in children?**

Enterobius vermicularis, or pinworm. A cheap and diagnostic test: apply a piece of scotch tape sticky-side down to the perineal area, than smooth it out (with a cotton swab) on a glass slide and examine under low power for eggs. Treatment is mebendazole, 100 mg in a single dose, repeated at 2 weeks.

❒ ❒ ❒ ➤ **What two stool studies are crucial in evaluating acute diarrhea?**

Statistically speaking, acute diarrhea is so common and typically self-limited that <u>most cases need no testing</u>, just oral rehydration. In sick patients or those at risk for complications (at the extremes of age, recently hospitalized, immunocompromised), <u>enteroinvasive infection should be ruled out</u> with a stool guaiac and test for fecal leukocytes (Gram or methylene blue stains are comparable).

❐ ❐ ❐ ➤ **Which diarrheal illnesses cause fecal leukocytes?**

Usual culprits:
　　Shigella.
　　Campylobacter.
　　Enteroinvasive E. coli.
Others:
　　Salmonella, Yersinia, Vibrio parahemolyticus, and C. difficile.

Fecal WBCs are absent in toxigenic and enteropathogenic infection, even with such a virulent organism as Vibrio cholera; viral and parasitic infections rarely produce fecal WBCs.

❐ ❐ ❐ ➤ **Name the most likely cause of diarrhea in a 6-mo old in day-care.**

Viral diarrhea is most common, with Rotavirus the most common virus; be on the lookout for Giardia and Cryptosporidia, recently added to the list of day-care-associated diarrheal illnesses.

❐ ❐ ❐ ➤ **The most common cause of bacterial diarrhea?**

E. coli (enteroinvasive, enteropathogenic, enterotoxigenic).

❐ ❐ ❐ ➤ **A former IV drug user with sickle-cell disease and a history of splenectomy presents with unremitting fever, crampy abdominal pain, and meningismus after recently acquiring a pet turtle. He has no diarrhea. What bacteria may be the culprit?**

Salmonella typhi, the causative agent of typhoid fever. The attack rate is remarkably high in patients with HIV, in those without spleens, and in those with sickle cell disease. Rose spots occur in 10-20%; relative bradycardia in the face of a high fever, and a low or normal WBC with a pronounced left shift are suggestive findings.

❐ ❐ ❐ ➤ **The treatment?**

Intravenous chloramphenicol and ampicillin, or TMP/SMX. Make sure to check blood cultures, which may suggest metastatic infection. Avoid antimotility agents.

❐ ❐ ❐ ➤ **Match the diarrheal syndrome with the culprit:**

(1) Aeromonas hydrophilia

(2) Bacillus cereus

(3) Campylobacter

(4) Clostridium difficile
(5) Clostridium perfringens

(6) Vibrio parahemolyticus

(7) Staph. aureus
(8) Yersinia

(9) Giardia
(10) Ciguatera toxin

___Diarrhea on the way to the car after eating fried rice at a Chinese buffet.
___Diarrhea followed by thigh myalgias, perioral dysesthesias, and pruritus.
___ Profuse, foul-smelling diarrhea with bloating and cramps after a fishing trip.
___Bloody diarrhea and fever in a child.
___Acute dysentery, fever, and pseudoappendicitis after getting a new puppy.
___Rice water diarrhea without fever or constitutional symptoms.
___Diarrhea from raw seafood.
___Diarrhea from contaminated meat; no nausea or vomiting.
___Diarrhea from antibiotic-associated enterocolitis.
___Diarrhea (enterocolitis) associated with either antibiotics *or* food.

(Answers: 2, 10, 9, 3, 8, 1, 6, 5, 4, 7)

Diarrhea on the way to the car after eating fried rice at a Chinese buffet - Bacillus cereus; treatment is symptomatic.
Diarrhea followed by thigh myalgias, perioral dysesthesias, and pruritus - Ciguatera toxin; no treatment.
Profuse, foul-smelling diarrhea with bloating and cramps after a fishing trip - Giardia; quinacrine or metronidazole.
Bloody diarrhea and fever in a child - Campylobacter; erythromycin; tetracycline in adults.
Acute dysentery, fever, and pseudoappendicitis - Yersinia; optimal tx unknown, chloramphenicol, tetracycline, TMP/SMX.
Rice water diarrhea without fever or constitutional symptoms - Aeromonas hydrophilia with sx due to enterotoxin; tx primarily symptomatic.
Diarrhea from raw seafood - Vibrio parahemolyticus; treat symptoms.
Diarrhea from contaminated meat; no nausea or vomiting - Clostridium perfringens; usually no therapy, rarely antitoxin antibodies.
Diarrhea from antibiotic-associated enterocolitis - Clostridium difficile; vancomycin.
Diarrhea (enterocolitis) associated with either antibiotics or food - Staph. aureus; treat symptoms.

METABOLIC AND ENDOCRINE

"...I don't want to live-I want to love first, and live incidentally..."

Zelda Fitzgerald, 1919.

❏ ❏ ❏ ➤ **What tissues do not use free fatty acids as the source of energy?**

Brain and formed blood elements.

❏ ❏ ❏ ➤ **A 36 y old female presents with a history of being difficult to arouse in the morning. Her husband says, "After she's had breakfast, she perks right up". Diagnosis?**

Fasting hypoglycemia. Fasting hypoglycemia may reflect serious organic disease. As a consequence, evaluation of this disorder typically requires hospitalization.

❏ ❏ ❏ ➤ **How do you distinguish between endogenously produced and exogenously administered insulin?**

Endogenous - Insulin and C peptide levels corresponds.
Exogenously - Insulin level elevated, C peptide level low.

❏ ❏ ❏ ➤ **In the first two years of life, what is the most common cause of <u>drug-induced</u> hypoglycemia?**

Salicylates. In the 2-8 y old group, alcohol is the most likely cause, and in the 11 to 30 y old group, insulin and sulfonylureas are the most likely cause.

❏ ❏ ❏ ➤ **What is the principle hormone protecting the human body against hypoglycemia?**

Glucagon.

❏ ❏ ❏ ➤ **What drugs potentiate the hypoglycemic effects of sulfonylurea?**

Salicylates, alcohol, sulfonamides, phenylbutazone, and bis-hydroxycoumarin. Chlorpropamide is the sulfonylurea compound most likely to cause hypoglycemic events. It also causes the most prolonged hypoglycemia.

❏ ❏ ❏ ➤ **How is sulfonylurea-induced hypoglycemia treated?**

IV glucose alone may be insufficient. It may require diazoxide 300 mg slow IV over 30 min repeated every four h.

❏ ❏ ❏ ➤ **What effect does propranolol have on blood sugar in diabetic patients?**

Propranolol is thought to precipitate hypoglycemia.

❏ ❏ ❏ ➢ **What is the most common cause of hypoglycemia in a child?**

Ketotic hypoglycemia. Attacks usually occur when the child is stressed with caloric deprivation. Most common in boys, typically between 18 mo and 5 y of age. Attacks may be episodic, vomiting may occur, and are more frequent in the morning or during periods of illness.

❏ ❏ ❏ ➢ **What are the neurologic signs and symptoms of hypoglycemia?**

Hypoglycemia may produce mental and neurologic dysfunction. Neurologic manifestations may include paresthesias, cranial nerve palsies, transient hemiplegia, diplopia, decerebrate posturing, and clonus.

❏ ❏ ❏ ➢ **What lab findings are expected with diabetic ketoacidosis?**

Elevated ß-hydroxybutyrate, acetoacetate, acetone and glucose. Ketonuria and glucosuria are present. Serum bicarbonate level, PCO_2, and pH are decreased. Potassium may be initially elevated but falls if the acidosis is corrected.

❏ ❏ ❏ ➢ **What is the treatment of DKA?**

Fluids, approximately 5-10 liters of normal saline alternating with 1/2 normal saline. Potassium 100-200 mEq in the first 12-24 h. Insulin 20 unit bolus followed by 5-10 U/h. Add glucose to the IV fluid when glucose levels fall below 250 mg/dl. Phosphate supplement when level drops below 1.0 mg/dl.
Peds : NS 20 ml/kg/h for 1-2 h.
Insulin 0.1 U/kg bolus followed by 0.1 U/kg/h drip.

❏ ❏ ❏ ➢ **A 42 y old female presents with a history of palpitations, sweating, diplopia, blurred vision, and weakness. The family indicates she has been confused. Symptoms usually occur before breakfast. Diagnosis?**

Islet cell tumor of the pancreas can be a cause of a fasting hypoglycemia.

❏ ❏ ❏ ➢ **What sulfonylurea compound most commonly causes hypoglycemia?**

Chlorpropamide.

❏ ❏ ❏ ➢ **What are the key features of nonketotic hyperosmolar coma?**

Hyperosmolality, hyperglycemia, and dehydration. Blood sugar should be greater than 800 mg/dl, serum osmolality should be greater than 350 mOsm/kg, and serum ketones should be negative.

❏ ❏ ❏ ➢ **What is the treatment of nonketotic hyperosmolar coma?**

Fluids (normal saline), potassium 10-20 mEq/h. Insulin 5-10 U/h, and glucose should be added to the IV when the blood sugar drops below 250 mg/dl.

❏ ❏ ❏ ➢ **What is the most consistent finding with lactic acidosis?**

Kussmaul's respirations or hyperventilation.

❏ ❏ ❏ ➤ **Distinguish between type A and type B lactic acidosis.**

Type A lactic acidosis is often seen in the Emergency Department. It is most commonly due to shock. Type A lactic acidosis is associated with inadequate tissue perfusion and resultant anoxia, with subsequent lactate and hydrogen ion accumulation. Type B lactic acidosis includes all forms of acidosis in which there is no evidence of tissue anoxia.

❏ ❏ ❏ ➤ **What are the pathognomonic findings as well as confirmatory lab tests diagnostic of thyroid storm?**

Trick question. Thyroid storm is based on clinical impression. There are no findings or confirmatory tests available.

❏ ❏ ❏ ➤ **What is the most common cause of thyroid storm?**

Infections, typically pulmonary infections, are the most common precipitating event.

❏ ❏ ❏ ➤ **What clinical clues might help in the diagnosis of thyroid storm?**

Eye signs of Graves' disease, a history of hyperthyroidism, widened pulse pressure, and a palpable goiter.

❏ ❏ ❏ ➤ **What are the diagnostic criteria for thyroid storm?**

Tachycardia, CNS dysfunction, cardiovascular dysfunction, GI system dysfunction, and temperature greater than 37.8 °C (100 °F).

❏ ❏ ❏ ➤ **What are the signs and symptoms of thyroid storm?**

Tachycardia, fever, diaphoresis, increased CNS activity, emotional lability, heart failure, coma, and death.

❏ ❏ ❏ ➤ **What are the complications of bicarbonate therapy in DKA?**

Paradoxical CSF acidosis, cardiac arrhythmias, decreased oxygen delivery to tissue, and fluid and sodium overload.

❏ ❏ ❏ ➤ **What is the approximate overall mortality of nonketotic hyperosmolar coma?**

Approximately 50%.

❏ ❏ ❏ ➤ **What is the <u>most</u> <u>common</u> cause of hypothyroidism?**

Primary thyroid failure. The most common etiology of hypothyroidism in adults is the use of radioactive iodine or subtotal thyroidectomy in the treatment of Graves' disease. The second most common cause is autoimmune thyroid disorders.

❏ ❏ ❏ ➢ **In a patient receiving anticoagulation therapy with heparin, when is adrenal hemorrhage most likely to strike?**

Typically between the 3rd and 18th d of anticoagulation. Patients present with sudden hypotension and flank or epigastric pain. Nausea, vomiting, fever, and a change in sensorium may be associated.

❏ ❏ ❏ ➢ **What is the most common cause of secondary adrenal insufficiency and adrenal crisis?**

Iatrogenic adrenal suppression from prolonged steroid use. Rapid withdrawal of steroids may lead to collapse and death.

❏ ❏ ❏ ➢ **An <u>increase</u> of PCO$_2$ of 10 mmHg will lead to an expected decrease in pH of about:**

pH increases 0.08.

❏ ❏ ❏ ➢ **A <u>decrease</u> of PCO$_2$ of 10 mm Hg will lead to an expected increase in pH of about:**

pH increases 0.13.

❏ ❏ ❏ ➢ **What is the expected increase in pH associated with a rise in HCO$_3$ of 5.0 mEq/l?**

pH increases 0.08.

❏ ❏ ❏ ➢ **What is the expected decrease in pH associated with a decrease in HCO$_3$ of 5.0 mEq/l?**

pH decreases 0.10.

❏ ❏ ❏ ➢ **Discuss the implications of Ebden-Meyerhof pathway disruption on phospho-fructokinase enhanced glycolysis. Contrast these implications with those of the Van Leeuwen modifications and to Fast Fourier Transform (FFT) analysis of titration/buffering rates in acute acidosis.**

Just kidding! This is why God makes Internists! Let's review some metabolic pearls that may be useful in sorting out some disorders.

❏ ❏ ❏ ➢ **How is the anion gap calculated from electrolyte values?**

Anion gap = Na - Cl - CO$_2$ The normal gap is 12 $^+$/- 4 mEq/l.

❏ ❏ ❏ ➢ **Acidosis is closely related to anion gap measurement. Name the causes of an increased anion gap acidosis.**

A MUDPILE CAT

A   = alcohol,

M   = methanol,
U   = uremia,
D   = DKA,
P   = paraldehyde,
I   = iron and isoniazid,
L   = lactic acidosis,
E   = ethylene glycol,

C   = carbon monoxide,
A   = aspirin,
T   = toluene.

❏ ❏ ❏ ➤ **That's a pretty big differential. History and physical can go a long way in narrowing this list down. The magnitude of the anion gap can also be useful; discuss.**

Anion gap > 35 mEq/l is usually caused by ethylene glycol, methanol or lactic acidosis.
Anion gap 23 - 30 mEq/l usually also because of increased organic acids.
Anion gap 16 - 22 mEq/l may be due to uremia, which must be quite advanced before it causes an increased gap.

❏ ❏ ❏ ➤ **There is another "gap" that can aid in diagnosing the cause of an anion gap acidosis - the osmolar gap. Let's distract ourselves for a momentary discussion of the osmolar gap and how it may be useful.**

Uh-oh. Osmolality is a measure of the concentration of particles in a solution, its units are osmoles per kg water. Osmolarity is a measure of osmoles per liter of solution - for dilute solutions, like body fluids, these two measures are roughly equivalent. An osmolar gap is a difference between measured osmolality and calculated osmolarity. The osmolar gap is calculated as follows:
Measured osmolality - calculated osmolarity = osmolar gap.

$$CalculatedOsmol(mOsm/l) = 2(Na) + \frac{glucose}{18} + \frac{BUN}{2.8}$$

(Normal = 275 - 285 mOsm/l)

❏ ❏ ❏ ➤ **Different substances contribute to varying degrees to the osmolar gap, these are listed below:**

Substance	mg/dl to increase serum osmol 1 mOsm/l	# mOsm/l increase due to each mg/dl
Methanol	2.6	0.38
Ethanol	4.3	0.23
Ethylene glycol	5.0	0.20
Acetone	5.5	0.18
Isopropyl alcohol	5.9	0.17
Salicylate	14.0	0.07

Thus, small amounts of methanol cause greater increases in osmolality. Large amounts of salicylate will eventually increase osmolar gap.
Note also that the contribution to an osmolar gap due to EtOH may be calculated; this can be useful in when a mixed alcohol ingestion is suspected (and your IM colleagues in the ED will be impressed!).

❏ ❏ ❏ ➣ **O.K., with that distraction now behind us, review some other pearls that can help narrow the d/dx of an anion gap acidosis.**

Methanol- visual disturbances and headache common. Can produce quite wide gaps as discussed above.

Uremia- advanced before it causes an anion gap.

Diabetic Ketoacidosis- usually has both hyperglycemia and glucosuria.

Alcoholic Ketoacidosis (AKA)- often has a lower blood sugar and mild or absent glucosuria.

Salicylates- high levels required to contribute to gap.

Lactic Acidosis- can check serum level. Itself has broad differential to be discussed in a question in the random section.

Ethylene glycol- causes calcium oxalate or hippurate crystals in urine.

❏ ❏ ❏ ➣ **What are the causes of the oxygen saturation curve shift to the right?**

A shift to the right delivers more O_2 to the tissue.
Right = Release to tissues.

"CADET! Right face!!"

      Hyper   Carbia,
               Acidemia,
        2,3 DPG,
               Exercise,
   increased Temperature.

The mnemonic CADET helps in remembering causes of an O_2 shift to the right.

❏ ❏ ❏ ➣ **When body waste materials (urine & stool) are enterally recycled, they can cause a normal anion gap metabolic acidosis. Thus, USED CRAP _does_ in fact cause a normal anion gap (hyperchloremic) metabolic acidosis; discuss.**

U = ureteroenterostomy
S = small bowel fistula
E = extra chloride (NH_4Cl or amino acid chlorides 2° TPN)
D = diarrhea

C = carbonic anhydrase inhibitors
R = renal tubular acidosis
A = adrenal insufficiency
P = pancreatic fistula

❏ ❏ ❏ ➣ **What are the two primary causes of metabolic alkalosis?**

Loss of hydrogen and chloride from the stomach.
Overzealous diuresis with loss of hydrogen, potassium and chloride.

❏ ❏ ❏ ➢ **What is central pontine myelinolysis, a.k.a. osmotic demyelination syndrome?**

The complication of brain dehydration following too rapid correction of severe hyponatremia. Correct hyponatremia slowly, less than 12 mEq/d in chronic hyponatremia.

PEDI PEARLS

"Somebody BOUNCED me. I was just thinking by the side of the river -
...when I received a loud BOUNCE."

Eeyore

❐ ❐ ❐ ➢ **What is the normal pulse rate of a newborn?**

120 - 160 bpm.

❐ ❐ ❐ ➢ **External chest compressions should be initiated for a newborn with assisted ventilation who has a heart rate less than _____ beats per minute.**

50 bpm.

❐ ❐ ❐ ➢ **Outline the Apgar scoring system.**

Index	0 points	1 point	2 points
Pulse	Ø	< 100	> 100
Resp. effort	Ø	Weak cry	Strong cry
Color	Cyanotic	Extremities cyanotic	Pink
Tone	Flaccid	Weak tone	Strong
Response	Ø	Motion	Cry

❐ ❐ ❐ ➢ **A normal appearing term neonate presents with tachypnea and cyanosis. Likely pathology?**

Congenital cardiac pathology.
CHF can be presenting symptomatology for VSD, severe aortic coarctation or transposition of the great vessels.
The "hyperoxia" test may help differentiate cardiac etiology - Place the infant in 100% O_2, the PaO_2 will increase less than 20 mmHg with R→L shunting of cardiac decrease.

❐ ❐ ❐ ➢ **Stridor in the neonate is usually caused by congenital anomalies. Is infection also a common cause of neonatal stridor?**

No.

❐ ❐ ❐ ➢ **What is the <u>most common</u> cause of neonatal stridor?**

Laryngotracheomalacia.

❐ ❐ ❐ ➢ **Define apnea.**

No respiration for > 20 s.

❏ ❏ ❏ ➤ **Does apnea always indicate a serious problem and require admission?**

True apnea represents serious pathology and always merits immediate appropriate intervention and admission.

❏ ❏ ❏ ➤ **Physiologic jaundice occurs at about 2-4 d. How high may the bilirubin level be expected to climb?**

5-6 mg/dl.

❏ ❏ ❏ ➤ **A neonate presents with a history of poor feeding, vomiting, respiratory distress, has abdominal distention and is found to have hyperbilirubinemia. What is the likely cause of this complex?**

This neonate is septic!

❏ ❏ ❏ ➤ **Name some causes of jaundice occurring at age less than 1 d.**

Sepsis, congenital infections, ABO/Rh incompatibility.

❏ ❏ ❏ ➤ **Jaundice due to breast feeding occurs after 7 d and can reach very high levels over weeks; how high?**

Levels of bilirubin near 25 mg/dl can be reached.

❏ ❏ ❏ ➤ **A cyanotic infant's SaO_2 & PaO_2 do not increase with oxygen therapy. What cause does this suggest?**

Intracardiac (R→L) shunting, not pulmonary disease.

❏ ❏ ❏ ➤ **Do not skip to the answer to this question, make a real attempt to answer it - Name 8 clinical presentations of pediatric heart disease.**

1. Cyanosis
2. CHF
3. Pathologic murmur
4. Cardiogenic shock
5. HTN
6. Tachyarrhythmias
7. Abnormal pulses
8. Syncope

❏ ❏ ❏ ➤ **Tetralogy of Fallot (TOF) consists of VSD, an "overriding" aorta, pulmonary stenosis and right ventricular hypertrophy. What type of intracardiac shunting occurs?**

Right-to-left shunting whose severity is related to the degree of pulmonary stenosis.

❏ ❏ ❏ ➤ **Describe the murmurs of TOF.**

1. Holosystolic murmur of VSD - 3rd ICS @ LSB.
2. Crescendo-decrescendo murmur of pulmonary stenosis - 2nd ICS @ LSB.

N.B. - If you can differentiate these two murmurs in a sick cyanotic infant in a busy ED, go directly to Pediatric Cardiology, do not Pass Go, do not collect $200.

❏ ❏ ❏ ➢ **Describe the three aspects of acute treatment of TOF.**

Positioning -   Place in knee-chest position. Keep patient unstimulated (i.e., upright on lap in parent's arms).
Oxygenation -   Deliver high FIO_2.
Pharmacologic - Morphine 0.1 mg/kg.

❏ ❏ ❏ ➢ **SVT in adults usually occurs with a ventricular rate of about 150 - 200. What is the range of ventricular rates in children?**

220 - 360 bpm.

❏ ❏ ❏ ➢ **What is the dose of adenosine given to a pediatric patient with SVT?**

0.1 mg/kg.

❏ ❏ ❏ ➢ **Verapamil should not be used to treat infants of less than what age?**

Do not use verapamil in infants less than two years of age (can lead to asystole).

❏ ❏ ❏ ➢ **If cardioversion is necessary to treat an infant with unstable SVT, what is the appropriate energy to use?**

0.25 - 1 J/kg.

❏ ❏ ❏ ➢ **Differentiate sepsis from bacteremia.**

Bacteremia is the symptom of fever with a positive blood culture; sepsis is bacteremia with focal findings identified.

❏ ❏ ❏ ➢ **What are the two <u>most common</u> organisms causing bacteremia?**

S. pneumoniae and H. influenzae.

❏ ❏ ❏ ➢ **What are the two <u>most common</u> organisms causing sepsis in the neonate?**

Group B streptococcus and E. coli.

❏ ❏ ❏ ➢ **What are the three <u>most common</u> organisms causing sepsis after the newborn period?**

H. influenzae, N. meningitidis and S. pneumoniae.

❏ ❏ ❏ ➢ **There is much controversy surrounding the question of when to check a WBC** in a pediatric patient with suspected bacteremia and if results of this test should be used to decide whether or not to draw a blood culture or decide to initiate treatment with antibiotics. What is the current recommendation of when to draw a WBC for suspected bacteremia (Tintinalli, 3rd Ed.)?

Draw a WBC for patients 3 mo to 2 y old with temperature ≥ 39.4 °C (102.9 °F) and no clear source.
Draw a WBC for patients 3 mo to 2 y old who appear toxic with fever < 39.4 °C.

❏ ❏ ❏ ➢ What is the current recommendation, from the same source, of what level of WBC and absolute polymorphonuclear cell count should then lead to drawing blood for culture?

WBC ≥ 15,000/mm^3 or absolute polymorphonuclear cell count > 9,000/mm^3 should lead to drawing blood for culture.
N.B. Answers to these two questions are controversial.

❏ ❏ ❏ ➢ A septic pediatric patient is in shock. An initial bolus of normal saline at 20 ml/kg has been given. Urine output should be maintained at what level by delivery of appropriate fluid?

1 ml/kg/h.

❏ ❏ ❏ ➢ What is the appropriate dose of diazepam to be administered to a seizing pediatric patient with suspected meningitis?

0.3 mg/kg. Load with phenytoin or phenobarbital after termination of seizure activity.

❏ ❏ ❏ ➢ Many authors believe in giving methylprednisolone to pediatric patients with meningitis to decrease sequelae, especially deafness. What is the appropriate dose of methylprednisolone in meningitis?

30 mg/kg.

❏ ❏ ❏ ➢ What are the two most common organisms causing meningitis in the first month of life?

Group B streptococci and E. coli.

❏ ❏ ❏ ➢ Describe antibiotic selection to treat meningitis in patients aged < 1 mo.

Use ampicillin plus an aminoglycoside*.

❏ ❏ ❏ ➢ What is the most common organism causing meningitis after the second mo of life?

H. influenzae.

❏ ❏ ❏ ➢ Describe antibiotic selection to treat meningitis in patients aged > 1 mo.

Ampicillin and chloramphenicol*.
This change in antibiotic choice is due to the increasing rate of H. influenzae as the

causative organism during the second mo of life and the resistance of some of these organisms.

*N.B. Answers to above 2 questions on antibiotic choices based on information from Tintinalli, 3rd Ed.; many physicians currently feel there is a role for third-generation cephalosporins in treatment of meningitis.

❑ ❑ ❑ ➣ **What percentage of children with asthma are likely to have symptoms that persist into adulthood?**

50%.

❑ ❑ ❑ ➣ **What is the <u>most common</u> cause of bronchiolitis?**

RSV.

❑ ❑ ❑ ➣ **What is the most common organism causing epiglottitis?**

H. influenzae.

❑ ❑ ❑ ➣ **What is the usual age range for presentation of <u>retropharyngeal abscess</u>?**

6 mo - 3 y.

❑ ❑ ❑ ➣ **Surprisingly, extrinsic asthma is the <u>most common</u> form in children. Does extrinsic asthma involve IgE production?**

Yes, extrinsic asthma involves IgE production in response to allergens.

❑ ❑ ❑ ➣ **Current recommendations include obtaining a CXR on all pediatric patients with first presentation of symptoms of reactive airway disease or asthma who are less than one y of age. Name some of the etiologies of these symptoms that may be discovered by CXR.**

Foreign body aspiration, bronchiolitis, parenchymal pulmonary disease and heart disease.

❑ ❑ ❑ ➣ **What is the common age range for <u>bronchiolitis</u>?**

Though it may occur in patients up to age 2 y, bronchiolitis commonly occurs between ages 2 - 6 mo.

❑ ❑ ❑ ➣ **Sympathomimetic agents are used to treat asthma. What enzyme is activated by these agents?**

Adenyl cyclase.

❑ ❑ ❑ ➣ **What reaction is catalyzed by adenyl cyclase?**

Adenyl cyclase catalyzes ATP to cyclic AMP.

❏ ❏ ❏ ➢ **What effect does increased levels of cyclic AMP have on bronchial smooth muscle and on the release of chemical mediators (histamine, proteases, platelet activation factor and chemotactic factors) from airway mast cells?**

Smooth muscle relaxation and decreased release of mediators.

Recall that the effects of cyclic AMP are opposed by cyclic GMP - this provides another treatment approach by *decreasing* levels of cyclic GMP which is achieved via anticholinergic (antimuscarinic) agents such as ipratropium bromide.

❏ ❏ ❏ ➢ **As discussed above, stimulation of ß-adrenergic receptors increases cyclic AMP availability and results in smooth muscle relaxation. Which flavor of ß-adrenergic receptors primarily control bronchiolar and arterial smooth muscle tone?**

ß$_2$-adrenergic receptors.

❏ ❏ ❏ ➢ **What is current understanding of the mechanism of action of the methylxanthines?**

The mechanism of action of these agents is not known.

❏ ❏ ❏ ➢ **Pediatric patients presenting with severe asthma may be treated with "high-dose" albuterol. What dose of nebulized albuterol is considered "high-dose," and how frequently may it be given?**

0.15 mg/kg (0.03 ml/kg of 0.5%) per dose to a maximum of 5 mg may be provided every 20 min up to six times.

❏ ❏ ❏ ➢ **How may albuterol dosing be changed if the patient has not responded to the above 6 doses?**

Consider switching to continuous delivery of albuterol nebulized at 0.5 mg/kg/h up to a rate of 15 mg/h. Monitor heart rate.

❏ ❏ ❏ ➢ **What makes albuterol the usual agent of choice?**

Of nebulized ß-adrenergic agonists it has the longest duration of action and the greatest degree of ß$_2$-adrenergic selectivity.

❏ ❏ ❏ ➢ **Terbutaline is given SQ for asthma in what dose?**

0.01 ml/kg (of 1 mg/ml) up to 0.25 ml (0.25 mg) which may be repeated once in 20 minutes.

❏ ❏ ❏ ➢ **Is theophylline of use in the emergency management of severe asthma in pediatric patients?**

No. It has not been shown to cause further bronchodilatation in patients fully treated with ß-adrenergic agents. Theophylline does have a role in inpatient management of asthma and may be started in the ED.

❐ ❐ ❐ ➤ **If corticosteroids are given, how should prednisone be dosed?**

1 - 2 mg/kg/d in two divided doses; no tapering is necessary if duration of therapy is 5 d or less.

❐ ❐ ❐ ➤ **What effect can acidosis have on treatment with ß-adrenergic agonists?**

Decreased efficacy.

❐ ❐ ❐ ➤ **What percentage of aminophylline is theophylline?**

85%.

❐ ❐ ❐ ➤ **If one prefers the most simplified algorithm for determining loading dose of theophylline, what are the appropriate doses for:**
   a. A patient who has not taken any theophylline recently,
   b. A patient who has taken a recent theophylline dose?

a.   No recent dose - load with 7 mg/kg theophylline.
b.   Recent dose - load with 5 mg/kg theophylline.

❐ ❐ ❐ ➤ **What is the appropriate parenteral dose of methylprednisolone (Solu-Medrol) to give a pediatric patient with status asthmaticus?**

1 - 2 mg/kg every 6 h.

❐ ❐ ❐ ➤ **If mechanical ventilation is required for such a patient, what is an appropriate setting for initial tidal volume?**

10 ml/kg.

❐ ❐ ❐ ➤ **Parents of a child who has suffered a febrile seizure often want to know what the risk of a recurrence is. What is it?**

Risk of recurrence is the chance that the same thing will happen again.
About 35%.

❐ ❐ ❐ ➤ **Is LP usually an appropriate component of the evaluation of a first febrile seizure?**

Yes. Many clinicians prefer LP in this situation only if a prolonged postictal period or clinical symptoms such as lethargy are present.

❐ ❐ ❐ ➤ **Treatment of febrile seizures is primarily directed at gradual cooling and treatment for the source of the fever. If anticonvulsant therapy is begun, which medication is best?**

Phenobarbital.

❐ ❐ ❐ ➤ **Phenobarbital is also the drug of choice in neonatal seizures. Its half-life in children over one mo of age is about 65 h. The half-life is even longer in newborns up to** one week of age. How long is it in this age group?

100 h.

❏ ❏ ❏ ➤ Neonatal seizures have a broad range of presentations. What are the two frequent causes of myoclonic seizures?

Metabolic disorders and hypoxia.

❏ ❏ ❏ ➤ The initial treatment of neonatal seizures is directed initially at reversible causes; insure adequate oxygenation, provide pyridoxine (B$_6$), glucose, calcium and magnesium. Following these measures, pharmacologic intervention can be considered. Outline this treatment.

Phenobarbital load, 10 - 15 mg/kg IV.
Phenytoin load, 10 - 15 mg/kg IV.
Diazepam, 0.2 mg/kg IV, may repeat.
Lorazepam, 0.05 mg/kg IV, may repeat.
Clonazepam, 0.1 mg/kg NG.

❏ ❏ ❏ ➤ Infantile spasms are usually first noted in children of about 6 months of age. Is it true that these patients have a high rate of developmental disorders, and if so, what percentage of patients have such disorders?

Yes, it is true; 85%.

❏ ❏ ❏ ➤ Are infantile spasms a form of seizures?

Yes.

❏ ❏ ❏ ➤ Infantile spasms represent a significant disorder and require aggressive evaluation and management. In addition to anticonvulsants, what hormone plays a role in management of infantile spasms?

Adrenocorticotropic hormone.

❏ ❏ ❏ ➤ Febrile seizures occur relatively commonly; about what percentage of children will experience such a seizure?

3.5%; about 35% of these patients will experience a recurrence.

❏ ❏ ❏ ➤ Phenobarbital is probably the most efficacious drug used to treat febrile seizures. Should all patients with a febrile seizure receive phenobarbital as prophylaxis against future similar seizures?

Probably not, though its use may be warranted in patients who are particularly ill, who have had repeated febrile seizures or who have underlying neurologic disease.

❏ ❏ ❏ ➤ Posttraumatic seizures that occur immediately are associated with a very low rate of subsequent epilepsy. About what are the rates of subsequent epilepsy in patients suffering early (within 1 wk) and late (after 1 wk) posttraumatic seizures?

Early ≈ 25%.
Late ≈ 70%.

❒ ❒ ❒ ➢ **For how long must a continuous seizure last to be defined as status epilepticus?**

30 min.

❒ ❒ ❒ ➢ **You appropriately elect to administer diazepam to a patient in "status" at a loading dose of 0.3 mg/kg and a rate of 1 mg/min. This dose should be repeated prn up to a total of how many mg/kg?**

2.6 mg/kg maximum dose of diazepam.

❒ ❒ ❒ ➢ **The Valium given above does not break the seizure and phenytoin is appropriately selected as the next agent. Dose and rate of administration?**

Phenytoin load 15 mg/kg at 25 mg/min (cf. adults ≈ 17 mg/kg @ 50 mg/min!).

❒ ❒ ❒ ➢ **Your patient is *still* seizing!@#! What is the dose of phenobarbital to load?**

10 - 15 mg/kg.

❒ ❒ ❒ ➢ **The seizure has stopped! What three alternative treatments remained?**

Paraldehyde, lidocaine and general anesthesia.

❒ ❒ ❒ ➢ **Hepatic failure is associated with which anticonvulsant?**

Valproic acid.

❒ ❒ ❒ ➢ **What antibiotic can cause carbamazepine to accumulate quickly?**

Erythromycin.

❒ ❒ ❒ ➢ **Bronchopulmonary dysplasia (BPD) is commonly caused by hyaline membrane disease, prematurity and/or mechanical ventilation. BPD is treated with O_2, hydration and time. Describe the clinical features of BPD.**

Tachypnea, reactive airways, hypoxia, and hypercarbia, on occasion with pulmonary edema and cor pulmonale.

❒ ❒ ❒ ➢ **Patients with BPD may have chronic hypercarbia; does administering O_2 blunt respiratory drive in such patients?**

No.

❒ ❒ ❒ ➢ **A youngster presents with signs and symptoms that suggest a pneumonia. She describes chest pain that is pleuritic. Is such pain more commonly associated with viral or with bacterial pneumonia?**

Bacterial.
Strep. pneumoniae in particular is the most common cause in this age group, and is often associated with pleuritic pain and a pleural effusion.

❏ ❏ ❏ ➢ **The spectrum of likely etiology of a pneumonia changes with patient age. What are likely agents causing pneumonia in neonates?**

Bacterial -
  Group B streptococci (Lancefield group B, mostly S. agalactiae).
  Listeria monocytogenes.
  Enteric Gram negative bacilli.
Chlamydia.
Viral -
  Rubella.
  CMV.
  Herpes.

❏ ❏ ❏ ➢ **A neonate presents at 2 wk of age febrile with tachypnea and a history of poor feeding. Your suspicion of a pneumonia is confirmed by a CXR revealing diffuse homogenous infiltrates. You correctly presume a bacterial origin, likely with group B Strep., given the young age and fever (Chlamydia usually presents between about 4 - 10 wk and afebrile, RSV presents between 1 - 6 mo). Though group B Strep. is always susceptible to penicillin G, you are aware that some strains require higher doses of penicillin G and that other less common causes still need to be considered, such as Listeria monocytogenes and Gram negative enteric bacteria. Thus you wish to add a second agent to this patient's treatment, one that is synergistic with penicillin G and will help cover these pathogens. Treat with:**

Penicillin G and gentamycin.

❏ ❏ ❏ ➢ **Causes of pneumonia in patients aged 1 mo to 5 y?**

Bacterial - Streptococcus pneumonia and Hemophilus influenzae.
Viral - RSV, parainfluenza, adenovirus. RSV occurs primarily in patients less than 6 mo of age.

❏ ❏ ❏ ➢ **Hemophilus influenzae is the second most common cause of pediatric pneumonia; what percentage of cases of H. influenzae occur in patients of less than 1 y of age?**

50%, half of remaining cases occur between ages 1 - 2 y.
H. influenzae pneumonia is common primarily in young infants.

❏ ❏ ❏ ➢ **Causes of pneumonia in patients greater than 6 y old?**

Strep. pneumonia, Mycoplasma pneumoniae and influenza virus.

❐ ❐ ❐ ➢ **Mycoplasma pneumoniae is the second most common cause of pneumonia in children greater than 6 y old. Contrast pneumonia due to Mycoplasma with that due to Strep. pneumoniae.**

Characteristic	S. pneumoniae	M. pneumoniae
Prodrome	Little	Mild fever, malaise, cough, HA.
Onset	Rapid	Gradual
URI sx	Tachypnea, cough, occasional pleuritic pain.	Little
Associated findings	High fever.	Exanthem, arthritis, GI complaints, neurologic complications.
Pleural effusion	Occasional	Rare
Lab	Leukocytosis	WBC normal or sl. elevation.
Tx	Penicillin	Erythromycin

❐ ❐ ❐ ➢ **What are the three stages of pertussis?**

Catarrhal stage - rhinorrhea, cough, conjunctivitis.
Paroxysmal stage - after 1 wk of above, paroxysms of continuous coughing. Lasts up to 6 wk.
Convalescent stage - Coughing decreases. (NSS).

Dangerous pneumonias are usually superinfections; treat patient and household contacts with erythromycin (provide broader coverage if pneumonia present), immunize household contacts who are less than 7 y old.

❐ ❐ ❐ ➢ **SIDS is the <u>most common</u> cause of death of infants between 1 mo and 1 y of age (incidence 2 per 1000 = 10,000/y). What are the four risk factors that increase an infant's risk of SIDS?**

Prematurity with low birth weight.
Previous episode of apnea or apparent life threatening event (ALTE).
Mother is a substance abuser.
Sibling of infant who died of SIDS.

❐ ❐ ❐ ➢ **SIDS has a bimodal distribution. At what ages do the peaks occur?**

2.5 & 4 mo.

❐ ❐ ❐ ➢ **What is the <u>most common</u> cause of neonatal conjunctivitis?**

A trick question, as chemical conjunctivitis due to silver nitrate is most common. Chlamydia trachomatis is the <u>most common</u> clinically significant cause in the first 14 d with a usual incubation period of at least 5 d. Gonococcal conjunctivitis has a shorter incubation and may present as soon as 2 d.

❐ ❐ ❐ ➢ **What is the name of the condition of fluid collected in the middle ear that is usually painless, is without sign of infection and that may result in a hearing deficit?**

Serous otitis media, aka otitis media with effusion (OME). An underused diagnosis.

❐ ❐ ❐ ➢ **Which type of agent is the most common cause of acute otitis media (AOM), found in about 70% of cases, bacteria or viruses?**

Bacteria, most commonly S. pneumoniae and H. influenzae.

❐ ❐ ❐ ➢ **How useful is the light reflex in evaluation of suspected AOM?**

It is useless. TM mobility is very valuable.

❐ ❐ ❐ ➢ **Describe the use of topical steroids, midazolam, antihistamines or decongestants in the management of AOM.**

All these agents are of no use in AOM. Antihistamines may decrease Kleenex® use.

❐ ❐ ❐ ➢ **What solution is appropriate treatment of otitis externa?**

Acetic acid ear drops. Treat for ≥ 7 d.

❐ ❐ ❐ ➢ **Among pediatric emergency patients, what is the <u>most common</u> skin infection?**

Impetigo.
Impetigo is a bacterial infection of the dermis, most commonly caused by group A ß-hemolytic streptococcus; it comes in two flavors - impetigo contagiosa and the bullous form.

❐ ❐ ❐ ➢ **What is the recommended treatment for impetigo?**

Erythromycin, 50 mg/kg/d.
Some authors recommend penicillin.
Dicloxacillin and cephalexin in the same dose as erythromycin and topical mupirocin may also be used.

❐ ❐ ❐ ➢ **Impetigo is the most common skin infection affecting children presenting to the emergency department. Honey-colored serous fluid from ruptured vesicles and similarly colored crusts are typical. Erysipelas (St. Anthony's fire) is another pediatric exanthem that represents a primary bacterial infection. What organism causes this uncommon cellulitis that is usually characterized by pain at the affected site, malaise and fever?**

Erysipelas is also caused by group A, ß-hemolytic streptococci.
Penicillin or, in penicillin allergic patients, erythromycin usually cause rapid improvement.
Recurrences are common and can lead to irreversible lymphedema (termed elephantiasis nostras).

❐ ❐ ❐ ➢ **"Strawberry tongue" is a physical finding associated with what systemic bacterial infection also caused primarily by group A, ß-hemolytic streptococci?**

Scarlet fever. Also seek characteristic Pastia's lines found in the antecubital area.
Recall the scarlet rash that spares the perioral area usually has onset 1 - 2 d after high

fever, sore throat, headache and occasional vomiting and abdominal pain. Mucocutaneous lymph node syndrome (Kawasaki disease), a disorder of unclear etiology, may also present with this finding.

❏ ❏ ❏ ➢ **Speaking of rashes...Dermacentor andersoni is a vector for Rickettsia rickettsii which cause Rocky Mountain spotted fever. The rash of RMSF usually begins on the wrists and ankles and spreads centripetally. What is the underlying pathologic lesion that causes the serious sequelae of this disease, as well as the hemorrhagic rash?**

Vasculitis 2° to rickettsial invasion of endothelial cells in small blood vessels, including arterioles.

❏ ❏ ❏ ➢ **Cellulitis in childhood is <u>most commonly</u> caused by S. aureus. The *least common* causative organism is responsible for most of the dangerous forms of this disease - striking younger children in more dangerous locations (e.g.. periorbital cellulitis), causing fever and bacteremia. What is the *least common* cause (overall) of pediatric cellulitis?**

H. influenzae.

❏ ❏ ❏ ➢ **A pediatric patient presents with cellulitis. As this patient does not have a violaceous lesion, nor a fever, nor a markedly elevated WBC, H. influenzae is not considered likely and discharge is planned. What antibiotic selection is appropriate in such a case?**

Dicloxacillin or cephalexin.

❏ ❏ ❏ ➢ **H. influenzae is the <u>most common</u> cause of periorbital cellulitis. What is the <u>most common</u> cause of *orbital* cellulitis?**

S. aureus.

❏ ❏ ❏ ➢ **Group A ß-hemolytic streptococcus is the most common cause of pharyngitis in older children. About what percentage of such patients with pharyngitis will have GABHS?**

≈ 50 %.

❏ ❏ ❏ ➢ **T/F - GABHS is a *frequent* cause of pharyngitis in patients less than 3 y of age.**

False.

❏ ❏ ❏ ➢ **We all know that the streptococcal antigen sampling tests for pharyngitis have a high false-negative rate (sensitivity variable, generally > 50%). What is the false-negative rate for a single throat culture?**

≈ 10 %.

❏ ❏ ❏ ➢ **For how long should a school-age child receive antibiotic treatment for GABHS before being allowed to return to school?**

1 d.

76

❏ ❏ ❏ ➢ **Rheumatic fever is preventable if antibiotic therapy is begun prior to how many days after the start of GABHS?**

9 d.

❏ ❏ ❏ ➢ **Poststreptococcal glomerulonephritis is preventable if antibiotic therapy is begun prior to how many days after the start of GABHS?**

TRICK QUESTION! Poststreptococcal glomerulonephritis is not an infectious complication of GABHS and is not preventable with antibiotic therapy.

❏ ❏ ❏ ➢ **What is the maximum dose of lidocaine for infiltration, a.) without epi and b.) with epi?**

a.) 5 mg/kg without epinephrine.
b.) 7 mg/kg with epinephrine.

❏ ❏ ❏ ➢ **Midazolam (Versed) may be given IV, IM, PO, PR and intranasally. The usual IV or IM dose is 0.15 mg/kg. What is a usual PR dose?**

0.25 mg/kg.

❏ ❏ ❏ ➢ **A child presents in DKA. On average, how dehydrated is this patient likely to be (give answer in ml/kg)?**

≈ 125 ml/kg average fluid volume deficit.

❏ ❏ ❏ ➢ **You are managing a child in DKA. After initial 20 ml/kg bolus with 0.9% NS and careful fluid replacement with 0.45% NS for maintenance and replacement you are considering switching to D5 0.45% NS. At about what glucose level should this change in fluid selection occur?**

250 mg/dl.

❏ ❏ ❏ ➢ **What is the dose of insulin to be used for low-dose continuous infusion therapy?**

0.1 unit/kg/h of regular insulin.

❏ ❏ ❏ ➢ **Insulin is usually mixed in NS at 1 unit/5 ml NS. How much of this fluid should be run through the tubing to saturate binding sites in the plastic?**

50 ml = 10 units!

❏ ❏ ❏ ➢ **A child known to have IDDM presents unconscious. What is the correct amount of D50W (expressed in ml/kg) to administer to this patient?**

0.5 ml/kg.

❏ ❏ ❏ ➢ **You have given the dose of medication from the previous question with no real improvement after 5 min. Now what should you do?**

Try to sit tight, clinical response to glucose often takes 10 min. Use the time to think of other causes in this patient's d/dx, including sepsis, meningitis, metabolic abnormalities, poisoning, head injury, postictal state.

❏ ❏ ❏ ➢ **Is intestinal intussusception associated with GI bleeding?**

Yes, though the classic history of sudden onset of severe pain that often is relieved as quickly as it arose and is recurrent is more sensitive. The currant jelly stool associated with this disorder is present in about half of cases.

❏ ❏ ❏ ➢ **About how old is the average patient presenting with intussusception?**

One year, +/- 6 mo.

❏ ❏ ❏ ➢ **Pyloric stenosis usually presents at about what age?**

4 wk.

❏ ❏ ❏ ➢ **What is the eponym for congenital aganglionic megacolon (the disease in which a portion of the distal colon lacks ganglion cells impairing the normal inhibitory innervation in the myenteric plexus impairing coordinated relaxation which can in turn cause clinical symptoms of obstruction, and that presents 85% of the time _after_ the newborn period)?**

Hirschsprung's disease.

❏ ❏ ❏ ➢ **Acute enterocolitis with development of "toxic" megacolon is the life-threatening complication of Hirschsprung's disease. Between what range of ages does this complication most frequently present?**

2 - 3 mo.

❏ ❏ ❏ ➢ **What signs and symptoms are associated with increased probability of a bacterial pathogen causing diarrhea?**

Fever, acute onset of multiple diarrhea stools/day and blood in the stool.

❏ ❏ ❏ ➢ **T/F - Antibiotic therapy for gastroenteritis is limited in utility to children with high or prolonged fevers, those with inflammatory cells present in stool, those with protracted diarrhea and infants of less than 6 mo of age.**

True.

❏ ❏ ❏ ➢ **Among infants less than 3 mo of age, are UTI's more common in males or in females?**

Males.

❏ ❏ ❏ ➢ **Dysuria among female pediatric patients; more common cause - vulvovaginitis or UTI?**

Vulvovaginitis.
Maternally acquired - Candida, Trichomonas, condyloma.
Prepubertal -
    No cause determined (most common).
    Enterobius vermicularis, characterized by nocturnal pruritus.
    Candida, associated with antibiotics, IDDM.
    Foreign body.
    STDs - suggests sexual contact.

❏ ❏ ❏ ➤ **About what percentage of injuries in children less than 5 y of age seen in the ED are due to child abuse?**

10%.

❏ ❏ ❏ ➤ **Of abused children seen in the ED, about what percentage will be killed by future abuse?**

5%.

❏ ❏ ❏ ➤ **What is the most concerning aspect of the definition of Reye's syndrome provided by the CDC?**

Two of the criteria required may be determined at autopsy. Mortality is about 25% or less overall and varies with age of patient and clinical stage. The underlying abnormality is one of mitochondrial morphology and function, affecting primarily brain and liver.

❏ ❏ ❏ ➤ **Signs and symptoms of Reye's syndrome:**

Patient age usually between ages 6 - 11 y with prior viral illness, possible use of ASA, followed by intractable vomiting. Patient may present irritable, combative, or lethargic, and may c/o right upper quadrant tenderness. Seizures may occur, check for papilledema.
Lab findings would include hypoglycemia, and an elevated ammonia level greater than 20 times normal. Bilirubin level is NORMAL.

❏ ❏ ❏ ➤ **Describe stage I and stage II of Reye's syndrome.**

Stage I - Vomiting, lethargy and liver dysfunction.
Stage II - Disorientation, combativeness, delirium, hyperventilation, increased deep tendon reflexes, liver dysfunction, hyperexcitable, tachypnea, fever, tachycardia, sweating and pupillary dilatation.

❏ ❏ ❏ ➤ **Treatment of stages I and II?**

Supportive.

❏ ❏ ❏ ➤ **Describe Stages III, IV, and V of Reye's syndrome.**

Stage III - coma, decorticate rigidity, increased respiratory rate, mortality rate of 50%.
Stage IV - coma, decerebrate posturing, no ocular reflexes, loss of corneal reflexes, and liver damage.
Stage V - loss of DTRs, seizures, flaccid, respiratory arrest, 95% mortality.

❐ ❐ ❐ ➤ **Treatment for advanced stages of Reye's syndrome?**

Manage ICP - elevate HOB, paralyze, intubate and hyperventilate, furosemide, mannitol, dexamethasone, pentobarbital coma.
Also consider hypertonic glucose and bowel sterilization.

NEURON PEARLS

"Examinations are formidable even to the best prepared, for the greatest fool may ask more than the wisest man can answer."

Unknown

❏ ❏ ❏ ➢ **As you walk into the room, your patient gives you a BIG smile. What CN is intact?**

7th.

❏ ❏ ❏ ➢ **How can upper motor neuron (UMN) lesions of CN VII (facial nerve) be distinguished from peripheral lesions?**

UMN - Unilateral weakness of the lower half of the face.
Peripheral - Involve entire half of the face.

❏ ❏ ❏ ➢ **A 35 y old woman with a history of flu like symptoms (URI) one wk ago now presents with vertigo, nausea, and vomiting. No auditory impairment or focal deficits are noted. What is the most likely cause of her problem?**

Labyrinthitis or vestibular neuronitis.

❏ ❏ ❏ ➢ **A patient presents with facial droop on the left and weakness of the right leg. What is the most likely site of the lesion?**

Brainstem (for you neuro fans, specifically the left pons).

❏ ❏ ❏ ➢ **During a routine Romberg exam a patient is asked to stand with his eyes open. He falls to the left. Diagnosis?**

Cerebellar dysfunction. An unsteady, broad-based gait suggests cerebellar problems. If the patient only falls with their eyes closed, the problem is with sensation, usually as a result of abnormality in position sense, most commonly posterior column dysfunction.

❏ ❏ ❏ ➢ **A 30 y old presents with progressively severe intermittent vertigo for six mo and progressive unilateral hearing loss for 3 mo. Diagnosis?**

Cerebellopontine angle tumor. Confirm diagnosis with MRI scan.

❏ ❏ ❏ ➢ **Describe the key signs and symptoms of classic, common, cluster, ophthalmoplegic, and hemiplegic migraine headache.**

Classic -	Prodrome lasts up to 60 min. Most common symptom is visual disturbance, such as homonymous hemianopsia, scintillating scotoma, and photophobia. Lips, face, and hand tingling as well as aphasia and extremity weakness may occur. Nausea and vomiting may also occur.

Common -   Most common. Slow evolving headache over hours to days. A positive family history as well as two of the following: nausea or vomiting, throbbing quality, photophobia, unilateral pain, and increase with menses. Distinguishing feature from "Classic" migraine is the lack of visual symptoms.

Cluster -   Mostly males. Intense unilateral ocular or retroocular pain which lasts less than 2 hours and occurs several times a day for weeks or months. Symptoms include lacrimation, facial flushing, rhinorrhea, sweating, and conjunctival injection. Often awakes patient from sleep.

Ophthalmoplegic - Most commonly seen in young adults. Patient has an outwardly deviated, dilated eye, with ptosis. The 3rd > 6th > 4th nerves are typically involved.

Hemiplegic -   Unilateral motor and sensory symptoms, mild hemiparesis to hemiplegia.

❏ ❏ ❏ ➢ **Treatment of a cluster headache?**

100% O_2 and 5-10% cocaine solution, 4% lidocaine in the ipsilateral nostril, and a short course of steroids.

❏ ❏ ❏ ➢ **A 29 y old drunken male presents after having his head pounded into the concrete by his wife. The patient had a brief episode of LOC, but was then ambulatory and alert. Now he appears drowsy and just threw up on you. Diagnosis?**

Epidural hematoma.

❏ ❏ ❏ ➢ **A 25 y old presents with a history of being knocked unconscious for 10 seconds while playing touch football one week ago. Since then he has felt malaise, intermittent vertigo, nausea, vomiting, blurred vision, and a headache. Neuro exam and CT are normal. Diagnosis?**

Post-traumatic vertigo. Expect recovery to normal over 2 to 6 wk.

❏ ❏ ❏ ➢ **A 64 y old presents with a bilateral "burning" headache. She describes jabs of pain which are worse at night. Treatment?**

Temporal arteritis is treated with long-term steroids. Treatment should begin immediately, do not wait for biopsy confirmation. ESR over 50 mm/h is highly suggestive.

❏ ❏ ❏ ➢ **A 53 y old female presents with unilateral right sided sudden-onset lancinating pain in the distribution of the second and third branches of the fifth cranial nerve. Treatment?**

Carbamazepine treats trigeminal neuralgia. An MRI to rule out a brainstem process (tumor) is indicated.

❏ ❏ ❏ ➢ **A 28 y old woman raised in Minnesota complains of weakness and tingling in the right arm and leg for 2 d. She reports an episode of right eye pain and blurred vision which resolved over one mo that occurred 2 y ago. She also recalls a two wk episode of intermittent blurred vision one y ago. Diagnosis?**

Presumptive MS. Confirm with MRI and CSF (oligoclonal bands).

❏ ❏ ❏ ➢ **What artery is most commonly associated with epidural hematomas?**

Middle meningeal artery.

❏ ❏ ❏ ➢ **Which way do the eyes look with a major hemispheric abnormality?**

Toward the lesion.

❏ ❏ ❏ ➢ **Which way do the eyes look with a brainstem abnormality?**

Away from the lesion.

❏ ❏ ❏ ➢ **A 50 y old female presents with acute vertigo, nausea, and vomiting. She reports similar episodes over the last 20 y, sometimes but not always associated with hearing change and/or hearing loss and tinnitus. She has permanent right > left sensorineural hearing loss. Diagnosis?**

Ménière's Disease.

❏ ❏ ❏ ➢ **What is the most common cause of a subarachnoid hemorrhage?**

Saccular aneurysm.

❏ ❏ ❏ ➢ **For the following clinical presentations identify if each is most consistent with peripheral or central vertigo.**

1. Intense spinning, nausea, hearing loss, diaphoresis.
2. Swaying or impulsion, worse with movement, tinnitus, acute onset.
3. Unidirectional nystagmus inhibited by ocular fixation, fatigable.
4. Mild vertigo, diplopia, and ataxia.
5. Multidirectional nystagmus not inhibited by ocular fixation, nonfatigable.

    1,2, and 3 -   Peripheral.
    4 and 5 -   Central.

❏ ❏ ❏ ➢ **The Nylen-Barany maneuver is performed as follows: the patient is rapidly brought from the sitting to supine position and the head is turned 45°. Match the findings with peripheral and central vertigo:**

1. Nystagmus is multidirectional, nonfatiguing, has no latent period, and lasts over a minute.
2. Vertigo increased. Nystagmus is unidirectional, fatiguing, latent period is 2-20s, with duration less than a minute.

    1 - Central.
    2 - Peripheral.

❏ ❏ ❏ ➢ **A 42 y old air traffic controller presents with attacks of vertigo whenever he scans the skies for landing airplanes. Symptoms last about a minute. He is worried sick. What do you tell him about his disease?**

The patient has benign positional vertigo. Attacks usually subside in a few weeks.

❏ ❏ ❏ ➢ **A 50 y old female presents with hearing loss over the last 6 mo. She now presents at 2 A.M. with vertigo which has progressively become worse over the last 2 months. On exam, she is mildly ataxic. Diagnosis?**

8th nerve lesion, possibly an acoustic schwannoma or meningioma.

❏ ❏ ❏ ➢ **Dangerous diagnosis of a purpuric, petechial rash?**

Think meningococcemia. Other causes include Hemophilus influenzae, Streptococcus pneumoniae, and Staphylococcus aureus.

❏ ❏ ❏ ➢ **On LP, opening pressure is markedly elevated. What should be done?**

Close 3-way stopcock, remove only a small amount of fluid from manometer, abort LP and initiate measures to decrease intracranial pressure. Call your lawyer.

❏ ❏ ❏ ➢ **A patient presents with acute meningitis; when should antibiotics be initiated?**

Immediately. Do not wait. Patients should receive a CT prior to LP only if papilledema or focal deficit is present.

❏ ❏ ❏ ➢ **What is the most common presenting symptom of MS?**

Optic neuritis (about 25%).

❏ ❏ ❏ ➢ **A patient with MS presents with a fever. The nurse asks "should I give the patient Tylenol?" What is your response?**

YES! Lowering temperature is important in MS patients as small increases in temperature can worsen existing signs and symptoms.

❏ ❏ ❏ ➢ **What rhythm disturbance would make phenytoin relatively contraindicated?**

Second or third degree heart block. If the patient is in status, you may have no choice.

❏ ❏ ❏ ➢ **What three bacterial illnesses present with peripheral neurologic findings?**

Botulism, tetanus, and diphtheria.

TOX PEARLS

"Prepare for the difficult while it is still easy.
Deal with the big while it is still small.
Difficult undertakings have always started with what is easy,
And great undertakings have always started with what is small....
He who takes things too easily will surely encounter much difficultly.
For this reason even the sage regards things as difficult,
And therefore he encounters no difficulty."

Tao-te Ching, 63; Lao Tzu

❏ ❏ ❏ ➤ **A patient presents in shock, lethargic, bordering on comatose, with vomiting, hematemesis and diarrhea? What could cause this?**

Iron, stage III. Check an abdominal x-ray for concretions.

❏ ❏ ❏ ➤ **What iron level is toxic?**

Moderate OD is considered with serum level 350 µg/dl, measured 4 h after ingestion.
Alternatively, try to determine the amount of <u>elemental</u> iron ingested, 20-40 mg elemental iron/kg is toxic.
Treat symptomatic patients without waiting for lab test results.

❏ ❏ ❏ ➤ **Discuss the 4 stages of iron toxicity.**

I (h) - Abdominal pain, vomiting, diarrhea, possible GI bleeding and 2° lethargy and metabolic acidosis. Due to direct corrosive effect of iron.

II (3-12 h) - Resolution of GI symptoms, M.D. falsely reassured.

III (>12 h) - Iron makes it into cells, blocks oxidative phosphorylation, catalyzes formation of free radicals. Cellular and organ disruption ensue with edema and venous pooling. Hepatic dysfunction, renal and cardiac failure can occur. Stage III occurs earlier in severe poisoning.

IV (days-wk) - Small bowel and gastric outlet obstruction.

[N.B. - Some sources prefer to break this up into 5 stages.]

❏ ❏ ❏ ➤ **What is the treatment of iron ingestion?**

If patient has Ø symptoms for 6 h and is completely normal on exam, go home.
If patient has minimal symptoms and appears fine and has iron level close to maximum normal level (150 µg/dl) measured 4 h after ingestion, go home.
Cathartics for patients without diarrhea (controversial).
Hydration and treat GI hemorrhage.
Deferoxamine if:
    Moderate or severely symptomatic,
    Serum iron level > TIBC,
    Serum iron level > 350 µg/dl.

Deferoxamine is a specific agent for iron and will not chelate other metals.
Give 15 μg/kg/h IV x 8 h for serum iron > 500 μg/dl or 90 mg/kg IM q 8 h for serum iron < 500 μg/dl.

❐ ❐ ❐ ➤ **What are the symptoms and signs of cyanide overdose?**

Dryness and burning in the throat, air hunger, and hyperventilation.
If not removed from the toxic environment loss of consciousness, seizures, bradycardia and apnea occur prior to asystole.

❐ ❐ ❐ ➤ **What is the treatment for cyanide overdose?**

Oxygen, CPR prn.
Amyl nitrite perle inhaled.
Sodium nitrite 10 ml of 3% solution in an adult which is 300 mg, or 0.2 - 0.33 ml/kg in a child.
Sodium thiosulfate - give 5 times the volume of sodium nitrite; 12.5 mg in an adult which is 50 ml of a 25% solution or 1.0 - 1.5 ml/kg in a child.

❐ ❐ ❐ ➤ **Interesting treatment! The mechanism of action of nitrites is not completely clear, though formation of methemoglobin is probably important. Methemoglobin rapidly combines with cyanide to form cyanomethemoglobin. O.K., so now you've stripped the cyanide off it's binding to cytochrome A$_3$, but how is the cyanomethemoglobin handled?**

The intrinsic enzyme rhodanase catalyzes the transport of cyanide from cyanomethemoglobin to sulfur forming thiocyanate. This reaction is limited by sulfur availability. Sodium thiosulfate is given to act as a sulfur donor. Thiocyanate is excreted by the kidney.

❐ ❐ ❐ ➤ **What order are the kinetics of elimination of ASA overdose?**

Zero-order elimination with hepatic enzymatic clearance saturated and renal clearance becoming important.

❐ ❐ ❐ ➤ **What is the mechanism of ASA leading to respiratory alkalosis?**

Direct stimulation of brainstem respiratory centers.
When even greater levels of ASA are present, respiratory depression can occur.

❐ ❐ ❐ ➤ **By what mechanism does ASA lead to a metabolic acidosis?**

ASA uncouples oxidative phosphorylation.
ASA enhances lipolysis leading to ketoacid production.

❐ ❐ ❐ ➤ **We all remember to think of ASA poisoning when a patient presents with mental status changes associated with respiratory alkalosis and metabolic acidosis. Many of us may recall that salicylate toxicity may be associated with elevated, normal, or decreased glucose levels. By what mechanisms are hyperglycemia and hypoglycemia caused?**

Hyperglycemia is caused by salicylate induced mobilization of glycogen.

Hypoglycemia is caused by salicylate inhibition of gluconeogenesis.

❑ ❑ ❑ ➢ **Is ARDS more likely to be a complication of acute or chronic ASA poisoning?**

Chronic.

❑ ❑ ❑ ➢ **ARDS is <u>not</u> a common complication of acute ASA OD. However, with acute ingestion, does ARDS occur more often in adults or children?**

Adults.

❑ ❑ ❑ ➢ **What is the "magic number" for the dose of non-enteric coated ASA which must be exceeded to cause toxicity (mg/kg)?**

150 mg/kg.

❑ ❑ ❑ ➢ **What is the "magic number" for the dose of enteric coated ASA which must be exceeded to require admission for observation and serial salicylate levels?**

150 mg/kg.

❑ ❑ ❑ ➢ **Metabolic acidosis favors formation of what form of salicylate, ionized or unionized?**

UN-IONIZED.
This is a KEY point because:
    a.) It is the reason to therapeutically produce an alkaline urine which then makes more of the free salicylate ionized, not reabsorbed by tubules, and excreted.
    b.) It is the reason for the large changes in amount of free drug able to diffuse into tissue. Small decreases in pH result in decreased protein binding and more salicylate in the un-ionized form able to diffuse into tissue thereby increasing its volume of distribution. [Thus, always treat the patient and not the level - serum levels can decrease as salicylate moves into tissue!!].

❑ ❑ ❑ ➢ **Under what circumstances is use of A.D. Done's nomogram O.K.?**

Only when the patient has an acute, single ingestion of non-enteric coated ASA without recent prior use.

❑ ❑ ❑ ➢ **Can a patient who is symptomatic with mental status changes from chronic salicylate poisoning have a level in the therapeutic range?**

Yes! Interestingly, patients taking acetazolamide are at particular risk for chronic salicylate poisoning because the carbonic anhydrase inhibitor results in acidified plasma (leading to increased V_d) and more alkalotic CSF, thereby encouraging salicylate concentration in the CNS.

❑ ❑ ❑ ➢ **Is hemodialysis used to treat salicylate toxicity?**

Yes, in severe poisoning (coma, ARDS, cardiac toxicity, serum level > 100 mg/dl), and for patients who are unresponsive to maximal therapy.

❑ ❑ ❑ ➤ **What is the "magic number" for the minimum ingestion of acetaminophen (N-acetyl-para-aminophenol, APAP) necessary to cause hepatic toxicity in an adult?**

7.5 gm.

❑ ❑ ❑ ➤ **In a child?**

140 mg/kg.

❑ ❑ ❑ ➤ **Let's review some aspects of hepatic anatomy and metabolism of APAP in the next few questions to help recall particulars of acetaminophen's toxicity.**

O.K.

❑ ❑ ❑ ➤ **What region of liver lobules contains the greatest amount of P_{450} related mixed-function oxidases (P450MFO)?**

The centrilobular regions, accounting for primarily centrilobular necrosis.

❑ ❑ ❑ ➤ **How is APAP usually metabolized under non-overdose conditions?**

Most APAP metabolism is by glucuronidation.
Some APAP metabolism is by conjugation with sulfate. This percentage increases with decreasing age.
4% or less is transformed into an extremely toxic intermediary compound by P_{450}MFO's. This toxic metabolite is likely immediately conjugated with glutathione and harmlessly excreted in the urine.

❑ ❑ ❑ ➤ **How does N-acetylcysteine (NAC, Mucomyst) work?**

Precise mechanism is still unknown. We know that NAC enters cells and is metabolized to cysteine which serves as a glutathione precursor.

❑ ❑ ❑ ➤ **Summarize, in the simplest possible outline, the 4 stages of APAP toxicity.**

I -   Primarily N, V; first d.
II-   N, V decrease, abdominal pain begins, LFT's increase; 1-2 d.
III-   N, V recur, LFT's peak; 3-4 d.
IV-   get better or die; 4 d - 2 wk.

❑ ❑ ❑ ➤ **Which measures of hepatic function are better indicators of prognosis, liver enzyme levels or bilirubin level and prothrombin time?**

Bilirubin level and prothrombin time.

❑ ❑ ❑ ➤ **Clonidine is a centrally acting presynaptic a_2-adrenergic agonist that results in decreased central sympathetic outflow. While its primary use is to treat hypertension, it has additional emergency utility in blunting withdrawal symptoms from opiates and EtOH. Clonidine overdose closely resembles OD with what other class of drugs?**

Opiates.

❒ ❒ ❒ ➤ **Can clonidine ever cause hypertension?**

Yes; high serum levels can result in direct peripheral α–adrenergic stimulation. Such hypertension usually yields to ensuing hypotension.

❒ ❒ ❒ ➤ **Toxicity from clonidine (Catapres) usually occurs within what time period?**

4 h.

❒ ❒ ❒ ➤ **What agent may be useful as an "antidote" for clonidine OD.**

Naloxone.

❒ ❒ ❒ ➤ **Name a few substances that have anticholinergic properties.**

Antihistamines, cyclic antidepressants, phenothiazines, atropine, amanita sp., Jimson weed.

❒ ❒ ❒ ➤ **Sure, patients who suffer anticholinergic toxicity have mental status changes, mydriasis, urinary retention, cardiogenic pulmonary edema, dry skin, tachycardia and decreased salivation, but what is the <u>most common</u> ECG abnormality?**

Sinus tachycardia. Other, dangerous, arrhythmias include conduction problems and V-Tach.

❒ ❒ ❒ ➤ **What is "cornpicker's pupil?"**

Mydriasis from contact of Jimson weed with the eye. Jimson weed contains atropine, scopolamine and hyoscyamine. It is a common plant and is available through health food stores.

❒ ❒ ❒ ➤ **Intermediate-chain aliphatic hydrocarbons are responsible for most of the exposures to hydrocarbons. What is the <u>most common</u> complication from these liquids?**

Chemical pneumonitis caused by direct injury to pulmonary parenchyma after aspiration.

❒ ❒ ❒ ➤ **Which hydrocarbons carry the greatest risk of aspiration?**

Those with low viscosity, less than 60 SSU.
(We'll return to the SSU in the random question section.)

❒ ❒ ❒ ➤ **Aromatic hydrocarbons, such as toluene present in glue, may be sniffed. Resulting effects most closely resemble those of what other class of compounds?**

Effects are similar to those of inhalational anesthetic agents: initial excitatory response gives way to CNS depression.

❒ ❒ ❒ ➤ **Can solvent abusers be scared to death?**

Yes. Halogenated hydrocarbons can "sensitize" myocardium to catecholamines, thus exertion or fright can lead to fatal arrhythmias.

❏ ❏ ❏ ➢ **What is the relationship between toluene and A MUDPILE CAT?**

Toluene is the "T"!

❏ ❏ ❏ ➢ **Is charcoal useful in hydrocarbon ingestions?**

No.

❏ ❏ ❏ ➢ **Is gastric emptying useful in hydrocarbon ingestions?**

Yes and no.
Yes for the following:
    Halogenated hydrocarbons - Carbon tetrachloride, other solvents and dry-cleaning agents.
    Aromatic hydrocarbons - Toluene, benzene, xylene.

❏ ❏ ❏ ➢ **For what period of time should an asymptomatic patient with hydrocarbon ingestion be observed prior to discharge?**

6 h.

❏ ❏ ❏ ➢ **Sure, digitalis increases myocardial inotropy by inhibiting Na^+-K^+-ATPase, thereby allowing intracellular Na^+ to increase providing more substrate for the Na^+-Ca^{2+} membrane exchange that leads to increased intracellular (sarcoplasmic) Ca^{2+} concentration, but does it also increase vagal tone and slow conduction through the AV node?**

Yes.

❏ ❏ ❏ ➢ **Serum potassium can soar to very high levels with acute digitalis toxicity; is this also true for chronic digitalis poisoning?**

No, not really.

❏ ❏ ❏ ➢ **T/F- A patient with acute digitalis OD presents with frequent multifocal PVC's, peaked T-waves and a K^+ of 6.2 mEq/l; correct treatment is to first administer $CaCl_2$ as this is the fastest acting agent for reducing hyperkalemia.**

No, no, this is a trick question! Yes, $CaCl_2$ is the fastest acting agent for decreasing hyperkalemia, but you don't want to give any more Ca^+ to a patient with digitalis induced cardiac toxicity.

❏ ❏ ❏ ➢ **Phenytoin has an appropriate role in the treatment of digitalis induced arrhythmias. For which arrhythmias is consideration of use of phenytoin appropriate?**

Digitalis induced ventricular arrhythmias.

❏ ❏ ❏ ➤ **Signs and symptoms of phenytoin toxicity?**

Seizure, heart blocks, bradyarrhythmias, hypotension, coma. All dangerous cardiovascular complications of phenytoin OD result from parenteral administration; high levels after PO doses do not cause such signs in a stable patient.

❏ ❏ ❏ ➤ **Treatment of phenytoin overdose?**

Systemic support, charcoal, atropine for bradyarrhythmias, and phenobarbital 20 mg/kg IV for seizures.

❏ ❏ ❏ ➤ **At what serum level of phenytoin do nystagmus, ataxia, and lethargy generally occur?**

Nystagmus -   20 µg/ml.
Ataxia -   30 µg/ml.
Lethargy -   40 µg/ml.

❏ ❏ ❏ ➤ **What rhythm and ECG findings are expected with phenytoin toxicity?**

Bradycardia, AV block, ventricular tachycardia, VF, and asystole. ECG findings might include increased PR interval and a wide QRS.

❏ ❏ ❏ ➤ **What is the treatment of phenytoin toxicity?**

Charcoal. Seizures are treated with benzodiazepine or phenobarbital. Extravasation may be limb threatening, consult an orthopedic or plastic surgeon. Hemodialysis and hemoperfusion are not helpful.

❏ ❏ ❏ ➤ **How many vials of digoxin-specific Fab should be administered to a patient in critical condition from digitalis toxicity in whom neither the ingested dose nor the serum level is known?**

10 vials = 400 mg Fab.

❏ ❏ ❏ ➤ **Is charcoal useful in treating digitalis toxicity?**

Right again.

❏ ❏ ❏ ➤ **ß-adrenergic antagonists have 3 main effects on the heart - name them.**

Negative chronotropy.
Negative inotropy.
Decrease AV nodal conduction velocity.

❏ ❏ ❏ ➤ **T/F - ß-adrenergic antagonists can cause mental status changes and seizures.**

True.

❏ ❏ ❏ ➤ **What is the agent of choice to counteract the effects of ß-adrenergic antagonists, and how does it work?**

Glucagon should be given in boluses of 3 - 5 mg q 5 min until response is obtained or 10 -15 mg has been administered. It has rapid onset and short-lived effect ($\approx$ 15 min), therefore administer a continuous infusion at the same number of mg/hr as the number of mg initially provided in boluses to obtain a response. The initial dose is 50 - 150 μg/kg in children.

Glucagon works by increasing intracellular cAMP by direct glucagon (non-adrenergic) receptors, bypassing ß-adrenergic receptors.

❐ ❐ ❐ ➤ **Activated charcoal?**

Sure.

❐ ❐ ❐ ➤ **Calcium channel blocking agents (CCB's) come in several flavors and all have the potential to be lethal. Which CCB has the most depressing effect on sinus nodal activity and AV nodal conduction?**

Verapamil.

❐ ❐ ❐ ➤ **Which CCB causes the greatest degree of systemic vasodilation?**

Nifedipine.

❐ ❐ ❐ ➤ **Describe the dosing of calcium for CCB OD.**

$CaCl_2$ 10 - 20 ml of 10% solution.
$CaCl_2$ 10 - 30 mg/kg for children.
Calcium gluconate 0.2-0.5 ml/kg/dose up to 10 ml/dose.

❐ ❐ ❐ ➤ **Charcoal; Yes.**

❐ ❐ ❐ ➤ **What is the <u>most common</u> cause of acute heavy metal poisoning?**

   a.) Twisted Sister
   b.) Metallica
   c.) Arsenic

❐ ❐ ❐ ➤ **Arsenic is initially housed in RBC's, WBC's and bound to serum proteins. From there it is distributed to major organs, bone, hair and nails. What is the primary mechanism of toxicity of arsenic?**

It blocks the conversion of a cofactor necessary for oxidative phosphorylation (Krebs cycle).
Arsenic also substitutes for phosphate, disrupting high-energy phosphates.

❐ ❐ ❐ ➤ **What is the resultant pathology of arsenic intoxication?**

N, V, D, cerebral edema, cerebral hemorrhage, arrhythmias, encephalopathy associated with mental status changes, and seizures, pulmonary edema, ARF, rhabdomyolysis.

❐ ❐ ❐ ➤ **T/F- Chronic arsenic poisoning tends to present less dramatically with constitutional symptoms and peripheral neuropathy.**

True.

❏ ❏ ❏ ➣ **Charcoal probably doesn't absorb arsenic much. What chelating agents are appropriate?**

Play BAL with a DMSAl named MAG!

This means that Mercury, Arsenic and Gold (MAG) can be chelated with BAL and with DMSA. D-Penicillamine can also be used.

❏ ❏ ❏ ➣ **Arsine is a gaseous form of arsenic; is chelation also used to treat arsine?**

No.

❏ ❏ ❏ ➣ **What are the effects of arsine poisoning?**

Binds to hemoglobin; causes anemia with jaundice, ARF.
Manage with transfusions and dialysis for ARF.

❏ ❏ ❏ ➣ **Which two antidepressants tend to cause less problems when taken in large quantities?**

Trazodone (Desyrel) and Fluoxetine (Prozac).

❏ ❏ ❏ ➣ **Describe the signs and symptoms of cyclic overdose.**

Anticholinergic toxicity. CNS depression. Cardiac depression of contractility and conduction. The earliest signs of toxicity tend to be lethargy, slurred speech, and tachycardia. Other signs include myoclonic jerks, seizures, and coma.

❏ ❏ ❏ ➣ **A patient with a history of CA overdose is found by paramedics awake and alert. Prognosis?**

25% of patients who die from cyclic overdose are awake and alert at the scene. Treat with O_2, IV, monitor, multiple doses of 50 to 100 grams of activated charcoal q 2 h and alkaline diuresis. The drug has a high tissue binding, thus once absorbed, it is poorly removed.

❏ ❏ ❏ ➣ **Is degree of toxicity in CA overdose closely related to QRS duration?**

NO! QRS > 100 ms has a specificity of 75 percent and a sensitivity of 60% for serious complications. A normal ECG will not rule out serious overdose!

❏ ❏ ❏ ➣ **What electrolytes should be followed closely in a CA overdose?**

Potassium increases toxic effects. Sodium antagonizes CAs.

❏ ❏ ❏ ➣ **How should seizures be treated in a patient with cyclic overdose?**

Most patients do not need treatment as seizures tend to be brief. Diazepam, 5-10 mg IV has been used but its efficacy is questionable. Phenytoin is used to treat conduction defects and seizures, it will not treat myoclonic jerks. Alkalinize with IV sodium bicarbonate 1-5 mEq/kg.

❏ ❏ ❏ ➢ **What agent should be used as part of the intubation protocol in a cyclic overdose patient.**

A nondepolarizing agent, such as vecuronium. Succinylcholine (the depolarizing agent) has potent vagal effects and should be avoided.

❏ ❏ ❏ ➢ **How should cardiac complications of cyclic overdose be treated?**

Alkalinize the blood to a pH of 7.5. Either hyperventilate the patient or administer sodium bicarb IV 1-5 mEq/kg over several minutes. For hypotension, epinephrine, norepinephrine, and phenylephrine may be tried. Dobutamine is contraindicated.

❏ ❏ ❏ ➢ **What IV fluid should be used in a patient with cyclic overdose?**

Isotonic saline.

❏ ❏ ❏ ➢ **For how long should an asymptomatic CA overdose patient be monitored?**

6 h.

❏ ❏ ❏ ➢ **A schizophrenic patient presents to the ED with muscular rigidity, confusion, and a high temperature. Diagnosis and treatment?**

Neuroleptic malignant syndrome. Treat by supportive care, IV diazepam for skeletal muscle relaxation, and with hyperthermia treatment. Dantrolene and bromocriptine are also effective. Consider paralysis with a non-depressing agent.

❏ ❏ ❏ ➢ **What lithium level is considered toxic?**

2.0 mEq/l.

❏ ❏ ❏ ➢ **Signs and symptoms of lithium toxicity?**

Confusion, lethargy, tremor, and muscle jerking are early signs. GI symptoms are frequent. Stupor, seizures, and coma in severe toxicity. Bradycardia, conduction defects, and ST-T wave changes may occur. Hypotension secondary to volume depletion may also occur.

❏ ❏ ❏ ➢ **Treatment of lithium toxicity?**

Gastric lavage, IV NS, alkalinize the urine, and supportive care. **Charcoal does not bind lithium**. Hemodialysis is effective and should be used if urine output decreases or renal failure is present, severe poisoning is present, or for deteriorating clinical condition.

❏ ❏ ❏ ➢ **Clinical signs and symptoms of barbiturate overdose?**

Emotional lability, lethargy, impaired thinking, slurred speech, decreased coordination, and nystagmus. Hypotension, hypothermia, vasodilation, shock, and skin bullae may also occur.

❏ ❏ ❏ ➤ **Treatment of barbiturate overdose?**

Systemic support, gastric lavage, charcoal q 6 h, and diuresis. Alkalinization of the urine for long-acting barbiturates.

❏ ❏ ❏ ➤ **A narcotic addict presents to the ED with bone and joint pain. Two causes that should be considered are _____ and _____.**

Osteomyelitis and septic arthritis. Pseudomonas aeruginosa and Serratia marcescens. In a patient with back pain, think of osteomyelitis.

❏ ❏ ❏ ➤ **What is the most frequent neurologic complication of narcotic abuse?**

Non-traumatic mononeuropathy (painless weakness occurring 2 to 3 h post injection). Other CNS complications include traumatic mononeuritis, seizures, subarachnoid hemorrhage, and spinal epidural abscess (Staphylococcus aureus is the most common).

❏ ❏ ❏ ➤ **What are the common causes of bacterial pneumonia in narcotic addicts?**

Streptococcus pneumoniae, Haemophilus, Staphylococcus aureus, and Klebsiella.

❏ ❏ ❏ ➤ **How is pulmonary edema associated with heroin use treated?**

Naloxone and ventilatory support. Diuretics, digitalis, and rotating tourniquets are not effective.

❏ ❏ ❏ ➤ **What valve is most commonly infected in narcotic IV drug abusers?**

Tricuspid valve, usually with Staphylococcus aureus.

❏ ❏ ❏ ➤ **What is the treatment of narcotic overdose?**

Naloxone, 0.4 to 2.0 mg in an adult, and 0.01 mg/kg in a child. Naloxone's duration of action is about 1 h.

❏ ❏ ❏ ➤ **What signs and symptoms are expected with cocaine overdose?**

Tachycardia, hyperthermia, hypertension, seizures, and agitation may occur. Extremely high doses cause depressant effects, bradycardia, hypotension, and coma.

❏ ❏ ❏ ➤ **A cocaine addict presents with chest pain. The ECG is normal. What are the odds they will have abnormal CPK and CPK-MB isoenzymes?**

19%.

❏ ❏ ❏ ➣ **Treatment of cocaine overdose?**

Sedation with benzodiazepine to control hypertension and tachycardia, phentolamine to treat remaining hypertension, and nitroprusside if hypertension persists.

❏ ❏ ❏ ➣ **What is the treatment of amphetamine overdose?**

Gastric lavage, charcoal, diazepam for seizures, haloperidol for hyperactivity, and nitroprusside for hypertension.

❏ ❏ ❏ ➣ **What type of nystagmus is expected with PCP overdose?**

Vertical, horizontal, and rotary. Vertical nystagmus is not common with other conditions/ingestions. The most common findings of PCP overdose are hypertension, tachycardia, and nystagmus.

❏ ❏ ❏ ➣ **What are the two most common complications of PCP intoxication?**

Hyperpyrexia and rhabdomyolysis. Urine acidification as a treatment is no longer recommended.

❏ ❏ ❏ ➣ **What type of necrosis does lye produce?**

Base = Liquefaction necrosis. Lye is the most common cause of severe caustic injuries. Bases tend to cause esophageal strictures.
Acids = Coagulation necrosis. Acids tend to cause pyloric strictures.

❏ ❏ ❏ ➣ **Evaluation and treatment of a button battery ingestion?**

If button is in the esophagus, immediate endoscopy. If in the stomach, follow to make sure the battery passes within seven days.

❏ ❏ ❏ ➣ **Principle signs and symptoms of NSAID toxicity?**

Nephrotoxicity, tinnitus, headache, GI intolerance, platelet dysfunction, and peripheral edema. Toxic ingestions most commonly cause drowsiness and GI upset. Seizures can occur.

❏ ❏ ❏ ➣ **What respiratory complication can occur in children who ingest NSAIDS?**

Apnea. NSAIDs can cause toxic respiratory symptoms ranging from rhinitis to bronchospasm.

❏ ❏ ❏ ➣ **What effect do NSAIDs have on lithium?**

They can increase serum lithium concentrations.

❏ ❏ ❏ ➣ **Should charcoal be given for an NSAID overdose?**

Yes.

❏ ❏ ❏ ➢ **For how long should an asymptomatic patient with NSAID overdose be observed in the ED?**

4 to 6 h.

❏ ❏ ❏ ➢ **Treatment for benzodiazepine overdose?**

Gastric lavage and charcoal. Hemodialysis, hemoperfusion, and forced diuresis have not been found to be effective.

❏ ❏ ❏ ➢ **Treatment of mercury salt ingestion?**

Egg whites or milk to bind the mercury, lavage, and charcoal. BAL and D-penicillamine for chelation therapy. DMSA can be used for mercury.
PLAY BAL!

❏ ❏ ❏ ➢ **What is the most common cause of chronic heavy metal poisoning?**

Lead.

❏ ❏ ❏ ➢ **A patient presents with neurologic dysfunction and abdominal complaints. Lab studies reveal a hemolytic anemia. Diagnosis?**

Lead toxicity. Diagnosis is confirmed by finding an elevated PbB level. If indication of PB are found on abdominal x-ray, initiate whole-bowel irrigation with Golytely. Chelate with BAL followed by EDTA. Oral chelating agents , D-penicillamine and DMSA, may also be considered.

ID PEARLS

"Nobody will fly for a thousand years!"

Wilbur Wright, 1901, in a fit of despair.

❏ ❏ ❏ ➤ **Describe the pathophysiologic features of HIV:**

HIV attacks the T4 helper cells. HIV genetic material consists of single-stranded RNA. HIV has been found in saliva, urine, cerebrospinal fluid, tears, alveolar fluid, synovial fluid, breast milk, and amniotic fluid.

❏ ❏ ❏ ➤ **How quickly do patients infected with HIV become symptomatic?**

5-10% develop symptoms within three years of seroconversion. Predictive characteristics include low T4 count, and hematocrit less than 40.
Mean incubation time is about 8 y for adults and 2 y for children less than 5 y. When AIDS develops, survival is about 9 mo.

❏ ❏ ❏ ➤ **Name the most common causes of fever in HIV infected patients:**

HIV-related fever, Mycobacterium avium-intracellular, CMV, non-Hodgkin's and Hodgkin's lymphoma.

❏ ❏ ❏ ➤ **An HIV positive patient presents with a history of weight loss, diarrhea, fever, anorexia, and malaise. They are also dyspneic. Lab studies reveal abnormal LFTs and anemia. Diagnosis?**

Mycobacterium avium-intracellular. Lab confirmation is made by acid-fast stain of body fluids or by blood culture.

❏ ❏ ❏ ➤ **What is the most common cause of retinitis in AIDS patients?**

CMV. GI involvement is also common.

❏ ❏ ❏ ➤ **What is the second most common complication of AIDS?**

Kaposi's sarcoma. PCP is the <u>most</u> <u>common</u>.

❏ ❏ ❏ ➤ **What drugs are used to treat CNS toxoplasmosis in AIDS patients?**

Pyrimethamine plus sulfadiazine.

❏ ❏ ❏ ➢ **What is the most common cause of focal encephalitis in AIDS patients?**

Toxoplasmosis.
Symptoms include focal neurologic deficits, headache, fever, altered mental status, and seizures. Ring enhancing-lesions are seen on CT.

❏ ❏ ❏ ➢ **The differential diagnosis of ring-enhancing lesions in AIDS patients is:**

Lymphoma, cerebral tuberculosis, fungal infection, CMV, Kaposi's sarcoma, toxoplasmosis, and hemorrhage.

❏ ❏ ❏ ➢ **What are the signs and symptoms of CNS cryptococcal infection in an AIDS patient?**

Headache, depression, lightheadedness, seizures, and cranial nerve palsies.
Diagnosis is made by India ink prep, fungal culture, or by cryptococcal antigen in the CSF.

❏ ❏ ❏ ➢ **Presentation of an AIDS patient with tuberculous meningitis:**

Fever, meningismus, headache, seizures, focal neurologic deficits, and altered mental status.

❏ ❏ ❏ ➢ **On physical exam, what is the most common eye finding in AIDS patients?**

Cotton-wool spots thought to be associated with PCP. These may be hard to differentiate from fluffy-white, often perivascular retinal lesions that are associated with CMV.

❏ ❏ ❏ ➢ **An AIDS patient presents with complaints of decreased visual acuity, photophobia, redness, and eye pain. Diagnosis?**

Retinitis or malignant invasion of the periorbital tissue or eye.

❏ ❏ ❏ ➢ **What is the most common cause of retinitis in AIDS patients?**

Cytomegalovirus.
Findings include photophobia, redness, scotoma, pain, or change in visual acuity. On exam, findings include fluffy white retinal lesions.

❏ ❏ ❏ ➢ **Most common opportunistic infection in AIDS patients?**

PCP.
Symptoms may include non-productive cough and dyspnea. Chest x-ray may show diffuse interstitial infiltrates or be negative. Gallium scanning is more sensitive but results in false positives. Initial treatment includes TMP-SMX. Pentamidine is an alternative.

❏ ❏ ❏ ➢ **How is Candida of the esophagus diagnosed in the ED?**

Air-contrast barium swallow will show ulcerations with plaques. In contrast, herpes esophagitis will produce punched-out ulcerations with no plaques.

❏ ❏ ❏ ➢ **What is the most common gastrointestinal complaint in AIDS patients?**

Diarrhea.
Hepatomegaly and hepatitis are also common. Jaundice is an uncommon finding.

❏ ❏ ❏ ➢ **A patient is infected with Treponema pallidum, what is the treatment?**

Syphilis is treated with benzathine penicillin G, 2.4 million units IM or tetracycline 500 mg qid po for 15 d or erythromycin 500 mg qid po for 15 d.

❏ ❏ ❏ ➢ **Describe lesions associated with lymphogranuloma venerecum:**

LV caused by Chlamydia presents as painless skin lesions with lymphadenopathy. Lesions may be papular, nodular or herpetiform vesicles. Sinus formation involving the vagina and rectum are common in women.

❏ ❏ ❏ ➢ **What is the cause of chancroid?   Describe the lesions.**

Hemophilus ducreyi.
Presents with one or more <u>painful</u> necrotic lesions. Suppurating inguinal lymphadenopathy may also be present.

❏ ❏ ❏ ➢ **What is the cause of granuloma inguinale; describe the lesions?**

Calymmatobacterium granulomatis.
Typically begins with small papular, nodular, or vesicular lesions that develop slowly into ulcerative or granulomatous lesions. Lesions are PAINLESS and are located on mucous membranes of the genital, inguinal, and anal areas.

❏ ❏ ❏ ➢ **What is the incubation period in tetanus?**

Hours to over one month. The shorter the incubation the more severe the disease. Most patients in the U.S. who get the disease are over 50.

❏ ❏ ❏ ➢ **What is the most common presentation of tetanus?**

"Generalized tetanus" with pain and stiffness in the trunk and jaw muscles. Trismus develops and results in risus sardonicus (sardonic smile).

❏ ❏ ❏ ➢ **What cranial nerve is most commonly involved in cephalic tetanus?**

Cephalic tetanus usually occurs after injuries to the head and typically involves the 7th cranial nerve.

❏ ❏ ❏ ➤ **Outline tetanus treatment.**

1. Respiratory -	Succinylcholine for immediate intubation if required.
2. Immunotherapy -	Human tetanus immune globulin will neutralize circulating tetanospasmin and toxin in the wound (it will not neutralize toxin fixed in the nervous system). Dose TIG 3000 to 5000 units. Tetanus toxoid, 0.5 ml IM at 1 and 6 wk and 6 mo.
3. Antibiotics -	Clostridium tetani is sensitive to cephalosporins, tetracycline, erythromycin, and penicillin. Pen G is the drug of choice.
4. Muscle Relaxants -	Diazepam or dantrolene.
5. Neuromuscular blockade -	Pancuronium bromide, 2 mg plus sedation.
6. Autonomic dysfunction -	Labetalol 0.25-1.0 mg/min IV or magnesium sulfate 70 mg/kg IV load then 1-4 g/h continuous infusion is used to treat autonomic dysfunction. MS, 5-30 mg IV infusion q 2-8 h. Clonidine, 300 µg q 8 h per NG.

NOTE: FATAL CARDIOVASCULAR COMPLICATIONS HAVE OCCURRED IN PATIENTS TREATED WITH ß-ADRENERGIC BLOCKING AGENTS ALONE. ADRENERGIC BLOCKING AGENTS USED TO TREAT AUTONOMIC DYSFUNCTION MAY PRECIPITATE MYOCARDIAL DEPRESSION.

❏ ❏ ❏ ➤ **What is the most common tapeworm in the U.S.?**

Hymenolepis nana.

❏ ❏ ❏ ➤ **A patient presents with fever, dyspnea, cough, hemoptysis and eosinophilia. Diagnosis?**

Ascaris lumbricoides. This helminth is a roundworm. Serologic tests: ELISA, bentonite flocculation, and indirect hemagglutination. Treat with pyrantel pamoate (pyrimidine pamoate) or mebendazole. Obstruction of the intestine may require surgery.

❏ ❏ ❏ ➤ **How is hookworm infection acquired?**

In areas where human fertilizer is used and people don't wear shoes.
Patients present with chronic anemia, cough, low-grade fever, diarrhea, abdominal pain, weakness, weight loss, eosinophilia and guaiac positive stools.
Diagnosis is made by finding ova in the stool. Treatment is mebendazole or pyrantel pamoate [This is not a zebra - SHP].

❏ ❏ ❏ ➤ **What are the signs and symptoms of Trichuris trichiura?**

This hookworm lives in the cecum. Complaints include anorexia, abdominal pain especially RUQ, insomnia, fever, diarrhea, flatulence, weight loss, pruritus, eosinophilia, and microcytic hypochromic anemia.
Diagnosis is made by ova in the stool.
Mebendazole is the treatment.

❐ ❐ ❐ ➢ **A patient presents with a history of attending a walrus, bear, and pork roast. He now has N/V/D/F, urticaria, myalgia, splinter hemorrhages, muscle spasm, headache, and a stiff neck. What physical finding will clinch the diagnosis?**

Periorbital edema is pathognomonic of infection with Trichinella spiralis.
Patients may have acute myocarditis, nonsuppurative meningitis, catarrhal enteritis, or bronchopneumonia.
Lab studies may reveal leukocytosis, eosinophilia, ECG changes, and elevated CPK.
Diagnosis is confirmed with latex agglutination, skin test, or complement fixation or bentonite flocculation test.
Stool exam is not helpful after the initial GI phase in confirming the diagnosis.

❐ ❐ ❐ ➢ **Explain the pathophysiology of rabies:**

Infection occurs within the myocytes for the first 48 to 96 h. It then spreads across the motor endplate, ascends and replicates along peripheral nervous axoplasm into the dorsal root ganglia, the spinal cord, and CNS. From the gray matter, the virus spreads by peripheral nerves to tissues and organ systems.

❐ ❐ ❐ ➢ **What is the characteristic histologic finding in rabies?**

Eosinophilic intracellular lesions found within cerebral neurons called **Negri** bodies are the site of CNS viral replication. They are found in 75% of rabies cases; although pathognomonic for rabies, their absence does not rule out rabies.

❐ ❐ ❐ ➢ **What are the signs and symptoms of rabies?**

Initial - fever, headache, malaise, anorexia, sore throat, nausea, cough, and pain or paresthesias at the bite site.

CNS stage - agitation, restlessness, altered mental status, painful bulbar and peripheral muscular spasms, bulbar or focal motor paresis, and opisthotonos. Similar to Landry-Guillain-Barré syndrome, 20% develop ascending, symmetric flaccid and areflexic paralysis. Hypersensitivity to water and sensory stimuli (light, touch, and noise) may occur.

Progressive stage - lucid and confused intervals with hyperpyrexia, lacrimation, salivation, and mydriasis may occur along with brainstem dysfunction, hyperreflexia and extensor plantar response.

Final stage - coma, convulsions, and apnea, followed by death at days 4 to 7 in the untreated patient.

❐ ❐ ❐ ➢ **What is the diagnostic procedure of choice in rabies?**

Fluorescent antibody testing (FAT).

❐ ❐ ❐ ➢ **How is rabies treated?**

RIG 20 IU/kg, half at wound site and half in the DELTOID muscle. HDCV 1-ml doses

IM on days 0,3,7,14, and 28 also in the DELTOID muscle.

❐ ❐ ❐ ➤ **What is the <u>second</u> <u>most</u> <u>common</u> tick borne disease?**

Rocky Mountain spotted fever.
Causative agent - Rickettsia rickettsii.
Vector - Female Ixodi ticks, Dermacentor andersonii (wood tick) and D. variabilis (American dog tick).

❐ ❐ ❐ ➤ **A patient presents with fever up to 40 °C followed by a rash which is erythematous, macular, and blanching. The rash progresses to deep red, dusky, papular and becomes petechial. The patient also complains of a headache, vomiting, myalgias, and cough. Where did the rash begin?**

RMSF rash typically begins on the flexor surfaces of the ankles and wrists and spread centripetally and centrifugally.

❐ ❐ ❐ ➤ **Confirmatory tests for RMSF?**

Immunofluorescent antibody staining of skin biopsy or serologic fluorescent antibody titer. The Weil-Felix reaction and complement fixation tests are no longer recommended.

❐ ❐ ❐ ➤ **Antibiotics for RMSF?**

Tetracycline or chloramphenicol. Antibiotic therapy should not be withheld pending serologic confirmation.

❐ ❐ ❐ ➤ **What is the most deadly form of malaria?**

Plasmodium falciparum.

❐ ❐ ❐ ➤ **What is the vector for malaria?**

The female anopheline mosquito.

❐ ❐ ❐ ➤ **What lab findings are expected in a patient with malaria?**

Normochromic normocytic anemia, normal or depressed leukocyte count, thrombocytopenia, an elevated sed rate, abnormal kidney and LFTs, hyponatremia, hypoglycemia, and false-positive VDRL.

❐ ❐ ❐ ➤ **How is the definitive diagnosis of malaria established?**

Visualization of parasites on Giemsa-stained blood smears. In early infection, especially with P. falciparum, parasitized erythrocytes may be sequestered and be undetectable.

❏ ❏ ❏ ➢ **How is P. falciparum diagnosed on blood smear?**

1. Small ring forms with double chromatin knobs within the erythrocyte.
2. Multiple rings infected within red blood cells.
3. Rare trophozoites and schizonts on smear.
4. Pathognomonic crescent-shaped gametocytes.
5. Parasitemia exceeding 4%.

❏ ❏ ❏ ➢ **What is the drug of choice for treating P. vivax, ovale, and malariae?**

Chloroquine.

❏ ❏ ❏ ➢ **How is uncomplicated chloroquine-resistant P. falciparum treated?**

Quinine + pyrimethamine-sulfadoxine + doxycycline or mefloquine.

❏ ❏ ❏ ➢ **How is complicated chloroquine-resistant P. falciparum treated?**

Quinidine gluconate IV + doxycycline IV.

❏ ❏ ❏ ➢ **What complication of quinine and quinidine therapy should be considered?**

Insulin release which may result in hypoglycemia.

❏ ❏ ❏ ➢ **What are the adverse effects of chloroquine?**

N/V/D/F, pruritus, headache, dizziness, rash, and hypotension.

❏ ❏ ❏ ➢ **What type of parasitic infection commonly presents with a papular pruritic rash?**

Schistosoma.

❏ ❏ ❏ ➢ **What type of parasite infections do not typically result in eosinophilia?**

Protozoa infections such as amebas, Giardia, Trypanosoma, and Babesia.

❏ ❏ ❏ ➢ **What is the most common intestinal parasite in the U.S.?**

Giardia. Cysts are obtained from contaminated water or passed by hand-to-mouth transmission.
Symptoms include explosive foul smelling diarrhea, abdominal distention, fever, fatigue, and weight loss. Cysts reside in the duodenum and upper jejunum.
Treatment is quinacrine.

❏ ❏ ❏ ➢ **How is Chagas disease transmitted?**

The blood-sucking Reduviid (kissing) bug, blood transfusion, or breast feeding. A nodule or chagoma develops at the site of the bite.
Symptoms include fever, headache, conjunctivitis, anorexia, and <u>myocarditis</u>. CHF and ventricular aneurysms can occur. The myenteric plexus is involved and may result in megacolon.
Lab findings include anemia, leukocytosis, elevated sed rate, and ECG changes (PR interval, heart block, T-wave changes, and arrhythmias).

❏ ❏ ❏ ➢ **What two diseases does the deer tick, Ixodes dammini transmit?**

Lyme disease and Babesia.

❏ ❏ ❏ ➢ **How do patients present with Babesia infection?**

Intermittent fever, splenomegaly, jaundice, and hemolysis. The disease may be fatal in patients without spleens. Treatment is with clindamycin and quinine.

❏ ❏ ❏ ➢ **What is the most frequently transmitted tick-borne disease?**

Lyme disease.
Causative agent - spirochete Borrelia burgdorferi.
Vector - Ixodes dammini (deer tick) also I. pacificus, Amblyomma americanum, and Dermacentor variabilis.

❏ ❏ ❏ ➢ **When are patients most likely to acquire Lyme disease?**

Late spring and late summer, peaks in July.

❏ ❏ ❏ ➢ **How is Lyme disease diagnosed?**

Immunofluorescent and immunoabsorbent assays diagnose the antibodies to the spirochete.
Treatment includes doxycycline or tetracycline, amoxicillin, IV penicillin V in pregnant patients, or erythromycin.

❏ ❏ ❏ ➢ **What type of paralysis does tick paralysis cause?**

Ascending paralysis. The venom which causes paralysis is probably a neurotoxin which causes a conduction block at the peripheral motor nerve branches. This prevents acetylcholine release at the neuromuscular junction. 43 species of ticks are implicated as causative agents.

❏ ❏ ❏ ➢ **What is the most common sign of tularemia?**

Lymphadenopathy, usually cervical in children and inguinal in adults. It is caused by Francisella tularensis and is transmitted by the vectors Dermacentor variabilis and A. americanum.

❐ ❐ ❐ ➤ **What two tick born diseases are transmitted by the tick vector I. dammini? FEEL the Force, Luke...**

Lyme disease and babesiosis.

❐ ❐ ❐ ➤ **A patient presents with sudden-onset of fever, lethargy, headache, myalgias, anorexia, nausea and vomiting. They describe the headache as retro-orbital and are extremely photophobic. They have been on a camping trip in Wyoming. What tick borne disease might cause these symptoms?**

Colorado tick fever is caused by a virus of the genus Orbivirus of the family Reoviridae. The vector is the tick D. andersoni. The disease is self-limited and treatment is supportive.

RHEUM/IMMUNOLOGY

"SUCCESS FOUR FLIGHTS THURSDAY MORNING ALL AGAINST TWENTY ONE MILE WIND STARTED FROM LEVEL WITH ENGINE POWER ALONE AVERAGE SPEED THROUGH AIR THIRTY ONE MILES LONGEST 57 SECONDS INFORM PRESS HOME CHRISTMAS."

Telegram from Orville Wright to his father, 12/17/1903

❏ ❏ ❏ ➢ **What is the treatment of choice for a patient in anaphylactic shock?**

Epinephrine 0.3-0.5 mg IV of 1:10,000 solution. If no IV access, then inject into the venous plexus at base of the tongue.

❏ ❏ ❏ ➢ **What is the most common cause of anaphylactoid reactions?**

Radiographic contrast agents.

❏ ❏ ❏ ➢ **For how long should a patient with a generalized anaphylactic reaction be observed?**

24 h. Recurrence and delayed reactions are possible. Patients should be treated with oral antihistamines and corticosteroids for at least 72 h.

❏ ❏ ❏ ➢ **What percentage of patients with relapsing polychondritis can be expected to have airway involvement?**

Approximately 50% have airway involvement. They frequently present with acute onset of pain, oropharyngeal tenderness over cartilaginous structures, and hoarseness. Erythema and edema of the nose and oropharynx is also common.

❏ ❏ ❏ ➢ **What is the appropriate treatment of a patient presenting with acute onset of relapsing polychrondritis with airway involvement?**

Admit for observation and high dose steroids. These patients may develop dyspnea, stridor, or cough. Repeated exacerbations may lead to asphyxiation .

❏ ❏ ❏ ➢ **A RA patient presenting with painful speaking or swallowing, hoarseness, or stridor requires what type of diagnostic procedure?**

Urgent laryngoscopy to evaluate involvement of the paired cricoarytenoid joints. These may become fixed in the closed position, resulting in airway compromise.

❏ ❏ ❏ ➢ **What percentage of SLE patients will develop signs and symptoms of pleurisy during the course of their disease?**

Approximately half. Pleurisy is also common in RA, but is often asymptomatic. All pulmonary effusions in patients with rheumatic disease require thoracentesis to distinguish from infectious processes.

❏ ❏ ❏ ➢ **Myocardial infarction can be related to which two rheumatic diseases?**

Kawasaki disease and polyarteritis nodosa.

❏ ❏ ❏ ➢ **What percentage of patients with Kawasaki disease who do not receive proper therapy will develop coronary artery aneurysms?**

20%. 2-3% will go on to die from MI during the resolution phase of the disease.

❏ ❏ ❏ ➢ **A patient presents with fever, acute polyarthritis, or migratory arthritis a few weeks after a bout of Streptococcal pharyngitis, they should be evaluated for what disease?**

Rheumatic fever. Approximately 30% will have subcutaneous nodules, erythema marginatum, or chorea.

❏ ❏ ❏ ➢ **What is the Rx of choice for the fever and arthritis of rheumatic fever?**

Salicylates and bedrest until signs and symptoms return to normal.

❏ ❏ ❏ ➢ **What clinical sign do the following often have in common; rheumatic fever, bacterial endocarditis, Schonlein-Henoch-purpura, prodromal pulmonary Mycoplasma, or fungal infections?**

Migratory arthritis.

❏ ❏ ❏ ➢ **What pathological process should be considered in a patient treated with steroids, who presents with weakness, depression, fatigue, and postural dizziness?**

Adrenal insufficiency. Treatment consists of stress steroids - dexamethasone is preferred because it does not interfere with testing of adrenal steroids levels.

❏ ❏ ❏ ➢ **Name a common complication of SLE, RA, & JRA.**

Pericarditis.

❏ ❏ ❏ ➢ **What is the normal atlantodental distance on lateral flexion views of the C-spine?**

3.5 mm in adults.
4 mm in the child under 12 y.

❏ ❏ ❏ ➢ **What might a change in bladder or bowel function, limb paresthesias, or new weakness indicate in a patient with RA or ankylosing spondylosis?**

Destruction of the C-spine ligamentous structures - this can lead to atlantoaxial subluxation.

❏ ❏ ❏ ➢ **What is Lhermitte's sign, found in patients with RA or ankylosing spondylosis?**

The sensation of an electric shock radiating down the back with neck flexion. A classic sign of C-spine instability.

❏ ❏ ❏ ➢ **What is another name for granulomatous arteritis of the thoracic aorta, and branches? (Hint: usually presents with tender scalp, new headache, fluctuating vision, reduced or lost brachial pulse, and pain in the tongue or jaw while talking or chewing).**

Temporal arteritis.

❏ ❏ ❏ ➢ **Polymyalgia rheumatica coexists in 10-30% of patients with which disease affecting the vascular system?**

Temporal arteritis.

❏ ❏ ❏ ➢ **What rheumatic syndrome may lead to corneal irritation, ulceration, and infection?**

Sjogren's syndrome.

❏ ❏ ❏ ➢ **What is the most common pathogen found in osteomyelitis and septic arthritis of the foot?**

Pseudomonas.

❏ ❏ ❏ ➢ **How does the time course of the onset of joint pain help differentiate between gout and pseudogout?**

Patients with gout develop joint pain over a few hours, while pseudogout usually evolves over a day.

❏ ❏ ❏ ➢ **The finding of rhomboid shaped crystals under a polarizing scope in an aspirate of a painful joint indicates what type of synovitis?**

Pseudogout (calcium pyrophosphate).
Blue needle shaped crystals indicate gout (urate).

❏ ❏ ❏ ➢ **What is the first priority in the workup of a patient suspected of having gout?**

Exclusion of septic arthritis.

❏ ❏ ❏ ➢ **Name a complication of RA that mimics a DVT?**

Ruptured Baker's cyst. The ruptured cyst may be differentiated from a DVT by absence of swelling in the foot, and a crescent sign (a purplish discoloration below the malleoli).

❏ ❏ ❏ ➢ **How may an olecranon bursitis be differentiated from arthritis of the elbow?**

Bursitis will not affect pronation or supination.

❐ ❐ ❐ ➢ **What is the treatment of choice if there is any clinical suspicion of a septic olecranon bursa?**

Appropriate antibiotic therapy should be started. Using a large bore needle the bursa should be drained completely.

❐ ❐ ❐ ➢ **What uncommon musculoskeletal disorder of children must be considered in a child that refuses to sit or walk, and holds themself rigidly stiff?**

Discitis. Any attempts to maneuver the child will elicit guarding, and plain films will often reveal an abnormal lordosis.

❐ ❐ ❐ ➢ **Toxic synovitis affects what age group of patients?**

School age children. Treatment is to rule out sepsis, and relieve synovial pressure through aspiration.

❐ ❐ ❐ ➢ **What disease entity should be investigated in a child with joint swelling following minor trauma.**

JRA. Minor trauma may cause intra-articular bleeding. The joint should not be immobilized.

❐ ❐ ❐ ➢ **What is the appropriate management for a child with normal x-rays and tenderness over the end of a long bone after trauma.**

Immobilization and orthopedic evaluation for Salter-Harris type I fracture. These fractures may be occult.

❐ ❐ ❐ ➢ **What pathologic process must be considered in a patient with painless progressive weakness in a C-spine distribution?**

Cervical ventral root compromise by a degenerative disk. The dorsal and ventral nerve roots remain discrete in the C-spine in over half the population.

❐ ❐ ❐ ➢ **Complaints of <u>bilateral</u> upper extremity pain may involve what pathologic process?**

A C6 spinal radiculopathy.

❐ ❐ ❐ ➢ **What pathological process is suggested in a patient with a reduction of the radial pulse when the shoulder is passively abducted? Hint - a patient with this syndrome may also have a subclavian bruit.**

Thoracic outlet syndrome.

❐ ❐ ❐ ➢ **Tenderness over the ulnar nerve at the elbow may indicate a cervical radiculopathy at what level?**

C8 - T1.

❑ ❑ ❑ ➤ **Numbness or tingling in the long finger may be the only presenting symptom of a radiculopathy at what level?**

C7.

❑ ❑ ❑ ➤ **Hyperreflexia and a Hoffman's sign in the upper extremities with neck pain indicate a lesion where?**

Above C5.

❑ ❑ ❑ ➤ **Where does cervical disk prolapse most often occur?**

C6-7 (on the left), and C5-6 (on the right). Most often in the fourth decade.

❑ ❑ ❑ ➤ **Angina-like chest pain, Horner's syndrome, painless upper extremity weakness, and severe radicular symptoms without neck pain may all be caused by what pathologic cervical process?**

Spurious cervical osteophytes.

❑ ❑ ❑ ➤ **What pathology should be presumed when there is a sudden loss of bladder control, onset of lumbosacral pain, and associated bilateral leg pain?**

Midline herniation of a thoraco-lumbar disk. With these symptoms comes the threat of paraparesis.

❑ ❑ ❑ ➤ **What constitutes immediate admission criteria for a patient with acute low back pain?**

Paraparesis, bowel or bladder incontinence, intractable L-S pain and spasticity, inability to sit or stand, upright sleeping position, metastatic cancer, 2nd ED visit, or X-ray film with defects.

❑ ❑ ❑ ➤ **An inability to walk on the toes indicates a radiculopathy where?**

S1. An L5 radiculopathy manifests as inability to walk on the heels.

❑ ❑ ❑ ➤ **A painful "strum" sign in the presence of a progressive inability to extend the knee on the affected side is pathognomic of what pathology?**

A herniated disk with nerve root impaction.

❑ ❑ ❑ ➤ **Compromise of which nerve roots can mimic the muscular calf pain of thrombophlebitis or the anterior tibial compartment pain of "shin splints"?**

L5 and S1 root compromise.

❑ ❑ ❑ ➤ **What are the two most common causes of fatal anaphylaxis?**

#1 = Drug reactions, 95% to penicillin. Parenteral most dangerous. 300 people/y.

#2 = Hymenoptera stings. 100 people/y.

❏ ❏ ❏ ➢ **Which type of hypersensitivity reaction is responsible for anaphylaxis?**

Type I, (IgE mediated).

Hypersensitivity Reaction	Mediator	Example
Type 1 - Immediate	IgE binds allergen, includes mast cells and basophils	Food allergy. **Asthma in children.**
Type 2 - Cytotoxic	IgG & IgM antibody reactions to antigen on cell surface activates complement and killers	Blood transfusion rxn. ITP, hemolytic anemia,
Type 3 - Immune complex, Arthrus	Complexes activate complement	Tetanus toxoid in sensitized persons. **Poststreptococcal glomeru- lonephritis.**
Type 4 - Cell mediated, delayed hypersensitivity	Activated T-lympho- cytes	Skin tests

❏ ❏ ❏ ➢ **Food mediated hypersensitivity reactions are due to what component of the immune system?**

IgE. Dairy products, nuts and eggs are the most common.

❏ ❏ ❏ ➢ **When do the clinical manifestations of a drug allergy reaction usually become apparent?**

The first or second week following administration of the drug.

❏ ❏ ❏ ➢ **Generalized malaise, fever, arthralgias, and urticaria are common to what type of allergic reaction?**

Drug allergy. Allergic reactions to drugs may involve any or all of the four types of hypersensitivity reactions.

PSYCHIATRIC PEARLS

"It is difficult to say what is impossible, for the dream of yesterday is the hope of today and the reality of tomorrow."

Robert H. Goddard, at his high school
graduation, 1904.

❏ ❏ ❏ ➤ **Describe a patient with generalized anxiety disorder.**

Patients appear apprehensive, restless, irritable and easily distracted. Patients may experience muscle tension and fatigue as well as various autonomic symptoms such as palpitations, shortness of breath, chest tightness, nausea or diffuse weakness and numbness.

❏ ❏ ❏ ➤ **Name a few substances that may mimic generalized anxiety when ingested.**

Nicotine, caffeine, amphetamines, cocaine, anticholinergics; alcohol and sedative withdrawal.

❏ ❏ ❏ ➤ **What is the epidemiologic difference between suicide attempters and suicide completers?**

Suicide completers tend to be older males with medical problems, living alone or with a poor social network.

❏ ❏ ❏ ➤ **Name 2 Axis I disorders commonly associated with suicidal ideation.**

Alcohol abuse and affective (mood) disorder.

❏ ❏ ❏ ➤ **What happens when one combines EtOH with an anxiolytic (benzodiazepine)?**

Death! (Due to their combined respiratory depressive effects).

❏ ❏ ❏ ➤ **Name another contraindication to benzodiazepine use.**

Known hypersensitivity, acute narrow angle glaucoma, pregnancy especially 1st trimester.

❏ ❏ ❏ ➤ **Why have mono-amine oxidase (MAO) inhibitors been prescribed less frequently?**

Why don't you try a tyramine-free diet sometime! Mmm Mmm good!
Tyramine containing substances can cause hypertensive crisis - such foods include pickled herring, snails, chicken liver, beer, red wine and cheese.

❏ ❏ ❏ ➤ **Name some drugs <u>contraindicated</u> for a patient taking MAO inhibitors.**

Toxic reactions that include excitation and hyperpyrexia can occur with meperidine (Demerol) and with dextromethorphan. The effects of indirect acting adrenergic drugs are potentiated, including ephedrine, sympathomimetic amines in cold remedies, amphetamines, cocaine and methylphenidate (Ritalin).

❒ ❒ ❒ ➤ **Name the three common MAO inhibitors (chemical and Brand name).**

Phenelzine (Nardil).
Isocarboxazid (Marplan).
Tranylcypromine (Parnate).

❒ ❒ ❒ ➤ **How does one treat hypertensive crisis caused by combining MAO inhibitors with a known toxin, cheese pizza?**

An α- and ß-adrenergic antagonist such as labetalol.
Also consider nifedipine or nitroglycerin. If unsuccessful, consider IV phentolamine or sodium nitroprusside.

❒ ❒ ❒ ➤ **A 27 y old male arrives somnolent with vitals of P 130, R 26, BP 170/80 T of 105 °F. You note diffuse muscular rigidity and intermittent focal muscle twitching/jerking lasting 1-2 seconds. As you 'work him up', your faithful nurse returns from the waiting area with news from the family that the patient has had a progressive decline of mental status for 2 d after seeing his psychiatrist. The patient has had a history of 'psychosis' for almost one year. What process should be included in your differential diagnosis at this time?**

Neuroleptic malignant syndrome.

❒ ❒ ❒ ➤ **Psychiatrists use a multiaxial diagnostic system to describe a particular patient's medical problem list; discuss.**

Axis I: Symptoms and syndromes comprising a mental disorder, includes substance abuse/addiction.
Axis II: Personality and developmental disorders (underlying the Axis I diagnosis).
Axis III: Physical medical problems/conditions which may or may not contribute to Axis I diagnosis.
Axis IV: Psychosocial factors.
Axis V: Adaptive ability/disability.

❒ ❒ ❒ ➤ **What is organic brain syndrome?**

Reversible or nonreversible mental condition thought to be caused by disease process or substance use which interrupts normal anatomical, physiological or biochemical brain functions.

❒ ❒ ❒ ➤ **Describe dementia.**

Disturbed cognitive function resulting in impaired memory, personality, judgment and/or language. Insidious onset, but may present as acute worsened mental state while facing other physical or environmental stressors.

❒ ❒ ❒ ➤ **Describe delirium.**

"Clouding of consciousness" resulting in disorientation, decreased alertness and impaired cognitive function. Acute onset, visual hallucinosis, fluctuating psychomotor activity; all symptoms variable and may change over hours.

❏ ❏ ❏ ➢ **Neuroleptic medications come in three flavors: low, medium and high potency. Can you name some of these meds and their category?**

Low potency: Chlorpromazine (Thorazine).
Medium potency: Perphenazine (Trilafon).
High potency: Haloperidol, droperidol (Inapsine), thiothixene (Navane),
                   fluphenazine (Prolixin), trifluoperazine (Stelazine).

❏ ❏ ❏ ➢ **So, what's the big deal?**

Neuroleptics act to block dopamine receptors. Receptor blockade within the mesolimbic area of the brain provides their antipsychotic effect. Dopaminergic receptor blockade throughout the CNS and anticholinergic effect produce many side effects observed in the ED.

❏ ❏ ❏ ➢ **Which neuroleptics produce which side effects?**

Low potency: Sedative, orthostatic hypotension, anticholinergic effects.

High potency: Less sedating, profound extrapyramidal reactions.

❏ ❏ ❏ ➢ **What are extrapyramidal reactions?**

Dopamine receptor blockade within the nigrostriatal system results in involuntary and spontaneous motor responses including: dystonia, akathisia and Parkinson's-like syndrome.

❏ ❏ ❏ ➢ **What is a dystonic reaction?**

Very common side effect of neuroleptics seen in the ED. Muscle spasm of tongue, face, neck and back are seen. Severe laryngospasm and extraocular muscle spasm may occur also. Patients may bite the tongue leading to potential airway compromise either by inability to open the mouth or by tongue edema or hemorrhage.

❏ ❏ ❏ ➢ **How do you treat a dystonic reaction?**

Diphenhydramine (Benadryl), 25-50 mg IM or IV or benztropine (Cogentin), 1-2 mg IV or PO.
Remember that dystonias can recur acutely.

❏ ❏ ❏ ➢ **Describe symptoms of alcohol withdrawal.**

Autonomic hyperactivity: tachycardia, hypertension, tremors, anxiety, agitation; 6-8 h after drinking.

Hallucinations: auditory, visual, tactile; 24 h after drinking.

Global confusion: 1-3 d after drinking.

❏ ❏ ❏ ➤ **List some life-threatening causes of acute psychosis.**

WHHHIMP: Wernicke's Encephalopathy, Hypoxia, Hypoglycemia, Hypertensive encephalopathy, Intracerebral hemorrhage, Meningitis/Encephalitis, and Poisoning.

❏ ❏ ❏ ➤ **Characteristics of schizophrenia?**

Delusional disorder, hallucinations, (usually auditory), disorganized thinking, loosening of associations, disheveled appearance, lack of insight in realizing thoughts and behavior are abnormal, onset age usually less than 40, and duration of symptoms longer than 6 mo.

❏ ❏ ❏ ➤ **What is the difference between schizophrenia and schizophreniform disorder?**

Very little. In schizophreniform disorder, schizophrenic symptoms have lasted less than 6 mo.

❏ ❏ ❏ ➤ **What is a brief reactive psychosis?**

Acute psychotic break, usually after an emotional or traumatic event. Short duration, usually less than 2 wk.

❏ ❏ ❏ ➤ **Signs and symptoms suggestive of organic source of psychosis.**

Acute onset, disorientation, visual or tactile hallucinations, evidence suggesting overdose or acute ingestion, such as abnormal vital signs, pupil size and reactivity, nystagmus, and age less than 10 or older than 60.

❏ ❏ ❏ ➤ **Name some symptoms of major depression.**

In sad cages: Interest, sleep, appetite, depressed mood, concentration, activity, guilt, energy, suicide.

❏ ❏ ❏ ➤ **Name some vegetative symptoms.**

Loss of appetite, lack of concentration, chronic fatigue, agitation, restlessness, inability to sleep, weight loss.

GU PEARLS

❐ ❐ ❐ ➤ **Describe acute glomerulonephritis (GN).**

Hematuria.
Proteinuria.
Oliguria or Anuria.
Edema.
Hypertension.

❐ ❐ ❐ ➤ **Let us mention some diseases that cause glomerular dysfunction (skip this one if you are in a hurry!)** -

Goodpasture's syndrome - pulmonary hemorrhage with hemoptysis followed by anti-glomerular basement membrane antibody induced glomerulonephritis.
Post-infectious GN - most commonly post-streptococcal (group A, ß- hemolytic) but may follow other infections with GN secondary to immune complex deposits in glomeruli.
Polyarteritis Nodosa (PAN)- A systemic necrotizing vasculitis affecting primarily medium and small caliber arteries particularly at bifurcations and branchings. PAN occurs from infancy to old age with a peak incidence near age 60. 90% of patients with PAN develop renal involvement.
Systemic Lupus Erythematosus - Autoimmune disorder resulting, in part, in necrotizing vasculitis of primarily small vessels complicated by direct immunoglobulin deposits in glomeruli; mortality range 18-58% depending on histologic type.
Henoch-Schönlein Purpura (HSP) - another systemic necrotizing vasculitis of small vessels with typical renal presentation of nephritic syndrome without edema or hypertension, or with hematuria.
Hemolytic Uremic Syndrome (HUS) - microangiopathic hemolytic anemia, thrombocytopenia and renal dysfunction with rapid onset in children about 1 wk after gastroenteritis or URI. May occur in adults, most commonly complicating pregnancy or postpartum period. Acute renal failure develops in ~ 60% of children with HUS, most of which resolve in weeks with only supportive therapy.
Thrombotic Thrombocytopenic Purpura (TTP) - closely related to HUS with higher occurrence in young adults and association with fevers, more neurologic problems and less renal involvement, usually with hematuria and proteinuria. TTP prognosis is much worse than HUS with 75% 3-mo mortality.

❐ ❐ ❐ ➤ **What is the mortality for patients with acute renal failure?**

About 65%.

❐ ❐ ❐ ➤ **ATN resulting from 2 different mechanisms is the <u>most</u> <u>common</u> cause of intrinsic renal failure. Name the 2 mechanisms.**

Ischemic injury and nephrotoxic agents.

❐ ❐ ❐ ➤ **Name some common drugs/substances that can contribute to renal failure.**

Aminoglycosides, NSAIDs, contrast agents, myoglobin.

❏ ❏ ❏ ➣ **Can a selected group of women with a UTI probably be treated safely with single dose or short-course (3 d) antibiotic therapy with TMP/SMX?**

Yes; those with few "priors", short period of UTI symptoms and no risk factors for subclinical pyelonephritis.

❏ ❏ ❏ ➣ **What are the risk factors for subclinical pyelonephritis?**

Those are the things that make someone more likely to have it. They include multiple prior UTIs, longer duration of sx, recent pyelonephritis, diabetes, anatomic abnormalities, immunocompromised patients and in those who are indigent.

❏ ❏ ❏ ➣ **The "rule of twos" is a wonderful pearl described by Dr. David S. Howes of the University of Illinois in Tintinalli, 3rd Ed. which explains outpatient management for appropriate women who present at that institution with uncomplicated pyelonephritis. Outline the "rule of twos."**

Give 2 L of IV fluid.
Give 2 Tylenol #3.
Give 2 g ceftriaxone.
If patient can tolerate 2 glasses of water and fever decreases by 2 degrees:
Give TMP/SMX Double strength bid for 2 weeks, plan f/u in 2 d for progress check.

Ed. note: <u>Gotta</u> love that one!!

❏ ❏ ❏ ➣ **About what percentage of patients with epididymitis will have pyuria?**

24%.

❏ ❏ ❏ ➣ **Contrast the pain associated with epididymitis to that of prostatitis.**

Epididymitis -pain begins in scrotum or groin radiates along spermatic cord, often intensifies quickly after onset, may be associated with dysuria and may be relieved by scrotal elevation.
Prostatitis -acute prostatitis is associated with more frequency, dysuria and urgency, bladder outlet obstruction and retention, low back and perineal area pain associated with fever and chills, and with arthralgias and myalgias.

Patients with either of these disorders may become toxic and require admission.

❏ ❏ ❏ ➣ **T/F - Incidence of testicular torsion is bimodal with peak occurrence rates in the first year of life and again near puberty.**

True.

❏ ❏ ❏ ➣ **T/F - Testicular torsion often occurs after exertion or during sleep.**

True.

❏ ❏ ❏ ➣ **T/F - About 40% of patients with testicular torsion have a history of a similar pain that resolved spontaneously.**

True.

❑ ❑ ❑ ➢ **With what condition is the "blue dot" sign associated?**

Torsion of the testicular appendage, also of epididymis.

❑ ❑ ❑ ➢ **What is the eponym for idiopathic scrotal gangrene?**

Fournier's gangrene.

❑ ❑ ❑ ➢ **A penile fracture is actually a rent of the tunica albuginea and requires surgery to appose the ends of the tunica and to evacuate the hematoma. Is a retrograde urethrogram necessary in the evaluation of a patient with this injury?**

Yes, though uncommon, the urethra can be disrupted.

❑ ❑ ❑ ➢ **What is the initial treatment for priapism?**

Terbutaline 0.25-0.5 mg SQ q 4 - 6 h.

❑ ❑ ❑ ➢ **What are most renal calculi made out of?**

70% of renal calculi are composed of calcium oxalate.

❑ ❑ ❑ ➢ **About what percentage of renal stones are radiopaque?**

90%.

❑ ❑ ❑ ➢ **About what percentage of renal calculi will pass spontaneously?**

90%.

EMS PEARLS

"Houston, Tranquility Base here. The Eagle has landed."

Neil Armstrong, radio transmission to Mission Control, at the moment of the first manned landing on the moon, 7/20/1969.

❏ ❏ ❏ ➢ **About what percentage of normal <u>coronary</u> blood flow is achieved during CPR?**

5%.

❏ ❏ ❏ ➢ **About what percentage of normal cardiac output is achieved during CPR?**

20-25%.

❏ ❏ ❏ ➢ **What is the currently favored theory explaining how CPR works?**

The thoracic pump theory - that blood flow is induced by a pressure gradient between the intrathoracic and extrathoracic compartments.

❏ ❏ ❏ ➢ **What is the favored theory explaining how MAST works?**

MAST increases peripheral vascular resistance (PVR).

❏ ❏ ❏ ➢ **What is the absolute contraindication to using MAST?**

Pulmonary edema.

❏ ❏ ❏ ➢ **Name relative contraindications to MAST.**

Pregnancy.
Impaled objects.
Evisceration.
Thoracic/diaphragmatic injuries.

❏ ❏ ❏ ➢ **About what percentage of patients who undergo cardiac resuscitation attempts recover and are neurologically intact?**

10%.

❏ ❏ ❏ ➢ **About what percentage of patients who undergo cardiac resuscitation attempts survive, but are not functionally and neurologically intact?**

25%.

❏ ❏ ❏ ➢ **Intracellular accumulation of what electrolyte is currently thought to initiate a** cascade of events that lead to cell death?

Calcium.

❏ ❏ ❏ ➢ EOA is contraindicated in patients less than how old?

16 y.

❏ ❏ ❏ ➢ Catheter over needle puncture/ventilation, rather than cricothyroidotomy is recommended for patients under how many years of age?

10 y.

❏ ❏ ❏ ➢ Uncuffed ET tubes should be selected for patients under how old?

6 y.

❏ ❏ ❏ ➢ What is the most common complication of EOA use?

Insertion into the trachea (about 10%).

❏ ❏ ❏ ➢ T/F- When a patient arrives in the ED with an EOA the first thing the ED physician should do is remove the EOA and replace it with an endotracheal tube.

False - an endotracheal tube should be placed with the EOA still in position.

❏ ❏ ❏ ➢ What recent development, in the pre-hospital setting, has been documented to show improvement in cardiac arrest outcome?

Automatic External Defibrillator.

❏ ❏ ❏ ➢ EMS systems had an emphasis in their development of managing cardiac arrests. What percent of EMS calls are cardiac arrests?

<5%.

❏ ❏ ❏ ➢ What percent of an EMS system's call are pediatric?

10%.

❏ ❏ ❏ ➢ What act or law authorized the U.S. Dept. of Transportation to fund ambulance communication & training programs for pre-hospital medical services?

1966 National Highway Safety Act. In 1973, Public Law 93-154 defined a goal to improve EMS services on a national scale. This law identified 15 elements.

❏ ❏ ❏ ➢ What are the 3 emergency medical technician levels recognized nationally?

EMT-A (ambulance), EMT-I (intermediate), EMT-P (paramedic).

❏ ❏ ❏ ➢ **What are the 3 main duties of EMS off-line medical director?**

Development of protocols, of medical accountability (quality assurance), and of ongoing education.

❏ ❏ ❏ ➢ **How does the American College of Emergency Physicians define a medical disaster?**

Destructive effects of natural or man-made forces that overwhelm the ability of a given area or community to meet health care demands.

❏ ❏ ❏ ➢ **What are the 3 phases of a disaster response?**

Activation, implementation, recovery.

❏ ❏ ❏ ➢ **What are the 4 categories for a typical triage system?**

Severe, Moderate, Minor, Dead or Expectant Death. Remember, triage is a dynamic process that is ongoing; each patient should be reassessed numerous times.

❏ ❏ ❏ ➢ **Who is in command of a disaster scene?**

The chief executive officer or commander. The EMS director acts in support, not command, of public safety agencies with overall scene control.

❏ ❏ ❏ ➢ **Who requires hospitals to have a disaster plan? How often should it be tested?**

The Joint Commission on Accreditation of Health Organizations (JCAHO). Test it twice per year.

❏ ❏ ❏ ➢ **What are the key points when dealing with a disaster?**

Do the most good for the most number of potential survivors. Don't become a victim yourself. Prioritize patient care. Triage is an ongoing process. Make your plan as close to every day operating procedures as possible. EMS is not in overall scene command.

ENVIRONMENTAL PEARLS

"He who possesses virtue in abundance may be compared to an infant. Poisonous insects will not sting him. Fierce beasts will not seize him. Birds of prey will not strike him....
He may cry all day without becoming hoarse,
This means that his natural harmony is perfect."

Tao-te Ching, 55; Lao Tzu

❏ ❏ ❏ ➢ **Above what altitude does acute mountain sickness typically develop?**

8,000 feet.

❏ ❏ ❏ ➢ **A near-drowning victim presents to the ED. What electrolyte abnormalities are expected?**

Electrolyte abnormalities are usually not significant.

❏ ❏ ❏ ➢ **What antibiotics and what steroid dose are indicated in the ED for a near-drowning victim?**

Trick question. Prophylactic antibiotics and steroids are not useful for preventing aspiration pneumonia or pulmonary edema. Steroids may be used for increased ICP.

❏ ❏ ❏ ➢ **A 14 y old football player presents to the ED with a history of light-headedness, headache, nausea, and vomiting. On exam, the patient has a HR of 110, RR 22, BP of 90/60, and is afebrile. Profuse sweating is noted. Diagnosis?**

Heat exhaustion. Treat with .9 NS IV fluid.

❏ ❏ ❏ ➢ **A 23 y old marathon runner presents confused and combative. Temperature is 105° C. Why must renal function be monitored?**

Patient has heatstroke. Rhabdomyolysis may occur 2-3 d post-injury. Recall that in heatstroke volume depletion and dehydration may not always occur.

❏ ❏ ❏ ➢ **Treatment of heatstroke?**

Cool sponging, ice packs to groin and axilla, fanning, and iced gastric lavage. Antipyretics are not useful.

❏ ❏ ❏ ➢ **A 12 y old male presents with complaints of fatigue, fever, headache, itching rash, and joint aches. Exam reveals multiple sites of lymphadenopathy. The patient cannot recall any past medical problems. Just as you are about to leave the room, scratching your head, mom says "Oh doctor, he was stung by a bee 2 wk ago. Is that important?" Diagnosis?**

Serum-sickness-like delayed reaction.

❐ ❐ ❐ ➢ **How should a honeybee's stinger be removed?**

Scrape it out. Squeezing with a tweezers or finger may increase envenomation.

❐ ❐ ❐ ➢ **A 4 y old presents with an itching lesion on the legs and waist. On exam, you find hemorrhagic puncta surrounded by urticarial and erythematous patches following a zig-zag pattern. Treatment?**

Starch baths at bedtime are used to treat pruritus of flea bites.

❐ ❐ ❐ ➢ **A 16 y old presents with intense itching of the penis and the web spaces of his hands. Diagnosis?**

Scabies frequently attacks the web spaces of the hands and feet. Small vesicles and papules may be present.

❐ ❐ ❐ ➢ **A 6 y old in Texas presents with a history of being bitten by a caterpillar. The child has tense rhythmic pain. Edema and a red blotchy rash are apparent at the site as well as a white vesicle. Diagnosis and treatment?**

Megalopyge opercularis larva (puss caterpillar) sting. Remove remaining spines with sticky-tape and treat with 10 ml of 10% calcium gluconate IV.

❐ ❐ ❐ ➢ **A color blind 36 y old Texan presents with a history of snake bite. He says the snake was as big as a telephone pole, had fangs like a lion, and was striped like a zebra. On exam, you find ptosis, slurred speech, dysphagia, myalgia, and dilated pupils. What snake bit this man?**

Most likely a coral snake (Micrurus sp.).

❐ ❐ ❐ ➢ **Should blisters be debrided for a burn victim?**

YES. They contain vasospastic agents and should be drained.

❐ ❐ ❐ ➢ **An Osborn (J) wave seen on ECG is associated with what disorder?**

Hypothermia.

❐ ❐ ❐ ➢ **Hypothermia is defined as a core temperature below:**

35 °C.

❐ ❐ ❐ ➢ **Heat loss can occur via radiation, convection, conduction and evaporation. Which of these accounts for the greatest loss?**

Radiation, followed by convection when not perspiring.
If immersed, conduction causes the greatest heat loss.

❐ ❐ ❐ ➤ **A 4 y old bites into an extension cord and receives a burn on the lips. What specific concern do you have?**

Delayed rupture of the labial artery may occur 3-5 d post-injury.

❐ ❐ ❐ ➤ **Compare the entrance and exit wounds of AC and DC.**

AC -   Entrance and exit wounds same size.
DC -   Small entrance and large exit.
NB. -   Not all texts agree!

❐ ❐ ❐ ➤ **How is a sodium metal wound debrided?**

Cover with mineral oil and excise retained metal fragments.

❐ ❐ ❐ ➤ **Is lightning AC or DC?**

DC. May cause asystole and respiratory arrest.

❐ ❐ ❐ ➤ **What type of arrhythmia is expected with AC shock?**

V-fib.

❐ ❐ ❐ ➤ **Can lightning strike twice in the same place?**

Yes. Yes.

❐ ❐ ❐ ➤ **Why should the ears be examined in a lightning strike victim?**

TM rupture (50%). Associated with basilar skull fracture.

❐ ❐ ❐ ➤ **For how long should an asymptomatic lightning strike victim be monitored?**

Several hours as CHF may be delayed. Serial enzymes if EKG changes or chest pain.

❐ ❐ ❐ ➤ **What neurologic injury may be expected in a lightning injury?**

Lower and upper extremity paralysis due to vascular spasm.

❐ ❐ ❐ ➤ **What lab work-up should be considered in a lightning victim?**

CBC, BUN/Cr, UA (Check myoglobin), CPK -MM & MB, EKG, and CT if change in sensorium.

❐ ❐ ❐ ➤ **What eye finding is associated with lightning strike?**

Cataracts.

❐ ❐ ❐ ➤ **A patient presents with a history of headache, nausea, vomiting, and weak-**

ness. They also feel lightheaded. In addition to gastroenteritis, what other diagnosis should always be considered?

CO poisoning.

❏ ❏ ❏ ➤ **What is the most common cause of death with CO poisoning?**

Cardiac arrhythmias.

❏ ❏ ❏ ➤ **How is topical phenol exposure treated?**

Water and olive oil can be useful in the field. Isopropyl alcohol, glycerol, or polyethylene glycol mixture in the ED for carbolic acid exposure.

❏ ❏ ❏ ➤ **In what two plant ingestions is ipecac contraindicated?**

Jequirity bean (alkaline) and hemlocks sp. (may induce seizures).

HEM/ONC PEARLS

"Nature does nothing without a purpose."

Aristotle

❏ ❏ ❏ ➢ **Vitamin K dependent factors of the clotting cascade include:**

X, IX, VII and II.   REMEMBER 1972.

❏ ❏ ❏ ➢ **An adult patient receives a major head injury. He also suffers from classic hemophilia, what treatment should be given?**

Give cryoprecipitate 35 U/kg.

❏ ❏ ❏ ➢ **What is von Willebrand's disease?**

It is an autosomal dominant disorder of platelet function.
It causes bleeding from mucous membranes, menorrhagia and increased bleeding from wounds.
Patients with vW disease have less (or dysfunctional) vW factor.
vW factor is a plasma protein secreted by endothelial cells. vW factor serves two functions - it is required for platelets to adhere to collagen at the site of vascular injury (initial step in forming a hemostatic plug) and it forms complexes in plasma with factor VIII which are required to maintain normal factor VIII levels.

❏ ❏ ❏ ➢ **Describe the laboratory features of von Willebrand's disease (PT, PTT, Plt Ct, BT, and Factors).**

PT	- Normal.
PTT	- Prolonged (usually slightly reflecting low factor VIII level).
Plt Ct	- Normal.
BT	- Prolonged.
Factors	- Levels low of VIII-C (coagulation activity), vWF:Ag (immunologic activity) and vWF: activity (platelet aggregation).

❏ ❏ ❏ ➢ **What is the treatment for a bleeding patient with von Willebrand's disease (usual type 1 form)?**

vW factor may be replaced by giving cryoprecipitate.
Some texts now recommend using a strong vasopressin analog, D-amino-8, D-arginine vasopressin (DDAVP) that stimulates release of vW factor from endothelial stores.
This results in increased serum factor VIII levels. (DDAVP is not effective in severe vW disease and is not indicated for the rare type II form).

❏ ❏ ❏ ➢ **What lab abnormalities does DIC cause?**

Increased PT, elevated fibrin split products, decreased fibrinogen and thrombocytopenia.

❏ ❏ ❏ ➢ **What type of hemophilia results from a deficiency of factor 9, is sex linked and has a positive family history?**

Christmas disease or hemophilia B.

❏ ❏ ❏ ➢ **What type of hemophilia has a factor 8 deficiency, is sex linked and may present without a family history?**

Classic hemophilia.
Also called hemophilia A, about 1/2 have a family hx!

❏ ❏ ❏ ➢ **What type of hemophilia is autosomal dominant and has a deficiency in factor 8?**

von Willebrand's.

❏ ❏ ❏ ➢ **What are the two most common tumors causing ischemic dysfunction of the spinal cord?**

Lymphoma and multiple myeloma.

❏ ❏ ❏ ➢ **What is the most effective way to control the bleeding induced by warfarin therapy?**

Fresh frozen plasma provides fast response.
Also give vitamin K, intramuscularly. May want to check test dose first.

❏ ❏ ❏ ➢ **What laboratory abnormalities would be expected in a patient with platelet dysfunction?**

Abnormal bleeding time with normal PT, normal PTT and normal platelet count.
NSAIDs are a common cause of abnormal platelet function.

❏ ❏ ❏ ➢ **What are common features of thrombocytopenic purpura?**

Thrombocytopenia, micro-angiopathic hemolytic anemia, fever, renal failure and fluctuating neurologic symptoms. Coagulation studies are typically normal.

❏ ❏ ❏ ➢ **What clotting study is typically abnormal with thrombocytopenia?**

Bleeding time.
Usually thrombocytopenia is an acquired disorder secondary to infections, drugs or autoimmune disease. As platelets are not involved in the intrinsic or extrinsic clotting pathways, both PT and PTT remain normal.

❏ ❏ ❏ ➢ **Name four conditions that may cause reactive thrombocytosis.**

Iron deficiency, post-splenectomy, malignancy and infection.

❏ ❏ ❏ ➢ **Name a special feature of von Willebrand's disease which allows differentiation**

from classic hemophilia.

von Willebrand's disease has both a prolonged bleeding time and prolonged PTT, whereas classic hemophilia has only prolonged PTT.

❑ ❑ ❑ ➢ **What electrolyte abnormalities are seen in acute tumor lysis syndrome?**

Hyperuricemia secondary to breakdown of nucleic acids.
Hyperkalemia from massive cell lysis.
Hyperphosphatemia because of protein breakdown.
Hypocalcemia secondary to hyperphosphatemia.

❑ ❑ ❑ ➢ **What is the treatment for acute tumor lysis syndrome?**

Hydration, alkalinization, allopurinol, and hemodialysis.
The hypocalcemia associated with acute tumor lysis syndrome is secondary to increased phosphate, and should not be treated with calcium. Additional calcium could cause widespread precipitation of calcium phosphate.

❑ ❑ ❑ ➢ **A patient with lung cancer presents with complaints of nausea, vomiting, weakness, anorexia, and is also experiencing polydipsia and polyuria. What diagnosis is suspected?**

Hypercalcemia. The patient has GI, CNS, and renal symptoms which are commonly associated with hypercalcemia in a cancer patient.

❑ ❑ ❑ ➢ **A cancer patient presents with a history of constipation, decreased mental status, and back pain. What diagnosis is suspected?**

Hypercalcemia.

Remember - the signs and symptoms of hypercalcemia include nausea, vomiting, anorexia, constipation, polyuria, hypertension and decreased mentation.

❑ ❑ ❑ ➢ **What is appropriate treatment for a life threatening level of hypercalcemia of 16 mg per deciliter?**

Start giving the patient 0.9 NS at 5 to 10 liters per day. In addition, administer furosemide. A typical dose of Lasix would be 80 mg IV every 1 to 2 h. Watch out for hypokalemia.

The admitting internist may also administer agents to counteract parathyroid hormone which include calcitonin and mithramycin.

❑ ❑ ❑ ➢ **What factors are deficient in Classic hemophilia, Christmas disease, and von Willebrand's disease, respectively?**

Classic hemophilia -   Factor VIII.
Christmas disease -   Factor IX.
Willebrand's disease -   Factor VIIIc + von Willebrand's cofactor.

❑ ❑ ❑ ➢ **Which pathway involves factors VIII and IX?**

Intrinsic pathway.

❐ ❐ ❐ ➢ **What effect does deficiency of factors VIII and IX have on PT and on PTT?**

Deficiency leads to increase in PTT.

❐ ❐ ❐ ➢ **What pathway does the PT measure and what factor is unique to this pathway?**

Extrinsic, factor VII.

❐ ❐ ❐ ➢ **How may hemophilia A be clinically distinguished from hemophilia B?**

Hemophilia A is not clinically distinguishable from Christmas disease (Hemophilia B).

❐ ❐ ❐ ➢ **Which blood product is given when the coagulation abnormality is unknown?**

FFP.

❐ ❐ ❐ ➢ **What agent can be used for treating mild hemophilia A and von Willebrand's disease type 1?**

D-Amino-8, D-arginine vasopressin (DDAVP) induces a rapid rise in factor VIII levels.

❐ ❐ ❐ ➢ **Major cause of death in hemophiliacs?**

Blood component infections.

❐ ❐ ❐ ➢ **What diagnostic tests are available to distinguish SSA from sickle cell trait in the ED?**

None.
Sickledex, Sik-L-Stat, SickleScrene, and SCAT are unable to distinguish between trait and disease.

OB/GYN PEARLS

"A great part, I believe, of the Art is to be able to observe."

Hippocrates (460 - 370 B.C.)

❏ ❏ ❏ ➢ **How much blood does a standard size pad absorb?**

20 - 30 ml blood.

❏ ❏ ❏ ➢ **How soon after implantation can ß-HCG be detected?**

2-3 d.

❏ ❏ ❏ ➢ **What percentage of pregnancies are ectopic?**

1.5%. Ectopic pregnancies are the leading cause of death in the first trimester.

❏ ❏ ❏ ➢ **What is the most common presentation of ectopic pregnancy?**

Amenorrhea followed by pain.

❏ ❏ ❏ ➢ **How does a spontaneous abortion most commonly present?**

Pain followed by bleeding.

❏ ❏ ❏ ➢ **What is the <u>most</u> <u>common</u> finding on pelvic exam in a patient with an ectopic pregnancy?**

Unilateral adnexal tenderness.

❏ ❏ ❏ ➢ **Does a negative culdocentesis rule out an ectopic pregnancy?**

No. It only rules out hemoperitoneum.

❏ ❏ ❏ ➢ **When can abdominal ultrasound find an intrauterine gestational sac?**

5th week. Fetal pole, 6th week. Embryonic mass with cardiac motion, 7th week.

❏ ❏ ❏ ➢ **A 3 mo pregnant patient presents with pelvic pain. On exam, a retroverted and retroflexed uterus is found. What diagnosis should come to mind?**

Incarceration of the uterus. Patients typically complain of rectal and pelvic pressure . Urinary retention may also be found. The knee-chest position or rectal pressure may correct the problem.

❐ ❐ ❐ ➢ **What patients with PID should be admitted?**

Pregnant; temperature > 38 °C (100.4 °F); nausea and vomiting which prohibits po antibiotics; pyosalpinx or tubo-ovarian abscess; peritoneal signs; IUCD present; no response to oral antibiotics; and uncertain diagnosis.

❐ ❐ ❐ ➢ **What criteria are necessary for the diagnosis of PID?**

All three of the following: adnexal tenderness, cervical and uterine tenderness, and abdominal tenderness. Also one of the following: T >38 °C, endocervix gram stain positive for gram negative intracellular diplococci, leukocytosis greater than 10,000/mm^3, inflammatory mass on US or pelvic, and WBC and bacteria in the peritoneal fluid.

❐ ❐ ❐ ➢ **What is the most common cause of toxic shock syndrome?**

The most common cause is S. aureus. Other causes which are clinically similar include group A Streptococci, Pseudomonas aeruginosa, and Streptococcus pneumoniae.

❐ ❐ ❐ ➢ **What criteria are necessary for the diagnosis of toxic shock syndrome?**

All of the following must be present: T > 38.9 °C (102 °F), rash, systolic BP < 90 and orthostasis, involvement of three organ systems (GI, renal, musculoskeletal, mucosal, hepatic, hematologic, or CNS), and negative serologic tests for such diseases as RMSF, hepatitis B, measles, leptospirosis, VDRL, etc.

❐ ❐ ❐ ➢ **What type of rash is seen with TSS?**

Blanching erythroderma which resolves in 3 d and is followed by a desquamation (full thickness). This typically occurs between the 6th and 14th d with peeling prominent on the hands and feet.

❐ ❐ ❐ ➢ **How should a patient with toxic shock syndrome be treated?**

FLUIDS, pressure support, FFP or transfusions, vaginal irrigation with iodine or saline, and antistaphylococcal penicillin or cephalosporin with anti-ß-lactamase activity (nafcillin or oxacillin). Rifampin should be considered to eliminate the carrier state.

❐ ❐ ❐ ➢ **What anticoagulant should be used in pregnant patients?**

Heparin does not cross the placenta.

❐ ❐ ❐ ➢ **What antiemetic should be used in pregnant patients?**

Prochlorperazine (Compazine) or trimethobenzamide (Tigan).

❐ ❐ ❐ ➢ **What dose of radiation to a fetus increases the risk of inhibiting fetal growth?**

10 rad. A typical abdominal or pelvic film delivers 100 to 350 mrad. A shielded chest x-ray should deliver < 10 mrad to the fetus. Necessary x-rays should not be withheld.

❏ ❏ ❏ ➢ **Define preeclampsia.**

HTN after 20 wk EGA with generalized edema or proteinuria.

❏ ❏ ❏ ➢ **Define eclampsia.**

Preeclampsia plus grand mal seizures or coma.

❏ ❏ ❏ ➢ **Should BP be lowered acutely in a preeclampsia patient?**

Dangerous HTN (>170/110) should be gradually lowered with hydralazine 10 mg IV followed by a drip. Definitive treatment for preeclampsia and eclampsia is delivery.

❏ ❏ ❏ ➢ **What level of serum glucose warrants admission in a patient with gestational diabetes?**

Hyperglycemia (>200 mg %) which is persistent requires admission.

❏ ❏ ❏ ➢ **Can iodinated radiodiagnostic agents be used in a pregnant patient?**

They should be avoided as concentration in the fetal thyroid can cause permanent loss of thyroid function. Nuclear medicine scans, pulmonary angiography with pelvic shielding, and impedance plethysmography are preferred.

❏ ❏ ❏ ➢ **What viral or protozoal infections require extensive work-up during pregnancy?**

Herpes genitalis, rubella, cytomegalovirus, and Toxoplasma gondii. These patients require full work-ups and referral for genetic counseling.

❏ ❏ ❏ ➢ **What is the most common cause of vaginitis?**

Candida albicans.

❏ ❏ ❏ ➢ **A 26 y old female complains of dysuria and mild lower abdominal pain. On pelvic exam, punctate hemorrhages are noted on the cervix. Diagnosis?**

Trichomonas vaginitis. The cervix is called "strawberry cervix." The diagnosis can be confirmed by obtaining vaginal vault secretions using the "hanging drip" slide test. The sexual partner must be treated.

❏ ❏ ❏ ➢ **A wet prep of vaginal secretions reveals clue cells. Diagnosis?**

Gardnerella vaginitis. Male partners should be treated.
Sherlock Holmes looks for "clues" in the "Garden."

❏ ❏ ❏ ➢ **A pregnant patient presents in a coma. The husband indicates the patient has had been itching for a few days, seemed slightly yellow, and earlier in the day her daughter said "Mom was confused". Diagnosis?**

Acute fatty liver of pregnancy. Conjugated bilirubin and transaminase levels will be increased.

❑ ❑ ❑ ➢ **Is appendicitis more common during pregnancy?**

No (1/850). Outcome is worse. As pregnancy progresses, the appendix moves, at term it is near the right subcostal margin. The distal end is pointed toward the diaphragm. The WBC count usually does not increase beyond the normal value of 12-15,000. In a pregnant patient, pyuria with no bacturia suggest appendicitis. Pregnant patients may lack GI distress, fever may be absent or low grade.

❑ ❑ ❑ ➢ **3 d post-partem a patient presents with fever. On exam, a foul lochia and tender boggy uterus is present. Diagnosis?**

Endometritis typically occurs 1-3 d post-partem.

❑ ❑ ❑ ➢ **Why is Rh status important in a pregnant patient?**

Rh negative with Rh positive fetus can result in fetal anemia, hydrops, and fetal loss. Rh immunoglobulin should be given to all Rh negative patients. The usual amount of RhoGAM may be inadequate in the setting of trauma; a Kleihauer-Betke assay can quantitate fetomaternal hemorrhage.

❑ ❑ ❑ ➢ **What is the expected finding on culdocentesis in a patient with ectopic pregnancy?**

Non-clotting blood.

❑ ❑ ❑ ➢ **When can transvaginal and abdominal ultrasound identify an intrauterine sac?**

Transvaginal, 5 wk. Abdominal, 6 wk.

❑ ❑ ❑ ➢ **A 24 y old, 10 w pregnant patient presents with bleeding per vagina. She also complains of nausea, vomiting, and abdominal pain. Physical findings reveal a blood pressure of 150/100 and a uterus which is larger than dates. Lab studies reveal proteinuria. Diagnosis?**

Molar pregnancy. Uterus may be larger or smaller than expected dates.

❑ ❑ ❑ ➢ **An 8 mo pregnant patient presents to the ED with profuse bleeding. What must be ruled out with ultrasound before a pelvic exam is performed?**

Placenta previa.

❑ ❑ ❑ ➢ **Risk factors for placenta previa?**

Previous cesarean section, previous placenta previa, multiparity, multiple induced abortions, and multiple gestations.

❑ ❑ ❑ ➢ **Risk factors for abruptio placenta?**

Smoking, hypertension, multiparity, trauma, and previous abruptio placenta.

❐ ❐ ❐ ➢ **What effect does pregnancy have on: Cardiac output, BP, HR, coagulation, sed rate, leukocytes, blood volume, arterial blood gases, tidal volume, bladder, BUN/CR, and GI.**

Cardiac Output	Increases. Moving the uterus off the IVC increases CO 25%.
BP	Falls in second trimester. Returns to normal state in third trimester.
Heart Rate	Increases.
Coagulation	Factors 7, 8, 9, 10, and fibrinogen increase, the others remain unchanged.
Sed Rate	Elevated.
Leukocytes	Increase to as much as 18,000.
Blood volume	Increases, RBC unchanged, dilutional "anemia" is physiologic.
Tidal volume	Increases 40%.
Bladder	Displaced superiorly and anteriorly.
BUN/Cr	Decrease because of increased GFR and renal blood flow.
GI	Gastric emptying and GI motility decrease. Peritoneal signs such as rigidity and rebound are diminished or absent. Alkaline phosphatase is increased.

❐ ❐ ❐ ➢ **What are the presenting signs and symptoms of abruptio placentae?**

Placental separation before delivery is associated with vaginal bleeding (78%), abdominal pain (66%), as well as tetanic uterine contractions, uterine irritability, and fetal death.

❐ ❐ ❐ ➢ **How much fetomaternal hemorrhage does the standard dose of Rho (D) immune globulin (300 μg) protect against?**

Approximately 30 ml. A quantitative Kleihauer-Betke assay should be ordered to calculate the dose of Rho(D) immune globulin to administer. Fetomaternal hemorrhage is common following trauma and should always be considered.

❐ ❐ ❐ ➢ **What dose of oxytocin (Pitocin) should be administered following a postpartum hemorrhage?**

20 to 40 units of oxytocin added to 1000 ml normal saline or Ringer's lactate infused at 200 - 500 ml/h.

❐ ❐ ❐ ➢ **How can ruptured membranes be diagnosed?**

Nitrazine paper turns blue and a "ferning" pattern is seen under a microscope in the presence of amniotic fluid.

❐ ❐ ❐ ➢ **What are the indications for cardiotocographic monitoring in a trauma patient?**

All women past 20 w gestation with indirect or direct abdominal trauma require 4 h of monitoring. Loss of beat-to-beat variability, uterine contractions, or fetal brady- or tachycardia demands immediate obstetrical consultation.

❐ ❐ ❐ ➢ **Is life threatening hemorrhage due to trauma during pregnancy most often intra- or retroperitoneal?**

Retroperitoneal.

❏ ❏ ❏ ➢ **What type of incision should be used in a post-mortem cesarean section?**

Vertical (Classical) incision.

❏ ❏ ❏ ➢ **What is the normal fetal heart rate?**

120 to 160 beats per minute. If bradycardia is detected, position the mother on her left side, give oxygen and an IV fluid bolus.

❏ ❏ ❏ ➢ **A pregnant patient presents with fetal bradycardia and tetanic contractions. Delivery is not imminent. Treatment?**

Tocolytic agents to relax the uterus: magnesium sulfate 4 to 6 g IV over 20 min or terbutaline 0.25 mg subcutaneously.

❏ ❏ ❏ ➢ **What technique can be used to identify intravaginal semen?**

Semen will fluoresce with a Wood's Lamp.

❏ ❏ ❏ ➢ **How long after intercourse can acid phosphatase be detected?**

2-9 h.

❏ ❏ ❏ ➢ **How quickly must a patient be treated to provide pregnancy prevention after a being raped?**

72 h. Treatment is Ovral, 2 tablets po and 2 tablets 12 hours later.

DERM PEARLS

❏ ❏ ❏ ➤ **What type of reaction is erythema multiforme?**

Hypersensitivity.
Bullae are subepidermal, the dermis is edematous, and a lymphatic infiltrate may be present around the capillaries and venules. In children, infections are the most important cause and in adults, drugs and malignancies. EM is often seen during epidemics of adenovirus, atypical pneumonia, and histoplasmosis.

❏ ❏ ❏ ➤ **A patient presents with fever, myalgias, malaise, and arthralgias. On exam, findings include bullous lesions of the lips, eyes, and nose. The patient indicates eating is very painful. What should the family be told about the patient's prognosis?**

Stevens-Johnson syndrome has a mortality of 5 - 10% and may have significant complications including corneal ulceration, panophthalmitis, corneal opacities, anterior uveitis, blindness, hematuria, renal tubular necrosis, and progressive renal failure. Scarring of the foreskin and stenosis of the vagina can occur. Treatment in a burn unit is supportive; steroids may provide symptomatic relief but are not of proven value, and may be contraindicated.

❏ ❏ ❏ ➤ **What are the two distinct causes of toxic epidermal necrolysis (scalded skin syndrome)?**

Staphylococcal and drugs or chemicals. Both begin with appearance of patches of tender erythema followed by loosening of the skin and denuding to glistening bases. Staphylococcal scalded skin syndrome is commonly found in children less than 5y and is due to toxin that cleaves <u>within the epidermis</u> under the stratum granulosum.

❏ ❏ ❏ ➤ **What area does Staphylococcal scalded skin syndrome usually affect?**

The face around nose and mouth, neck, axillae, and groin. Disease commonly occurs after upper respiratory tract infections or purulent conjunctivitis. Nikolsky's sign is present when lateral pressure on the skin results in epidermal separation from the dermis.

❏ ❏ ❏ ➤ **How can SSSS be distinguished from scalded skin syndrome caused by drugs or chemicals?**

Pull out your microscopes and call in the pathologists trivia fans, in drug or chemical etiologies the skin separates at the dermoepidermal junction. This drug induced TEN carries up to 50% mortality as a result of fluid loss and secondary infection.
On microscopic exam of SSSS intraepidermal cleavage occurs with a few acantholytic keratinocytes will be seen.
In non-staphylococcal type, cellular debris, inflammatory cells, and basal cell keratinocytes are present.

❏ ❏ ❏ ➤ **Treatment of SSSS?**

Oral or IV penicillinase-resistant penicillin, baths of potassium permanganate or dressings soaked in 0.5% silver nitrate, and fluids. Corticosteroids and silver sulfadine are contraindicated.

❏ ❏ ❏ ➤ **Trivia buffs only - What percentage of the average turd by wet weight is bacteria?**

20 to 30 % is anaerobic bacteria, first discovered by Professor Monsignor Mal O. Dorus Turdophillis, late one night after a particularly heavy meal.

❏ ❏ ❏ ➤ **What is the most common gram-negative anaerobe found in human feces?**

Bacteroides fragilis. It is also the <u>most common</u> organism found in abscesses involving the perineal region. Its other claim to fame is being the only anaerobe resistant to penicillin.

❏ ❏ ❏ ➤ **Where are cutaneous abscesses caused by Escherichia coli and Neisseria gonorrhoeae commonly found?**

"Sorry about that chief," but they are <u>not</u> typically seen in cutaneous abscesses.

Staphylococcus aureus is the <u>most common</u> aerobe in cutaneous abscesses, two-thirds are found in the upper torso, 97% are resistant to penicillin G. It is most commonly isolated in axilla abscesses.

❏ ❏ ❏ ➤ **What is the most common gram-negative aerobe found in the upper torso?**

Proteus mirabilis, most commonly isolated in the axilla.

❏ ❏ ❏ ➤ **What is the most common aerobe seen in stool and intra-abdominal abscesses?**

Escherichia coli. The pus of E. coli is odorless. The "sweat succulent" smell of abscesses in the perirectal area is due to anaerobic bacteria.

❏ ❏ ❏ ➤ **How may the Toxicodendron species be recognized?**

Poison oak and ivy have leaves with 3 leaflets per leaf. They also have U- or V-shaped leaf scars. The milky sap becomes black when exposed to air.

❏ ❏ ❏ ➤ **How quickly will people react to the Toxicodendron antigen?**

Contact dermatitis typically develops within 2 d of exposure; cases have been reported in as quickly as 8 h to as long as 10d. Lesions appear in a linear arrangement of papulovesicles or erythema. Fluid from vesicles does not contain antigen and does not transmit the dermatitis.

❏ ❏ ❏ ➤ **How should steroids be prescribed in a patient with poison ivy?**

Prednisone 40 - 60 mg q d tapered over 2 to 3 wk. Short courses may result in rebound.

❏ ❏ ❏ ➤ **What are the causes of exfoliative dermatitis?**

Chemicals, drugs, and cutaneous or systemic diseases. Usually scaly erythematous dermatitis involves most or all of the surface skin. It can be recognized by erythroderma with epidermal flaking or scaling. Acute signs and symptoms may include low-grade fever, pruritus, chills, and skin tightness. The chronic condition may produce dystrophic nails, thinning of body hair, and patchy hyperpigmentation or hypopigmentation. Cutaneous vasodilation may result in increased cardiac output and high-output cardiac failure. Splenomegaly suggests leukemia or lymphoma.

❏ ❏ ❏ ➢ **What is a furuncle?**

Deeeeep-inflammatory nodule which grew out of superficial folliculitis.

❏ ❏ ❏ ➢ **What is a carbuncle?**

Deep abscess that interconnects and extends into the subcutaneous tissue. Commonly seen in patients with diabetes, folliculitis, steroid use, obesity, heavy perspiration, and areas of friction.

❏ ❏ ❏ ➢ **What is a Bartholin's cyst?**

Obstructed Bartholin's duct resulting in an abscess.

❏ ❏ ❏ ➢ **What is a pilonidal abscess?**

Abscess which occurs in the gluteal fold as a result of disruption of the epithelial surface. They do not originate from rectal crypts and bacteria are from the cutaneous surface.

❏ ❏ ❏ ➢ **Where does a perirectal abscess originate?**

Anal crypts and burrows through the ischiorectal space. They may be perianal, perirectal, supralevator, or ischiorectal.
Perianal abscesses which involve the supralevator muscle, ischiorectal space, or rectum require operative drainage.

❏ ❏ ❏ ➢ **What is hidradenitis suppurativa?**

Chronic suppurative abscesses found in the apocrine sweat glands of the groin and/or axilla. Proteus mirabilis overgrowth is common.

❏ ❏ ❏ ➢ **What is the cause of tetanus?**

Tetanospasmin, which is an exotoxin produced by a gram-positive anaerobic rod, Clostridium tetani.

❏ ❏ ❏ ➢ **What is the mechanism of action of tetanospasmin?**

Enters peripheral nerve endings and ascends the axons to reach the brain and spinal cord. At this point it binds four areas of the nervous system:

1. Anterior horn cells of the spinal cord - impairs inhibitory interneurons resulting in

neuromuscular irritability and generalized spasms.
2. Sympathetic nervous system - resulting in sweating, labile blood pressure, tachycardia, and peripheral vasoconstriction.
3. Myoneural junction - inhibits release of acetylcholine.
4. Binds to cerebral gangliosides - thought to cause seizures.

❒ ❒ ❒ ➢ **What is the treatment of a tetanus prone wound?**

Surgical debridement, 3,000 to 10,000 units of human tetanus immune globulin [TIG (h), (Hyper-tet)] IM (Do Not Inject Into Wound), penicillin G or metronidazole.

❒ ❒ ❒ ➢ **What is the danger of giving tetanus toxoid boosters in a pleonastic fashion (e.g., with only a 9 mo interval)?**

Arthus-type hypersensitivity reaction, with onset about 4 - 6 h after injection. History of a severe hypersensitivity reaction or of a severe neurologic reaction are the only contraindications to tetanus toxoid.

❒ ❒ ❒ ➢ **What is the most common cause of gas gangrene?**

C. perfringens. The first symptom is a sensation of weight or heaviness in the muscle followed by severe pain. The DOC is penicillin G, an alternative is chloramphenicol.

❒ ❒ ❒ ➢ **A patient presents with a raised, red, small, and painful plaque on the face. On exam, a distinct, sharp advancing edge is noted. What is the cause?**

Erysipelas is caused by group A streptococci. When the face is involved, the patient should be admitted.

EMERGENCY MEDICINE
PEARLS OF WISDOM

Errors, like straws, upon the surface flow;
He who would search for pearls must dive below.

John Dryden 1631-1700, Prologues and Epilogues:
Prologue, All for Love.

❏ ❏ ❏ ➤ **Cricothyroidotomy is not recommended in children of less than what age?**

10 years.

❏ ❏ ❏ ➤ **Name, in order, the 5 Kübler-Ross stages.**

1.) Denial.
2.) Anger.
3.) Bargaining.
4.) Depression.
5.) Acceptance.

❏ ❏ ❏ ➤ **Use of an EOA is contraindicated in patients of less than _____ years of age.**

16.

❏ ❏ ❏ ➤ **Is succinylcholine a depolarizing or a non-depolarizing neuromuscular blocking agent?**

It is the only commonly used depolarizing agent.
It binds to post-synaptic acetylcholine receptors causing depolarization.
It is enzymatically degraded by pseudocholinesterase.
Onset within 1 minute with duration of paralysis of 7-10 min.

❏ ❏ ❏ ➤ **What is the rationale for pre-treating a patient with a subpolarizing ("defasciculating") dose of a non-depolarizing agent prior to administration of succinylcholine?**

Attenuates fasciculations from succinylcholine induced depolarization - this may decrease subsequent muscle pain.
Blunts increased intragastric and intraocular pressure associated with succinylcholine.

❏ ❏ ❏ ➤ **What is the appropriate dose of midazolam (Versed) to cause loss of consciousness and amnesia during a rapid sequence induction?**

0.1 mg/kg.
5 mg seems to work for most people.

❏ ❏ ❏ ➢ **What is the appropriate dose of thiopental to induce anesthesia during a rapid sequence induction?**

4 mg/kg.

❏ ❏ ❏ ➢ **Onset of loss of consciousness with thiopental usually occurs within 15 s. What is the usual duration of action?**

2-30 min, depending on source.

❏ ❏ ❏ ➢ **What is the appropriate dose of vecuronium for "defasciculating" or "priming" dose?**

0.01 mg/kg.

❏ ❏ ❏ ➢ **What is the appropriate dose of vecuronium for paralysis (no "priming")?**

0.20 mg/kg.

❏ ❏ ❏ ➢ **What is the appropriate dose of pancuronium (Pavulon) for "defasciculating" or "priming" dose?**

0.015 mg/kg.
≈ 1 mg common adult dose.

❏ ❏ ❏ ➢ **Dermacentor andersoni (wood tick) is a pesky arthropod associated with <u>four</u> tick-borne illnesses! Name each and its cause.**

Rocky Mtn. Spotted Fever caused by Rickettsia rickettsii for which Dermacentor andersoni is a vector.

Tick paralysis caused by neurotoxin. Its ascending paralysis with decrease or loss of DTRs can be similar to symptoms of Guillain-Barré syndrome.

Q Fever caused by Coxiella burnetii (a rickettsiae).

Colorado Tick Fever from orbivirus.

❏ ❏ ❏ ➢ **What is the <u>most</u> <u>common</u> opportunistic infection of AIDS?**

PCP. It is the initial opportunistic infection in 60% of AIDS patients and eventually affects 80%.

❏ ❏ ❏ ➢ **What is appropriate initial treatment of PCP?**

TMP/SMX or pentamidine.

❑ ❑ ❑ ➢ **Describe "AIDS dementia" complex (aka HIV-I encephalopathy).**

A progressive disease caused directly by HIV-I present in 1/3 of AIDS patients characterized by impairment of recent memory, concentration deficit, increasing DTRs, seizures and frontal release signs.

❑ ❑ ❑ ➢ **What is the <u>most</u> <u>common</u> cause of *focal* encephalitis in AIDS patients?**

Toxoplasma gondii.

❑ ❑ ❑ ➢ **Ethylene glycol is <u>the</u> alcohol that may present with hypocalcemia (1/3 of cases). Where does the calcium go?**

Oxalic acid is one of the metabolites of ethylene glycol.
Calcium precipitates with oxalate and forms calcium oxalate crystals.
The + birefringent calcium oxalate dihydrate crystals are pathognomonic of this ingestion.

❑ ❑ ❑ ➢ **What is the LD_{50} for falling in adults?**

48 feet.

❑ ❑ ❑ ➢ **A laryngeal fracture is suggested by finding the hyoid bone elevated above what cervical level on x-ray?**

C3.

❑ ❑ ❑ ➢ **Describe the action and side effects of diazoxide.**

Diazoxide is a direct arterial vasodilator. The onset of action is within one to two min and lasts up to 12 h. Side effects may include nausea, vomiting, fluid retention and hyperglycemia. Diazoxide is contraindicated in patients with aortic dissection or angina.

❑ ❑ ❑ ➢ **What species of plasmodium are resistant to chloroquine?**

Falciparum.

❑ ❑ ❑ ➢ **In children greater than one year of age, where are foreign bodies in the airway usually located?**

In the lower airway.

❑ ❑ ❑ ➢ **In a child with malrotation, what is the most likely age of presentation, what is a common complication, and what signs and symptoms are usually present?**

Malrotation usually occurs in children under 12 months of age.
Volvulus is a common complication.
Signs and symptoms usually include vomiting, blood streaked stools, and abdominal pain.

❑ ❑ ❑ ➢ **Name 2 causes of Toxic Epidermal Necrolysis (aka scalded skin syndrome).**

1.) Drug or Chemical. Usually in adults. Cleavage at dermo-epidermal junction.

2.) Staphylococcal. Usually in children < 5 y. SSSS results in intraepidermal cleavage beneath stratum granulosum.

❏ ❏ ❏ ➢ **Describe the presentation of SSSS.**

Disease begins after URI or purulent conjunctivitis. First lesions are tender, erythematous and scarlatiniform, usually found on face, neck, axillae and groin. Skin peels off in sheets with lateral pressure, a + Nikolsky's sign.

❏ ❏ ❏ ➢ **What is appropriate treatment for Toxic Epidermal Necrolysis?**

Regardless of cause, treat skin loss similarly to partial thickness burns. Do not use silver sulfadiazine. Adults can have large fluid loss. Admit patients with >10% BSA to burn unit.
For SSSS treat with IV penicillinase-resistant penicillin.

❏ ❏ ❏ ➢ **In bullous impetigo, which of the following drugs may not be effective: erythromycin, amoxicillin, cefaclor, or doxycycline?**

Amoxicillin.

❏ ❏ ❏ ➢ **Methanol intoxication causes early death by what cause?**

Respiratory arrest. Unknown pathophysiology.

❏ ❏ ❏ ➢ **Reiter's syndrome diagnostic triad:**

Conjunctivitis, polyarthritis, and non-gonococcal urethritis.

❏ ❏ ❏ ➢ **Nerve most commonly injured in glenohumeral dislocation?**

Axillary nerve, numb area over lateral deltoid.

❏ ❏ ❏ ➢ **Permanent pacemakers have a coding system of 5 letters. The first letter signifies the Chamber Paced. What does the second letter signify?**

Chamber Sensed.

❐ ❐ ❐ ➤ **Describe and contrast regional enteritis and ulcerative colitis.**

Category	Regional Enteritis	Ulcerative Colitis
Name	Crohn's disease Regional enteritis Terminal ileitis Granulomatous ileocolitis	Ulcerative colitis
Area	**Stem-to-stern** = social to anti-social (mouth to anus) **Segmental** (skip areas) <u>Most common</u> area is ileum	95% rectosigmoid **Contiguous** (no skip areas)
Demographics	15 - 22 y 55 - 60 y Common in Europeans Jews White > Black 10-15 % have family hx	10 - 20 y 20 - 30 y 15 x greater risk with 1st° relative
Bowel	**ALL LAYERS** Thick Bowel Wall Narrow lumen Creeping fat - mesenteric fat over bowel wall "Cobblestone" mucosal appearance **Fissures** **Fistulas** **Abscesses**	**Mucosa and Submucosa** Mucosal ulceration Epithelial necrosis Mild - Mucosa is fine, granular and friable **Severe - Spongy, red, oozing ulcerations** **Crypt abscesses** **Toxic Megacolon**

❐ ❐ ❐ ➤ **Describe the mechanism and cause of a boutonniere deformity.**

Boutonniere deformity is secondary to rupture of the extensor apparatus of the PIP joint. The result of the injury is a PIP joint which is flexed and a DIP joint which is hyperextended. It is treated by splinting the PIP joint in full extension.

❐ ❐ ❐ ➤ **A cyanotic patient has a low oxygen saturation measured on ABG. What flavor of cyanosis does this patient have?**

Central.

❐ ❐ ❐ ➤ **What is a peripheral cyanosis?**

ABG reveals an oxygen saturation within normal; shunting or increased O_2 extraction is taking place.

❐ ❐ ❐ ➤ **Name the two primary causes (groups) of peripheral cyanosis.**

Cyanosis with a normal SaO_2 can be due to:
    Decreased cardiac output.
    Redistribution - may be $2°$ to shock, DIC, hypothermia, vascular obstruction.

❏ ❏ ❏ ➢ **Name the causes of central cyanosis.**

The causes of cyanosis with a decreased SaO_2 are:

Decreased PaO_2, or decreased O_2 diffusion.
Hypoventilation.
V-Q mismatch, pulmonary shunting.
Dysfunctional hemoglobin (includes sickle cell crisis, drug induced hemoglobinopathies).
NOTE: Hb-CO does not cause cyanosis (though the cherry red appearance of skin and mucous membranes could suggest a cyanosis).

❏ ❏ ❏ ➢ **A pulmonary embolism causes which flavor of cyanosis?**

Central cyanosis, although secondary shock and right-heart failure can lead to peripheral cyanosis.

❏ ❏ ❏ ➢ **What is a positive Chvostek's sign?**

Twitch in the corner of the mouth occurring when the examiner taps over the facial nerve in front of the ear.
It is present in approximately 10 to 30 percent of normal individuals. Eyelid muscle contraction with Chvostek's maneuver is generally considered to be diagnostic of hypocalcemia.

❏ ❏ ❏ ➢ **What is Trousseau's sign and when is it seen?**

Trousseau's sign is a carpal spasm induced when a blood pressure cuff on the upper arm maintains a pressure above systolic for approximately three minutes. Fingers become spastically extended at the interphalangeal joints and flexed at the metacarpophalangeal joints.
Trousseau's sign is generally a more reliable indicator of hypocalcemia than is Chvostek's sign.
Positive Trousseau's sign may also be found in hypomagnesemia, severe alkalosis, and strychnine poisoning.

❏ ❏ ❏ ➢ **Activated charcoal is not effective treatment for what substances?**

Alcohols, ions, and acids and bases.

❏ ❏ ❏ ➢ **Permanent pacemakers have a coding system of 5 letters. In this system the letter A refers to the Atrium and V to the Ventricle. What does the letter D refer to?**

D = Double, meaning both Atrium and Ventricle.

❏ ❏ ❏ ➢ **Describe a patient with Sjogren's syndrome.**

Sjogren's syndrome is usually seen in women more than 50 years of age. Symptoms often include diminished lacrimal and salivary gland secretions, salivary gland enlargement and arthritis. Sjogren's syndrome predisposes a patient to corneal irritation, ulceration and superimposed infection. It may complicate many rheumatic diseases or may occur independently. The likely cause of Sjogren's syndrome is lymphatic infiltration of the lacrimal and salivary glands, resulting in dry eyes and dry mouth.

❏ ❏ ❏ ➢ **Describe the DeBakey classification of regions of aortic dissection.**

(I) Ascending and descending aorta.
(II) Ascending aorta.
(III) Descending aorta distal to the left subclavian artery.

❏ ❏ ❏ ➢ **What is the <u>most</u> <u>common</u> conduction disturbance in acute myocardial infarction?**

First degree AV block.

❏ ❏ ❏ ➢ **What is the <u>most</u> <u>common</u> foot fracture?**

Calcaneus (60%). The talus is a distant second most common.

❏ ❏ ❏ ➢ **Where does the <u>most</u> <u>common</u> metatarsal fracture occur?**

At the base of the fifth metatarsal, a Jones fracture.

❏ ❏ ❏ ➢ **Which tendons are involved in de Quervain's tenosynovitis?**

The abductor pollicis and the extensor pollicis brevis tendons.
Diagnosis is confirmed with positive Finkelstein's test.

❏ ❏ ❏ ➢ **Describe Dupuytren's (Guillaume, 1777-1835) contracture.**

Contraction of the longitudinal bands of the palmar aponeurosis.

❏ ❏ ❏ ➢ **What is the <u>most</u> <u>common</u> form of anorectal abscess?**

Perianal abscess. Anorectal abscesses are usually mixed infections, both gram negative and anaerobic organisms. Fistula formation is a frequent complication.

❏ ❏ ❏ ➢ **What is the <u>most</u> <u>common</u> rhythm disturbance in a pediatric arrest?**

Bradycardia.

❏ ❏ ❏ ➢ **How long does it take to prepare type-specific saline cross-matched blood?**

Ten minutes.

❏ ❏ ❏ ➢ **Describe the common features of a slipped femoral capital epiphysis.**

Injury usually occurs in adolescence. The rupture typically presents with an insidious development of knee or thigh pain, and a painful limp. Frequently hip motion is limited, particularly that of internal rotation. Evaluation is aided by anteroposterior and frogleg lateral films of both hips.

❏ ❏ ❏ ➢ **A core temperature of less than 32 °C (90 °F) is commonly associated with:**

Poor prognosis, complications including arrhythmias resistant to treatment, and loss of the shivering reflex.

❏ ❏ ❏ ➢ **What is the treatment for torsade de pointes?**

Treatment includes techniques to accelerate the heart rate, shortening the duration of ventricular repolarization. This may be accomplished with isoproterenol, temporary pacing, or with magnesium sulfate.

Drugs which increase or prolong repolarization, and therefore exacerbate torsade de pointes, include: Class IA antiarrhythmics (quinidine, procainamide, disopyramide), tricyclic antidepressants and phenothiazines.

❏ ❏ ❏ ➢ **Dobutamine in moderate doses causes what cardiovascular effects?**

Decreased peripheral resistance and pulmonary occlusive pressure, and inotropic stimulation of the heart.

❏ ❏ ❏ ➢ **Permanent pacemakers have a coding system of 5 letters. The first letter refers to chamber Paced, the second to chamber Sensed. What does the third letter refer to?**

Mode or Response. It comes in several flavors including I = Inhibited, T = Triggered, D = Double, R = Reverse and O = nOne.

❏ ❏ ❏ ➢ **What are the common concerns with anterior dislocation of the shoulder?**

Axillary nerve injury, Hillsack's deformity and possible fractures of the proximal humerus and greater tuberosity.

❏ ❏ ❏ ➢ **Describe a Monteggia fracture/dislocation.**

A fracture of the proximal ulna with dislocation of the radial head.

Treatment usually requires open reduction and internal fixation. When a Monteggia fracture is suspected, x-rays should include the forearm, elbow and wrist.

<u>M</u>ichigan <u>U</u>niversity <u>P</u>olice <u>D</u>epartment = <u>MUPD</u>

<u>MUPD</u> = <u>M</u>onteggia, <u>U</u>lnar fracture, <u>P</u>roximal <u>D</u>islocation.

❏ ❏ ❏ ➢ **Describe a Galeazzi's fracture/dislocation.**

A radial shaft fracture with dislocation of the distal radioulnar joint.

<u>G</u>reat <u>R</u>ays <u>D</u>own <u>D</u>eep! = GRDD

<u>GRDD</u> = <u>G</u>aleazzi, <u>R</u>adius fracture, <u>D</u>istal <u>D</u>islocation

This is a little-known but true story. Galeazzi's fracture/dislocation is named for the famous orthopod who suffered this injury in a fatal diving accident. Dr. Galeazzi, it seemed, was following a large ray off the coast of Cozumel when he <u>smashed</u> his arm into an unseen coral outcropping. The pain caused him to hyperventilate and head up. His last words as he made the surface (before his dysbaric air embolism) were "Great Rays Down Deep!"

❏ ❏ ❏ ➢ **Describe the clinical characteristics of carboxyhemoglobin concentrations, specifically for ranges of near 10%, 10 - 20%, near 30%, 40%, 50%, 60% and 70%.**

Frontal headache usually becomes evident with CoHb levels of 10 percent.
At 10 to 20 % CoHb may produce symptoms of headache and dyspnea.
30 % causes nausea, dizziness, visual disturbance, fatigue, and impaired judgment.
40 % leads to syncope and confusion.
Levels of 50 % may produce coma and seizures.
60 % causes respiratory failure and hypotension.
70 % level may be lethal.

❏ ❏ ❏ ➢ **What is the appropriate treatment for cyanide poisoning?**

Amyl nitrite, sodium nitrite IV, followed by sodium thiosulfate IV.

❏ ❏ ❏ ➢ **Organisms which produce focal nervous system pathology via an exotoxin include:**

C. diphtheria.
C. botulinum.
C. tetani.
wood and dog tick (Dermacentor A&B).
Staph aureus.

❏ ❏ ❏ ➢ **Signs and symptoms of diphtheria infection include:**

Infection is heralded by acute onset of exudative pharyngitis, high <u>fever</u> and malaise. A pseudomembrane may form in the oropharynx with possible respiratory compromise.
Powerful exotoxin has direct effects on the heart, kidneys and nervous system.
Diphtheria infection may lead to paralysis of the intrinsic and extrinsic eye muscles. You will never see such paralysis in your practice, but you may need to differentiate it from bulbar palsy caused by C. botulinum on an exam. Botulism does not cause fever.

❏ ❏ ❏ ➢ **Describe botulism intoxication.**

Botulism exotoxin is elaborated by C. botulinum. It affects the myoneural junction and prevents the release of acetylcholine. In the United States, it is caused principally by ingestion of foods that have been inadequately prepared.
The most common neurologic complaints are related to the bulbar musculature.
Neurologic symptoms usually occur within 24 to 48 hours of ingestion of contaminated foods.
Muscle paralysis and weakness usually spread rapidly to involve all muscles of the trunk and extremities. It is important to distinguish between botulism poisoning and myasthenia gravis. This distinction can be made by using the edrophonium (Tensilon) test, usually performed by a neurologist.

❏ ❏ ❏ ➢ **What are some of the key features of Guillain-Barré syndrome?**

Guillain-Barré syndrome is a lower motor neuron disease which commonly affects persons in their 30's and 40's. It presents as an ascending weakness involving the legs more than the arms. A sensory component may be present.

Bulbar muscles are usually involved late in the course of the disease. Reflexes are affected early. Paralysis can progress rapidly and recovery is usually slow, but almost always complete.

Lower motor neuron.
Ascending.
Bulbar late.
Reflexes early.

❑ ❑ ❑ ➢ **What formula should be used to calculate fluid requirements for resuscitation of a burn victim?**

2-4 ml/kg / %TBSA / day.
One-half of this is given in the first 8 hours.

❑ ❑ ❑ ➢ **What percentage of total body surface area is burned in a man with a circumferential burn to both arms, the penis and the anterior chest wall?**

37%.

❑ ❑ ❑ ➢ **How did this man <u>get</u> this burn?!@#**

❑ ❑ ❑ ➢ **In a patient who is either less than 10 or greater than 50 years of age, with both deep partial thickness and full thickness burns, what percentage of total body surface area must be burned before referral to the burn center is indicated?**

10%.

❑ ❑ ❑ ➢ **In a patient who is <u>between</u> the ages of 10 and 50 years, with both deep partial thickness and full thickness burns, what percentage of total body surface area must be burned before referral to the burn center is indicated?**

20%.

❑ ❑ ❑ ➢ **In a patient who has full thickness burns, what percentage of total body surface area must be burned before referral to the burn center is indicated?**

5% - independent of age.
NB. - Above are guidelines from one text, burns to hand, face and perineum require extra caution and burn center referral may be appropriate.

❑ ❑ ❑ ➢ **Poor prognostic signs <u>on admission</u> of a patient whth pancreatitis include:**

Age over 55 years.
Glucose level greater than 200 mg/dl.
LDH level greater than 700 IU/l.
WBC count greater than 16,000.
SGOT level greater than 250 U/l.

NOTICE - <u>NO</u> <u>AMYLASE</u> INVOLVEMENT!

❏ ❏ ❏ ➣ **Poor prognostic signs <u>at 48° after admission</u> of a patient with pancreatitis include:**

Hematocrit fallen more than 10% with a rise in BUN more that 5 mg/dl, declining calcium level to less than 8 mg/dl, PaO_2 less than 60 mm Hg, large fluid accumulation and base deficit greater than 4 mEq/L.
NOTICE - <u>NO</u> <u>AMYLASE</u> INVOLVEMENT!

Great quotes series:

"That's just something for your trivia basket."

Professor John "Jack" Nolte, formerly of University of Colorado Health Sciences Center which could not retain this outstanding teacher and author of <u>The Human Brain - An introduction to its functional anatomy</u>.

"My trivia basket is full." Medical student response.

❏ ❏ ❏ ➣ **What test is considered to be the gold standard in establishing the diagnosis of acute cholecystitis?**

Radionuclide scan of the biliary tree.

❏ ❏ ❏ ➣ **What pain medicine is theoretically contraindicated in the treatment of pain from acute diverticulitis?**

Codeine and morphine are contraindicated, as their use may increase intraluminal colonic pressure. Meperidine (Demerol) is a good substitute as it inhibits segmental contraction of the colon.

❏ ❏ ❏ ➣ **What test is best to confirm the diagnosis of Boerhaave's syndrome?**

An esophagram using a water soluble contrast medium should be used in place of barium to confirm the diagnosis.

❏ ❏ ❏ ➣ **What pseudonyms are associated with regional enteritis (4)?**

Crohn's disease.
Terminal ileitis.
Regional enteritis.
Granulomatous ileocolitis.

❏ ❏ ❏ ➣ **What are the other terms used to refer to ulcerative colitis?**

NONE. If any other pseudonym is used it refers to that other similar disease.

❏ ❏ ❏ ➣ **A patient presents with Mallory-Weiss syndrome, and a Sengstaken-Blakemore tube is being considered to control hemorrhage. What problem could a patient have by history that would prevent its use?**

Hiatal hernia, since proper placement of the balloon, as well as proper traction, cannot be applied in such persons.

❐ ❐ ❐ ➤ **What are the signs and symptoms of a patient with Boerhaave's syndrome?**

Substernal and left sided chest pain with a history of forceful vomiting leading to spontaneous esophageal rupture.

❐ ❐ ❐ ➤ **What is the <u>most</u> <u>common</u> cause of intestinal obstruction?**

Adynamic ileus is the <u>most</u> <u>common</u> cause of intestinal obstruction.

❐ ❐ ❐ ➤ **What is the <u>most</u> <u>common</u> cause of small bowel obstruction?**

<u>Adhesions</u> (#1) and hernias are the <u>most</u> <u>common</u> causes of small bowel obstruction.

❐ ❐ ❐ ➤ **What is the <u>most</u> <u>common</u> cause of large bowel obstruction?**

<u>Carcinoma</u> (#1), volvulus and sigmoid diverticulitis are the most common causes of large bowel obstruction.

❐ ❐ ❐ ➤ **What is the single <u>most</u> <u>common</u> cause of upper GI tract hemorrhage?**

Duodenal ulcers.

❐ ❐ ❐ ➤ **Which layers of the bowel wall and mesentery are affected by regional enteritis (Crohn's disease, granulomatous ileocolitis)?**

Inflammatory reaction of regional enteritis involves all layers of the bowel wall.

REGIONAL enteritis involves ALL layers, of course!

❐ ❐ ❐ ➤ **What is the <u>most</u> <u>common</u> hernia in women?**

<u>Inguinal</u> <u>hernia</u>, as it is in men.
Though not as common overall, femoral hernias are more common in women than in men.

❐ ❐ ❐ ➤ **What are Kanavel's four cardinal signs of infectious digital flexor tenosynovitis?**

Tenderness along the tendon sheath,
finger held in flexion,
pain on passive extension of the finger,
edema.

❐ ❐ ❐ ➤ **What symptoms are associated with presentation of regional enteritis (Crohn's disease, granulomatous ileocolitis)?**

Patients with regional enteritis may present with fever, abdominal pain, weight loss and diarrhea. Fistulas, fissures and abscesses may be noted.

Ulcerative colitis, on the other hand, usually presents with bloody diarrhea.

❏ ❏ ❏ ➤ **The <u>most</u> <u>common</u> cause of subacute infectious endocarditis is:**

S. viridans.

❏ ❏ ❏ ➤ **Subacute bacterial endocarditis <u>most</u> <u>frequently</u> affects which valve?**

SBE usually involves the left side of the heart, specifically the <u>mitral</u> valve.
The aortic valve is the second most commonly involved valve. Rheumatic fever is the
most likely cause of valvular damage associated with SBE. Mitral stenosis is a very
common predisposing factor in SBE. Drug addicts tend to develop right-sided SBE, usually involving the tricuspid valve.

❏ ❏ ❏ ➤ **The <u>most</u> <u>common</u> cause of acute infectious endocarditis is:**

S. aureus.

❏ ❏ ❏ ➤ **A good initial antibiotic choice for empiric treatment of acute infectious endocarditis is:**

Gentamycin (1.0 - 1.5 mg/kg q 8° for normal adults) and oxacillin (12 gm/d).

❏ ❏ ❏ ➤ **A patient presents to your emergency department after being bitten by a wild
raccoon. What treatment would you provide?**

Wound care, tetanus prophylaxis, RIG 20 IU/kg (1/2 at bite site and 1/2 IM), and HDCV
1 cc IM.

❏ ❏ ❏ ➤ **Describe the skin lesions found in a patient with disseminated gonococcemia.**

Umbilicated pustule with a red halo.

❏ ❏ ❏ ➤ **Describe the skin lesions associated with Pseudomonas aeruginosa infection.**

Pseudomonas aeruginosa bacteremia typically produces pale, erythematous skin lesions
that are approximately 1 cm in size with an ulcerated necrotic center (ecthyma gangrenosum for you Zebe-hunters).

❏ ❏ ❏ ➤ **Defect of sickle cell disease?**

Valine is substituted for glutamic acid in the 6th amino acid of the ß-chain.

❏ ❏ ❏ ➤ **What is the appropriate treatment for a patient with gonorrhea?**

Ceftriaxone 250 mg IM.
Spectinomycin 2 gm IM for ceftriaxone allergy.
Doxycycline 100 mg PO bid x 10 d for associated Chlamydia.

❏ ❏ ❏ ➤ **Describe the intracorporeal travel of the rabies virus.**

The virus is spread centripetally up peripheral nerve into the CNS. The incubation period for rabies is usually 30 to 60 d with a range of 10 d up to one yr. Transmission is usually by infected secretions, saliva or infected tissue. Stages include the upper respiratory tract infection symptomatology followed by encephalitis, and the final stage involving the brainstem.

❐ ❐ ❐ ➢ **What animals are the <u>most</u> <u>common</u> vectors of rabies a.) in the world, b.) in the U.S.?**

Worldwide, the d<u>o</u>g is the most common carrier of rabies.
In the <u>U</u>nited States, the sk<u>U</u>nk has become the <u>most</u> <u>common</u> source of disease. Bats, raccoons, cows, dogs, foxes and cats (descending order) are also sources.

Recall, parenthetically, that your rodents (Rocky (the flying squirrel), Dale (the chipmunk), Micky and Ratfink) and your lagomorphs (wild wangy wabbits) , are <u>NOT</u> carriers of rabies.

❐ ❐ ❐ ➢ **A septic appearing adult has multiple 1 cm diameter skin lesions with a necrotic, ulcerated center and an erythematous surround. What is the likely pathogen?**

Pseudomonas aeruginosa.

❐ ❐ ❐ ➢ **What is the IM treatment for adult streptococcal pharyngitis?**

1.2 million units of benzathine penicillin G.
0.6 million units of benzathine penicillin G for kids under 27 kg.

Mercedes "Benz" last a long time.

❐ ❐ ❐ ➢ **What is the <u>most</u> <u>common</u> initial symptom in botulism poisoning?**

Visual disturbance.
Visual difficulties have been reported in up to 90 percent of cases. Abducent nerve (CN VI) palsy is common and severe cases may show third cranial nerve involvement with dilated and fixed pupils. Other common initial symptoms include headache, dizziness, weakness, malaise and a dry mouth. Nausea and vomiting is found in about 35% of cases. Symptoms usually appear within the first 24 to 72 hours after exposure.

❐ ❐ ❐ ➢ **Describe the signs and symptoms of spinal shock.**

Spinal shock represents complete loss of spinal cord function below the level of injury. Patients have flaccid paralysis, complete sensory loss, areflexia and loss of autonomic function.
Such patients are usually bradycardic, hypotensive, hypothermic and vasodilated.

❐ ❐ ❐ ➢ **Active adduction of the thumb tests which nerve?**

Ulnar nerve.

❐ ❐ ❐ ➢ **Positive birefringent crystals in synovial fluid analysis is suggest of:**

Pseudogout. If you are POSITIVE, it must be PSEUDOgout - of course!

Great quote series:

The life so short, the craft so long to learn.

Hippocrates, c. 460-357 B.C.

❏ ❏ ❏ ➢ **In a school aged child, where would a patch of atopic dermatitis typically be found?**

Elbows and knees.

❏ ❏ ❏ ➢ **Describe the rash found in exanthem subitum (roseola).**

The rash is usually found on the trunk and neck, and is maculopapular.

❏ ❏ ❏ ➢ **What is the most common cause of death among children between 1 and 12 months of age?**

SIDS.

❏ ❏ ❏ ➢ **Alkali causes what type of necrosis?**

Liquefactive necrosis.

❏ ❏ ❏ ➢ **What is the antibiotic of choice in the treatment of Rocky Mountain spotted fever in a patient allergic to tetracycline?**

Chloramphenicol.

❏ ❏ ❏ ➢ **A renal dialysis patient suffers a crush injury. She develops an arrhythmia after intubation using succinylcholine assisted rapid-sequence induction. What is the best treatment?**

Calcium and bicarbonate.

❏ ❏ ❏ ➢ **Describe the chest x-ray of Mycoplasma pneumonia.**

Patchy densities involving the entire lobe are most common. Pneumatoceles, cavities, abscesses and pleural effusions can occur, but are uncommon. Erythromycin.

❏ ❏ ❏ ➢ **What type of bacterial pneumonia is commonly seen with viral illness?**

Staphylococcal infection.

❏ ❏ ❏ ➢ **What two types of pneumonia are often seen in the summer months?**

Staph pneumonia and Legionella.

❏ ❏ ❏ ➤ **Describe the chest x-ray findings in Legionella pneumonia.**

Dense consolidation and bulging fissures. Expect elevated liver enzymes and hypophosphatemia.

❏ ❏ ❏ ➤ **What are the classic signs and symptoms of TB?**

Night sweats, fever, weight loss, malaise, cough, and a green/yellow sputum most commonly seen in the mornings.

❏ ❏ ❏ ➤ **What are the chest x-ray findings in tuberculosis?**

Right upper lobe cavitation is classic.
Lower lung infiltrates, hilar adenopathy, atelectasis, and pleural effusion are common.

❏ ❏ ❏ ➤ **Where is the most likely location of a Boerhaave's tear?**

Left posterolateral region of the mid-thoracic esophagus.

❏ ❏ ❏ ➤ **How does a coin appear on AP view of the trachea?**

On its side.

❏ ❏ ❏ ➤ **How does a coin in the esophagus appear on AP?**

Like a solid circle.

❏ ❏ ❏ ➤ **Is GI bleeding common with a perforated ulcer?**

No.

❏ ❏ ❏ ➤ **During which trimester is acute appendicitis most common?**

Second.

❏ ❏ ❏ ➤ **What is the most common cause of paralytic ileus?**

Surgery.

❏ ❏ ❏ ➤ **What is the second most common cause of small bowel obstruction?**

Incarcerated hernia. The most common cause is adhesions.

❏ ❏ ❏ ➤ **An elderly female patient presents with the complaint of pain in the knee and also the medial aspect of the thigh. What GI diagnosis might you entertain?**

An obturator hernia may produce pain in the knee and thigh.

❏ ❏ ❏ ➢ **What is the second most common cause of colonic obstruction?**

Diverticulitis. Cancer of the sigmoid is the <u>most</u> <u>common</u> cause. Volvulus is the third most common cause.

❏ ❏ ❏ ➢ **What is the most common site of volvulus?**

Sigmoid colon.

❏ ❏ ❏ ➢ **Describe the location of an indirect inguinal hernia.**

Found <u>lateral to the epigastric vessels</u>, protrudes through the inguinal canal.

❏ ❏ ❏ ➢ **Describe a femoral hernia.**

Through the femoral canal and below the inguinal ligament.

❏ ❏ ❏ ➢ **Describe the location of a Spigelian hernia.**

Located 3-5 cm above the inguinal ligament.

❏ ❏ ❏ ➢ **What is a Pantaloon hernia?**

A hernia with both direct and indirect inguinal hernia components.

❏ ❏ ❏ ➢ **What is a sliding hernia?**

A hernia in which one wall of the hernia sac includes viscus.

❏ ❏ ❏ ➢ **Describe a Richter's hernia.**

An incarceration which contains only one wall of viscus.

❏ ❏ ❏ ➢ **What is the single most common hernia in children?**

An indirect hernia. Direct inguinal hernia is more common in the elderly.

❏ ❏ ❏ ➢ **When do umbilical hernias typically close?**

Age two.

❏ ❏ ❏ ➢ **List three other names for regional ileitis.**

Crohn's disease, terminal ileitis, and granulomatous ileocolitis.

❏ ❏ ❏ ➢ **What are other names for ulcerative colitis?**

None.

❏ ❏ ❏ ➢ **What is the most common site of Crohn's disease?.**

The ileum. It can actually involve any part of the GI tract from the social end to the antisocial end. It is segmental, often involving granuloma formation along with inflammatory reactions. Crohn's disease has two incidence peaks, one in the 15-22 y old age group and a second in the 55-60 y old age group.

❏ ❏ ❏ ➢ **How many layers of the bowel does Crohn's disease involve?**

All layers. Associated with *fissures, abscesses and fistulas*.

❏ ❏ ❏ ➢ **What are the signs and symptoms of Crohn's disease?**

Fever, diarrhea, right lower quadrant pain with mass possible, *fistulas*, rectal prolapse, perianal *fissures*, and *abscesses*. Associated with arthritis, uveitis, and liver disease.

❏ ❏ ❏ ➢ **What is the <u>most</u> <u>common</u> <u>complication</u> of Crohn's disease?**

Perianal abscess.
Also ischiorectal *abscess*, *fissures*, rectovaginal *fistulas*, rectal prolapse, and strictures.

❏ ❏ ❏ ➢ **Is toxic megacolon commonly associated with Crohn's disease?**

No. Toxic megacolon <u>is</u> a complication of ulcerative colitis.
Cancer is also an uncommon complication of Crohn's disease.

❏ ❏ ❏ ➢ **Systemic diseases associated with Crohn's disease?**

Pyoderma gangrenosum, uveitis, episclerosis, scleritis, arthritis, erythema nodosum, and nephrolithiasis.

❏ ❏ ❏ ➢ **Patient's with inflammatory bowel disease have ankylosing spondylitis what percentage of the time?**

20%.

❏ ❏ ❏ ➢ **What are the expected contrast x-ray findings with Crohn's disease?**

Segmental involvement in the colon with abnormal mucosal pattern and fistulas, often without involvement of the rectum. May see small intestinal narrowing.

❏ ❏ ❏ ➢ **What is the chief clinical feature of ulcerative colitis?**

Bloody diarrhea and involvement of the colon and rectum.
Peak incidence is in 20-30 y olds. The most common site is the rectosigmoid colon.
Ulcerative colitis typically involves only the submucosal and mucosal layers. May see crypt abscesses and ulcerations present. Pseudopolyps are associated with ulcerative colitis.

❏ ❏ ❏ ➣ **What are the principal signs and symptoms of ulcerative colitis?**

Fever, weight loss, tachycardia, pancolitis, and six bloody bowel movements per day.

❏ ❏ ❏ ➣ **Is toxic megacolon more commonly seen in ulcerative colitis or Crohn's disease?**

Toxic megacolon is a very common, serious complication of ulcerative colitis.

❏ ❏ ❏ ➣ **What medications may be used in the treatment of Crohn's disease that are absolutely contraindicated in the treatment of ulcerative colitis?**

Antidiarrheal agents may be used in Crohn's disease, they should not be used to treat ulcerative colitis.

❏ ❏ ❏ ➣ **Is ulcerative colitis or Crohn's more commonly associated with perirectal fistulas and abscesses?**

Crohn's.

❏ ❏ ❏ ➣ **Is cancer more commonly seen in ulcerative colitis or Crohn's disease?**

Ulcerative colitis.
Remember, with ulcerative colitis, think of toxic megacolon and cancer. Avoid antidiarrheal agents.

❏ ❏ ❏ ➣ **What are the two most common causes of acute diarrhea?**

Rotavirus and Norwalk.

❏ ❏ ❏ ➣ **What is the most common cause of diarrhea in a child less than one year old?**

Rotavirus.

❏ ❏ ❏ ➣ **What type of diarrhea is most commonly associated with seizures?**

Shigella.

❏ ❏ ❏ ➣ **What type of diarrhea is associated with rose spots and watery diarrhea, as well as high fever and relative bradycardia?**

Salmonella. Particularly common in IV drug abusers with new pet turtles! Salmonella typhi may not have much diarrhea.

❏ ❏ ❏ ➣ **Treatment for Salmonella?**

Supportive care without antibiotics.
Severe fever may require antibiotic therapy.

❏ ❏ ❏ ➣ **What bacteria is associated with mesenteric adenitis and pseudoappendicitis?**

Yersinia.

❐ ❐ ❐ ➤ **What is the most common food born pathogen?**

Staphylococcus which presents 6-12 h post ingestion with diarrhea and vomiting. Enterotoxin.

❐ ❐ ❐ ➤ **What gastroenteritis with diarrhea is associated with oysters, clams, crabs, and seafood?**

Vibrio parahaemolyticus. Symptomatic treatment is most common.

❐ ❐ ❐ ➤ **What type of diarrhea is associated with perfuse, bloody diarrhea and no vomiting?**

Entamoeba histolytica.
Diarrhea that is not necessarily bloody and that is associated with contaminated meat could be due to Clostridium perfringens.

❐ ❐ ❐ ➤ **What is the most common parasite in the United States?**

Giardia. Presents with foul smelling floating stools, abdominal pain, and perfuse diarrhea. It may be diagnosed with a positive string test, or duodenal aspiration for trophozoites.

❐ ❐ ❐ ➤ **What type of diarrhea is commonly seen in AIDS patients?**

Cryptosporidiosis. Diagnosed with a positive acid fast stain. Presents with profuse, watery diarrhea, no blood.

❐ ❐ ❐ ➤ **What is the incubation period for Hepatitis A?**

30 days. It is caused by an RNA virus.

❐ ❐ ❐ ➤ **How is hepatitis A transmitted?**

Oral fecal route. No carrier state exists.

❐ ❐ ❐ ➤ **What does an elevated IgM anti-HBc mean?**

Exposure to hepatitis B with antibody to the core antigen. High titers associated with contagious disease, low titers with chronic hepatitis B. M = might have the disease.

❐ ❐ ❐ ➤ **What does elevated IgG anti-HAV mean?**

It confers immunity. G = gone.

In hepatitis **B**, IgG anti-HBc means gone only along with anti-HBs. IgG anti-HBc along with HBsAg (surface antigen) implies chronic hepatitis B.

❑ ❑ ❑ ➢ **What type of hepatitis is caused by a DNA virus?**

Hepatitis B. Incubation period is 90 days.

❑ ❑ ❑ ➢ **What does anti-HBs mean?**

Suggests prior infection and immunity. Pt. has antibodies to the surface antigen just waiting for a chance...S = stopped.

❑ ❑ ❑ ➢ **What type of defects cause left to right shunt murmurs?**

ASD, VSD, and PDA.

❑ ❑ ❑ ➢ **What type of defect produces diminished pulses in the lower extremities of a pediatric patient?**

Coarctation of the aorta.

❑ ❑ ❑ ➢ **What are two fairly common conditions in pediatrics which produce cardiac syncope?**

Aortic stenosis, which is not cyanotic and tetralogy of Fallot, which is cyanotic.

❑ ❑ ❑ ➢ **What are two unique clinical findings of tetralogy of Fallot?**

A boot shaped heart on x-ray and exercise intolerance which is relieved by squatting. TOF is treated by placing the patient in the knee chest position and giving morphine.

❑ ❑ ❑ ➢ **What would be the signs and symptoms of aortic stenosis in a child?**

Exercise intolerance, chest pain, and a systolic ejection click with a crescendo, decrescendo murmur, radiating to the neck with a suprasternal thrill. No cyanosis!

❑ ❑ ❑ ➢ **What are the signs of left sided heart failure in an infant?**

Increased respiratory rate, shortness of breath, and sweating during feeding.

❑ ❑ ❑ ➢ **What is the single most common cause of CHF in the second week of life?**

Coarctation of the aorta.

❑ ❑ ❑ ➢ **What is the most common cause of otitis media?**

Strep pneumonia.

❑ ❑ ❑ ➢ **What is the most common cause of impetigo?**

Group A ß-hemolytic streptococcus.

❐ ❐ ❐ ➤ **What is the most common cause of bullous impetigo?**

Staph aureus.

❐ ❐ ❐ ➤ **What is the <u>most common</u> cause of sinusitis?**

Streptococcus pneumoniae.

❐ ❐ ❐ ➤ **What is the <u>most common</u> cause of orbital infections?**

Staph aureus. Periorbital infections are most commonly caused by H flu.

❐ ❐ ❐ ➤ **What is the <u>most common</u> cause of pediatric bacteremia?**

Strep pneumonia.

❐ ❐ ❐ ➤ **What are the most common causes of an abscess or pneumatocele in a pediatric patient?**

Staphylococcal pneumonia or anaerobic pneumonia.

❐ ❐ ❐ ➤ **A patient presents with a staccato cough and a history of conjunctivitis in the first few weeks after birth, what type of pneumonia does this patient have?**

Chlamydia.

❐ ❐ ❐ ➤ **Most common cause of viral pneumonia in the pediatric patient?**

RSV.

❐ ❐ ❐ ➤ **What is the most common type of asthma in children?**

Extrinsic asthma which is a type I, immediate hypersensitivity reaction mediated by IgE. Common causes are molds and pet dander.

❐ ❐ ❐ ➤ **How do steroids function in the treatment of asthma?**

They increase cAMP, decrease inflammation, and help restore the function of ß-adrenergic responsiveness to adrenergic drugs.

❐ ❐ ❐ ➤ **What two viral illnesses are prodromes for Reye's syndrome?**

Varicella (chicken pox) and influenzae B.

❐ ❐ ❐ ➤ **Signs and symptoms of Reye's syndrome:**

Irritable, combative, and lethargic, right upper quadrant tenderness, history of influenzae B or recent chicken pox, papilledema, hypoglycemia, and seizures.
Lab findings would include hypoglycemia, and an elevated ammonia level greater than 20 times normal. Bilirubin level is NORMAL.

❏ ❏ ❏ ➢ **Describe stage I and stage II of Reye's syndrome.**

Stage I - vomiting, lethargy and liver dysfunction.
Stage II - disorientation, combativeness, delirium, hyperventilation, increased deep tendon reflexes, liver dysfunction, hyperexcitable, tachypnea, fever, tachycardia, sweating and pupillary dilatation.

❏ ❏ ❏ ➢ **Describe Stages III, IV, and V of Reye's syndrome.**

Stage III - coma, decorticate rigidity, increased respiratory rate, mortality rate of 50%.
Stage IV - coma, decerebrate posturing, no ocular reflexes, loss of corneal reflexes, and liver damage.
Stage V - loss of deep tendon reflexes, seizures, flaccid, respiratory arrest, 95% mortality.

❏ ❏ ❏ ➢ **What are the first, second, and third drugs of choice for treatment of seizures in children?**

The first is phenobarbital, second is phenytoin, and third is carbamazepine.

❏ ❏ ❏ ➢ **What is the drug of choice for absence (petit mal) seizures in a child?**

Ethosuximide, valproate, and acetazolamide. An EEG is usually obtained prior to initiating therapy.

❏ ❏ ❏ ➢ **What is the drug of choice to treat a febrile seizure?**

Phenobarbital.

❏ ❏ ❏ ➢ **Use of diazepam (Valium) is avoided in neonatal seizures. Is part of the reason for this because it may cause hyperbilirubinemia by uncoupling the bilirubin-albumin complex?**

Yes.

❏ ❏ ❏ ➢ **Serious complication of valproic acid?**

Hepatic failure.

❏ ❏ ❏ ➢ **Complications of phenytoin use?**

Folate deficiency, osteomalacia, neutropenia, neuropathies, lupus and myasthenia.

❏ ❏ ❏ ➢ **What is the most common viral gastroenteritis in children?**

Rotavirus.

❏ ❏ ❏ ➢ **What is the most common cause of bacterial gastroenteritis in the world?**

E. coli.

❐ ❐ ❐ ➤ **What is the most common cause of diarrhea in infants and young children in day care centers?**

Giardia.

❐ ❐ ❐ ➤ **What bacterium is associated with mesenteric adenitis or appendicitis?**

Yersinia.

❐ ❐ ❐ ➤ **What enteritis causing bacterium produces watery diarrhea, encephalopathies, and convulsions.**

Shigella = seizures.

❐ ❐ ❐ ➤ **A child presents with vomiting and a moderate amount of blood in the stool. What is the diagnosis?**

Malrotation of the mid-gut.

❐ ❐ ❐ ➤ **What is the most common cause of painless lower GI bleeding in an infant or child?**

Meckel's diverticulum.

❐ ❐ ❐ ➤ **A 16 mo old presents with bilious vomiting, a distended abdomen, and blood in the stool. Diagnosis?**

Malrotation of the mid-gut.

❐ ❐ ❐ ➤ **A child presents with abdominal cramps which come and go, current jelly stools, and a sausage like tumor mass in the right lower quadrant. Contrast x-ray shows a coil spring sign. Diagnosis?**

Intussusception.

❐ ❐ ❐ ➤ **A child presents with a history of drug ingestion; she now has convulsions, coma, and cardiac collapse. What drug might have caused this?**

Salicylate with secondary hypoglycemia.

❐ ❐ ❐ ➤ **What side effect of propranolol may be concerning for a diabetic patient?**

Hypoglycemia.

❐ ❐ ❐ ➤ **What are some possible complications of sodium bicarbonate therapy?**

Hypokalemia, paradoxical CSF acidosis, impaired O_2 dissociation, and sodium overload.

❏ ❏ ❏ ➤ **What type of lactic acidosis is associated with hypoxia and shock?**

Type A.

❏ ❏ ❏ ➤ **Differentiate between non-ketotic hyperosmolar coma and DKA.**

In non-ketotic hyperosmolar coma, glucose is very high, often > 800. The serum osmolality is also very high, with average about 380. Nitroprusside test is negative.
In DKA, glucose is more often in the range of 600, the serum osmolality is approximately 350, nitroprusside test is positive.

❏ ❏ ❏ ➤ **What focal signs may be present in a patient with non-ketotic hyperosmolar coma?**

These patients may have hemisensory deficits or perhaps hemiparesis. 10-15% of these patients have a seizure.

❏ ❏ ❏ ➤ **What is the most common cause of hyperthyroidism?**

Grave's disease (toxic diffuse goiter).

❏ ❏ ❏ ➤ **What is the most common precipitating cause of thyroid storm?**

Pulmonary infection.

❏ ❏ ❏ ➤ **What is another name for life threatening hypothyroidism?**

Myxedema coma. Commonly seen in elderly women in the winter months and is stimulated by infection and stress.

❏ ❏ ❏ ➤ **What is the most common cause of hypothyroidism?**

Overtreatment of Grave's disease with iodine or subtotal thyroidectomy.

❏ ❏ ❏ ➤ **What is the second most common cause of hypothyroidism?**

Autoimmune Hashimoto's thyroiditis.

❏ ❏ ❏ ➤ **How may primary hypothyroidism be distinguished from secondary?**

In primary hypothyroidism the TSH levels are high, patients often have a history of thyroid surgery and may have a goiter; in secondary the TSH levels are low or normal, no hx of surgery and no goiter.

❏ ❏ ❏ ➤ **What drugs may make myxedema worse?**

Propranolol and phenothiazines.

❏ ❏ ❏ ➣ **What ECG finding would you expect in myxedema coma?**

Bradycardia.

❏ ❏ ❏ ➣ **What is a common "surgical problem" in myxedema that should be treated conservatively?**

Acquired megacolon.

❏ ❏ ❏ ➣ **What is primary adrenal insufficiency?**

Addison's disease, that is, failure of the adrenal cortex.

❏ ❏ ❏ ➣ **What hormones are produced by the adrenal cortex?**

Mineralocorticoids, glucocorticoids and androgenic steroids.
Salt, sugar, sex.

❏ ❏ ❏ ➣ **What is the major mineralocorticoid?**

Aldosterone. Aldosterone is regulated by the renin angiotensin system. Aldosterone increases sodium reabsorption and increased K^+ excretion.

❏ ❏ ❏ ➣ **What is the major glucocorticoid?**

Cortisol.

❏ ❏ ❏ ➣ **What does the medulla of the adrenal gland produce?**

Epinephrine and norepinephrine.

❏ ❏ ❏ ➣ **A patient presents two weeks after suffering a myocardial infarction. The patient takes warfarin and has sudden onset of hypotension, right flank pain, right CVA pain, epigastric pain, fever, nausea, and vomiting. Diagnosis?**

Bilateral adrenal gland hemorrhage - adrenal apoplexy.

❏ ❏ ❏ ➣ **What is Waterhouse-Fredrickson syndrome?**

Septicemia secondary to meningococcemia with associated bilateral adrenal gland hemorrhage. The patient will have a petechial rash, purpura, shaking chills, and severe headache.

❏ ❏ ❏ ➣ **What effect does Addison's disease have on cortisol and aldosterone levels?**

Cortisol and aldosterone levels are low.
Low cortisol levels mean nausea, vomiting, anorexia, lethargy, hypoglycemia, water intoxication, and inability to withstand even minor stress without shock.
Low aldosterone levels means sodium depletion, dehydration, hypotension, and syncope.

❏ ❏ ❏ ➢ **What are the signs and symptoms of Addison's disease?**

Hyperpigmentation, hyperkalemia, alopecia, and ascending paralysis secondary to hyperkalemia.
Lab findings in Addison's disease include hypoglycemia, hyponatremia, hyperkalemia, and azotemia.

❏ ❏ ❏ ➢ **What ECG findings are expected in Addison's disease?**

Because of the hyperkalemia, expect peaked T-waves.

❏ ❏ ❏ ➢ **What are the principal signs and symptoms in adrenal crisis?**

Abdominal pain, hypotension and shock. The common cause is withdrawal of steroids. Treatment of adrenal crisis is hydrocortisone (Solu-Cortef), 100 mg IV bolus and 100 mg added to a the first liter of D_5 0.9 NS.

❏ ❏ ❏ ➢ **Does cyanide cause cyanosis?**

No, except secondarily when bradycardia and apnea precede asystolic arrest.
Consider cyanide in an acidotic comatose patient without cyanosis and no hypoxia on ABG.

❏ ❏ ❏ ➢ **What key lab findings are expected in SIADH?**

Serum sodium would be low and urine sodium would be high, greater than 30.

❏ ❏ ❏ ➢ **What is the most common cause of a cerebral infarct?**

Atherosclerosis, and the most common site is in the internal carotids.

❏ ❏ ❏ ➢ **What is the typical anatomic source of an epidural hematoma?**

The middle meningeal artery.

❏ ❏ ❏ ➢ **What is the most common anatomic source of a subdural hematoma?**

Bridging veins.

❏ ❏ ❏ ➢ **What is the most common source of a subarachnoid bleed?**

A saccular aneurysm.

❏ ❏ ❏ ➢ **If the lesion is in the right hemisphere, which way will the eyes deviate?**

Eyes will deviate toward the lesion.

❏ ❏ ❏ ➢ **If there is a lesion in the brain stem, which way will the eyes deviate?**

They will deviate away from the lesion in the brain stem.

❏ ❏ ❏ ➢ **What is the single most common intraparenchymal site of intracranial bleeding?**

The putamen.

❏ ❏ ❏ ➢ **In the pediatric esophagus, what is the most common site of a foreign body?**

Cricopharyngeal narrowing.

❏ ❏ ❏ ➢ **Most common hernia in population?**

Inguinal.

❏ ❏ ❏ ➢ **Do household pets transmit Yersinia?**

Yes.

❏ ❏ ❏ ➢ **What is the most common cause of conjunctivitis in the newborn?**

Chlamydia.

❏ ❏ ❏ ➢ **Most common cause of meningitis after the first month of life?**

H. influenzae.

❏ ❏ ❏ ➢ **Most common cause of urinary tract infection in a female child?**

E. coli.

❏ ❏ ❏ ➢ **First line of treatment of a seizure in a five year old?**

Phenobarbital.

❏ ❏ ❏ ➢ **What is the most common cause of intrinsic renal failure?**

Acute tubular necrosis.

❏ ❏ ❏ ➢ **What is the most common cause of cardiac arrest in an uremic patient?**

Hyperkalemia.

❏ ❏ ❏ ➢ **A "blue dot" sign suggests:**

Torsion of the epididymis or appendix testis.

❏ ❏ ❏ ➢ **What is the first cardiac finding in cyclic antidepressant overdose?**

Sinus tachycardia.

❏ ❏ ❏ ➢ **What is the most common cause of right sided endocarditis in IV drug addicts?**

Staph aureus.

❏ ❏ ❏ ➢ **What is the most common valve affected in IV drug addicts?**

Tricuspid.

❏ ❏ ❏ ➢ **What is the most common cause of osteomyelitis or septic arthritis in an IV drug addict?**

Serratia marcescens.

❏ ❏ ❏ ➢ **What is the most common cause of chronic heavy metal poisoning?**

Lead. Arsenic is most common acute.

❏ ❏ ❏ ➢ **What is the most commonly injured area of the mandible?**

Angle.

❏ ❏ ❏ ➢ **What is the most commonly fractured area of the maxilla or mandible?**

Alveolar process.

❏ ❏ ❏ ➢ **Most common cause of Erysipelas:**

Group A streptococci.

❏ ❏ ❏ ➢ **Are steroids effective in treatment of toxic epidermal necrolysis?**

No.

❏ ❏ ❏ ➢ **Erythema nodosa is associated with which type of gastroenteritis?**

Yersinia.
I've a particular <u>YEN</u> for this answer!!

❏ ❏ ❏ ➢ **Thyrotoxicosis may be treated with:**

Support and hydration, IV propylthiouracil 1 gram, sodium iodine IV 1 g q 12 h or IV propanolol 1 mg/min up to 10 mg.

❏ ❏ ❏ ➢ **What is the most reliable method of diagnosing a posterior shoulder dislocation?**

Physical exam. Order a "Y-view" x-ray - it may be helpful.

❐ ❐ ❐ ➤ **The mortise view of the ankle is important in the diagnosis of:**

Medial (deltoid) ligament disruption of the ankle.

❐ ❐ ❐ ➤ **A fracture of the proximal fibular shaft is commonly associated with:**

Medial ankle fracture or sprain.
This is a Maisonneuve fx, it may be present with a widened mortise and no fx seen in the ankle.

❐ ❐ ❐ ➤ **What is the best x-ray view for diagnosing lunate and perilunate dislocations?**

Lateral x-ray views of the wrist.

❐ ❐ ❐ ➤ **What is the formula for calculating the serum osmolarity?**

$$CalculatedOsmol(mOsm / l) = 2(Na) + \frac{glucose}{18} + \frac{BUN}{2.8}$$

❐ ❐ ❐ ➤ **What is a good way to remember the signs and symptoms of anticholinergic toxicity?**

Think of atropine, as most of the signs and symptoms of atropine use are similar. Tachycardia, hyperthermia, mydriasis, Ø sweat, dry mucosa, blurred vision for near objects (poor accommodation), decreased GI activity, urinary retention, aberration of mentation including delirium, lethargy and hallucinations, seizure and coma.

Dry as a bone,
Red as a beet,
Mad as a hatter,
Hot as a stone,
(Blind as a bat).

❐ ❐ ❐ ➤ **What are common anticholinergic compounds?**

Atropine, tricyclic antidepressants, antihistamines, phenothiazines, antiparkinsonian drugs, belladonna alkaloids, and some Solanaceae plants (eg. deadly nightshade , jimson weed).

❐ ❐ ❐ ➤ **For how long should a patient with TCA overdose demonstrating tachycardia and conduction disturbances be monitored?**

24 h.

❐ ❐ ❐ ➤ **For how long will naloxone typically reverse opioid toxicity?**

$T_{1/2}$ is 1 h with a duration of action of 2-3 h per Tintinalli 3rd Ed, pg. 566.
$T_{1/2}$ is 12-20 min with little effect after 45 min per Rosen 3rd Ed, pg. 2611.

❑ ❑ ❑ ➤ **A baby is brought to the emergency department with persistent crying for two hours and vomiting. On exam, a testicle is tender and enlarged. What is the most common cause?**

Testicular torsion.

❑ ❑ ❑ ➤ **A child is seen with bluish discoloration of the gingiva. What diagnosis do you suspect?**

Chronic lead poisoning. You would also expect erythrocyte protoporphyrin level to be elevated in chronic Pb poisoning.

❑ ❑ ❑ ➤ **What is the <u>most</u> <u>common</u> cause of periorbital cellulitis in a two year old child?**

The <u>most</u> <u>common</u> cause is H. influenzae. The second most common cause is S. aureus.

❑ ❑ ❑ ➤ **What is the most appropriate drug for a patient with low cardiac output and pulmonary congestion?**

Dobutamine.

❑ ❑ ❑ ➤ **Permanent pacemakers have a coding system of 5 letters.   Just kidding!**

❑ ❑ ❑ ➤ **What is the anatomical weakness of the esophagus?**

Lack of a serosa.

❑ ❑ ❑ ➤ **In a humeral shaft fracture, what nerve is most commonly injured?**

Radial nerve.

❑ ❑ ❑ ➤ **What is the most common hip dislocation?**

Posterior.

❑ ❑ ❑ ➤ **What disorder is most likely to be confused with erythema nodosum?**

Cellulitis.

❑ ❑ ❑ ➤ **What is erythema nodosum?**

An inflammatory disease of skin and subcutaneous tissue characterized by tender red nodules. Nodules are most commonly found in the pretibial area.
Most commonly affects young adults.
Most common cause in children - UTI, especially with streptococci.
Most common cause in adults - Streptococcal infections and sarcoidosis.
Other causes - leprosy, TB, psittacosis, ulcerative colitis, drug reaction.

❑ ❑ ❑ ➤ **Galeazzi's fracture implies:**

Fracture of the shaft of the radius with dislocation of the distal radioulnar joint. "GREAT RAYS DOWN DEEP!"

❏ ❏ ❏ ➤ **What is the <u>most</u> <u>common</u> dysrhythmia in a child?**

Paroxysmal atrial tachycardia.

❏ ❏ ❏ ➤ **On an upright chest x-ray, what is the earliest radiographic sign of left ventricular failure?**

Apical redistribution of the pulmonary vasculature.

❏ ❏ ❏ ➤ **What is the <u>most</u> <u>common</u> cause of hyponatremia?**

Dilution.

❏ ❏ ❏ ➤ **Of the following, which is <u>not</u> a common cause of <u>large</u> <u>bowel</u> obstruction: diverticulitis, adhesions, sigmoid volvulus or neoplasms?**

Adhesions.

❏ ❏ ❏ ➤ **A fracture of the acetabulum may be associated with damage to what nerve?**

The sciatic nerve.

❏ ❏ ❏ ➤ **What are some <u>common</u> causes of increased anion gap?**

Aspirin, methanol, uremia, diabetes, idiopathic (lactic), ethylene glycol and alcohol are reasonably common.

Numerous etiologies may produce the entity above listed demurely as "lactic." Lactic acidosis may be the result of shock, seizures, acute hypoxemia, INH, cyanide, ritodrine, inhaled acetylene, carbon monoxide and ethanol. Sodium nitroprusside, povidone-iodine ointment, sorbitol and xylitol can cause an anion gap acidosis.

Other causes of anion gap acidosis include toluene intoxication, iron intoxication, sulfuric acidosis, short bowel syndrome (D-lactic acidosis), formaldehyde, nalidixic acid, methanamine and rhubarb (oxalic acid). Inborn errors of metabolism such as methylmalonic acidemia and isovaleric acidemia may also cause a gap acidosis.

Recall some pearls for sorting out the differential diagnosis:

Methanol- visual disturbances and headache common. Can produce quite wide gaps as each 2.6 mg/dl of methanol contributes 1 mOsm/L to gap. Compare this with alcohol, each 4.3 mg/dl adds 1 mOsm/L to gap.

Uremia- is quite advanced before it causes an anion gap.

Diabetic Ketoacidosis- usually has both hyperglycemia and glucosuria; alcoholic ketoacidosis (AKA) often has a lower blood sugar and mild or absent glucosuria.

Salicylates- high levels contribute to gap.

Lactic Acidosis- can check serum level. Itself has broad differential as above.

Ethylene glycol- causes calcium oxalate or hippurate crystals in urine. Each 5.0 mg/dl contributes 1 mOsm/L to gap.

A reasonably comprehensive mnemonic device for recalling causes of anion gap acidosis is A MUDPILE CAT.

A MUDPILE CAT

A = alcohol,

M = methanol,
U = uremia,
D = DKA,
P = paraldehyde,
I = iron and isoniazid,
L = lactic acidosis,
E = ethylene glycol,

C = carbon monoxide,
A = ASA (aspirin),
T = toluene.

❏ ❏ ❏ ➢ **What are the causes of <u>normal</u> anion gap metabolic acidosis?**

Causes include diarrhea, ammonium chloride, renal tubular acidosis, renal interstitial disease, hypoadrenalism, ureterosigmoidostomy, and acetazolamide.

❏ ❏ ❏ ➢ **What are some common causes of respiratory alkalosis?**

Respiratory alkalosis is defined as a pH above 7.45 and a pCO_2 less than 35. Common causes of respiratory alkalosis include any process that may cause hyperventilation including shock, sepsis, trauma, asthma, PE, anemia, hepatic failure, heat stroke and exhaustion, emotion, salicylate poisoning, hypoxemia, pregnancy and inappropriate mechanical ventilation. Alkalosis shifts the O_2 disassociation curve to the left. It also causes cerebrovascular constriction. Kidneys compensate for respiratory alkalosis by excreting HCO_3^-.

❏ ❏ ❏ ➢ **Causes of right shift of O_2 disassociation curve:**

"<u>CADET</u>! <u>Right</u> face!!"

Right = Release to tissues.

Hyper <u>C</u>arbia,
       <u>A</u>cidemia,
2,3 <u>D</u>PG,
       <u>E</u>xercise,
and increased <u>T</u>emperature.

❏ ❏ ❏ ➢ **How should a patient with hypertrophic cardiomyopathy be treated who presents with chest pain and normal vital signs except for a heart rate of 140?**

ß-antagonists are the primary treatment for hypertrophic cardiomyopathy. ß-antagonists are first-line treatment for any symptomatic patient even without tachycardia present. Calcium channel blocking drugs are second-line therapeutics.

❏ ❏ ❏ ➢ **What is the adult dose of epinephrine in acute anaphylactic shock?**

0.3 - 0.5 mg of 1:10,000 IV.

❏ ❏ ❏ ➢ **How should neurogenic shock be best managed?**

Neurogenic shock is treated with replacement of volume deficit followed by vasopressors.

❏ ❏ ❏ ➢ **What is the most appropriate medication to treat a hypertensive patient with an acute aortic dissection?**

Trimethaphan.
Trimethaphan reduces hydraulic stress on the aortic wall and as a consequence, minimizes further dissection. The mechanism of action is via decreasing myocardial contractility. Trimethaphan also functions as a vasodilator and therefore reduces intra-aortic pressure and concomitant total peripheral resistance. Esmolol, a new titratable short acting ß-blocker, may also be a valuable alternative.

❏ ❏ ❏ ➢ **An elderly male presents to your emergency department with ataxia, confusion, amnesia and ocular paralysis. The patient is apathetic to his situation and has an otherwise normal neurologic exam. What is the likely cause of the patient's problem?**

Vitamin B deficiency associated with Wernicke-Korsakoff's syndrome.

❏ ❏ ❏ ➢ **How is SVR calculated?**

$$\frac{(MAP - CVP) \times 80}{CO} \qquad Nl = 800 - 1400 \ dyn \cdot s^{-1} \cdot cm^{-5}$$

❏ ❏ ❏ ➢ **What is the <u>most</u> <u>common</u> dysrhythmia associated with excess digitalis?**

PVC's.

❏ ❏ ❏ ➢ **What is the order of appearance of CHF on chest x-ray?**

Initially cephalization and redistribution of blood flow is seen, followed by interstitial edema with evident Kerley B lines, as well as a perihilar haze. This is followed by alveolar infiltrates in the typical butterfly appearance. Finally, flagrant pulmonary edema and effusions are present.

❏ ❏ ❏ ➢ **The most common cause of sporadic encephalitis?**

Herpes simplex virus.

❏ ❏ ❏ ➢ **What are the classic EKG findings of a patient with a posterior MI.**

A large R-wave and ST depression in V1 and V2.

❐ ❐ ❐ ➤ **What is the classic EKG finding in Wolff-Parkinson-White syndrome?**

A change in the upstroke of QRS, the delta wave.

❐ ❐ ❐ ➤ **The most common cause of endemic encephalitis?**

Arbovirus.

❐ ❐ ❐ ➤ **What is the best treatment for an unstable patient with Wolff-Parkinson-White syndrome presenting with rapid atrial fibrillation?**

Shock.

❐ ❐ ❐ ➤ **What is the <u>most</u> <u>common</u> dysrhythmia seen with digitalis?**

PVC's are the <u>most</u> <u>common</u>.
AV block and PSVT with block are second most common.
V-tach and junctional tachycardia are the least common arrhythmias associated with digitalis.

❐ ❐ ❐ ➤ **What is the best treatment for a verapamil induced bradycardia?**

Calcium chloride 10%, give 10 - 20 ml IV.

(This is about 10 - 20 mg/kg, use 10 - 30 mg/kg in children).

❐ ❐ ❐ ➤ **The <u>most</u> <u>common</u> cause of pelvic pain in adolescent females?**

Ovarian cyst.

❐ ❐ ❐ ➤ **What is the <u>most</u> <u>common</u> cause of valvular induced syncope in the elderly?**

Aortic stenosis is the most common valvular cause of syncope in the elderly.
Vasovagal mechanisms are the most common mechanism overall.

❐ ❐ ❐ ➤ **Describe the signs, symptoms and ECG finding associated with lithium toxicity.**

Tremor, weakness, and flattening of the T-waves.

❐ ❐ ❐ ➤ **How many days after a measles vaccine might a fever and a rash be expected to develop?**

Seven to ten days.

❐ ❐ ❐ ➤ **The most common complication of acute otitis media?**

Tympanic membrane perforation. Other complications include mastoiditis, cholesteatoma, as well as intracranial infections.

❐ ❐ ❐ ➢ **Compare and contrast the rashes and associated symptoms and signs of roseola and rubella.**

With roseola, a child usually develops a fever up to 40 °C (104 °F) which lasts for three to five days. The child does not look particularly ill during the symptoms, although adenopathy may be noted. As the fever falls, the child may develop a maculopapular rash which usually appears within 48 hours after the fever disappears and may last from a few hours to a few days.

Rubella (measles) usually begins with a prodrome of three to four days of fever, conjunctivitis and upper respiratory tract symptoms. The characteristic rash is also maculopapular, confluent, but distinctively begins on the face and moves down the body. Koplik's spots are diagnostic.

❐ ❐ ❐ ➢ **What is appropriate treatment for a non-immunized individual exposed to hepatitis B?**

Treat with immune globulin, specifically HBIG. Consider vaccination.

❐ ❐ ❐ ➢ **What is the most common cause of sigmoid volvulus in the elderly?**

Constipation.

❐ ❐ ❐ ➢ **The most common complications of Varicella infections in adults:**

Encephalitis, pneumonia, Staph and Strep cellulitis.

❐ ❐ ❐ ➢ **The anterior drawer test of the ankle is used to test what ligament?**

The anterior talofibular ligament.

❐ ❐ ❐ ➢ **A patient presents with a shortened, internally rotated right leg after an accident. What injury is suspected?**

Posterior hip dislocation.

❐ ❐ ❐ ➢ **Describe a mallet finger deformity.**

Mallet finger deformity is produced by forced flexion of the DIP joint when the finger is in full extension. The deformity is a result of either rupture of the distal extensor tendon, or an avulsion fraction of the tendon insertion on the distal phalanx with a dorsal plate avulsion.

❐ ❐ ❐ ➢ **The most common cause of laryngotracheitis?**

Parainfluenza virus type I.
Staph aureus is the most common bacterial pathogen.

❐ ❐ ❐ ➢ **A patient has a fracture of the proximal 1/3 ulna; what associated injury should be ruled out?**

Dislocation of the radial head. This is also known as a Monteggia fracture. Anterior dislocation is most common.

Michigan University Police Department = MUPD

MUPD = Monteggia, Ulnar fracture, Proximal Dislocation.

Little known fact, this fracture/dislocation is named after the now world-famous quarterback, Joe Monteggia who suffered this injury during a scuffle with the Michigan University PD.

❐ ❐ ❐ ➢ **A patient has an orbital floor fracture; what symptoms and signs might be seen?**

The most common symptom would be diplopia due to entrapment of the inferior rectus and inferior oblique muscles, and resultant paralysis of upward gaze. In addition, one would worry that the inferior orbital nerve could be damaged with paresthesia resulting to the lower lid, infraorbital area and side of the nose.

❐ ❐ ❐ ➢ **What gynecological infection presents with a malodorous, itchy, white to grayish sometimes frothy vaginal discharge?**

Trichomoniasis.

❐ ❐ ❐ ➢ **What are the signs of an upper motor neuron lesion?**

Upper motor neuron lesion involves the corticospinal tract. The lesion usually gives paralysis with:
1. initial loss of muscle tone and then increased tone, resulting in spasticity;
2. Babinski sign;
3. loss of superficial reflexes;
4. increased deep tendon reflexes.

A lower motor neuron lesion is associated with the anterior horn cells' axons. The lesion gives paralysis with decreased muscle tone and prompt atrophy.

❐ ❐ ❐ ➢ **What condition commonly presents with ocular bulbar deficits?**

Botulism poisoning.
Patients with myasthenia gravis may present similarly.
Diphtheria toxin may rarely produce similar deficits.

❐ ❐ ❐ ➢ **What is the best diagnostic procedure to diagnose ectopic pregnancy?**

Laparoscopy.

❐ ❐ ❐ ➢ **Describe the symptoms and signs of myasthenia gravis.**

Weakness and fatigability with ptosis, diplopia and blurred vision are the initial symptoms in 40 to 70 percent of patients. Bulbar muscle weakness is also common with dysarthria and dysphagia.

❏ ❏ ❏ ➢ **Describe the presenting symptoms of botulism poisoning.**

Botulism poisoning often presents with ocular bulbar deficits. Symmetrical descending weakness, usually with no sensory abnormalities, classically develops. Common associated symptoms include dysphagia, dry mouth, diplopia, dysarthria. Deep tendon reflexes may be decreased or absent.

❏ ❏ ❏ ➢ **Describe the signs and symptoms of Guillain-Barré disease.**

Guillain-Barré disease classically presents with symmetric weakness in the leg which ascends to include the arms or trunk. Distal weakness is usually greater than proximal. Onset rarely involves the cranial nerves.

❏ ❏ ❏ ➢ **Which nerve provides sensation to both dorsum and volar aspects of hand?**

Ulnar. Radial is primarily dorsum, and median is primarily volar.

❏ ❏ ❏ ➢ **Describe the key features of Ménière's disease, also known as endolymphatic hydrops.**

Vertigo, hearing loss and tinnitus are the hallmarks of Ménière's disease.
Ménière's disease typically presents with rapid onset of vertigo, often with associated nausea and vomiting that lasts for hours to one day. Nystagmus may be spontaneous during the critical stage. Tinnitus may be present and is louder during the attacks. Sensorineural hearing loss may be present. There may also be an aura with a sensation of fullness in the ear during the attack. Symptoms are unilateral in over 90 percent of patients, and recurring attacks are typical.

❏ ❏ ❏ ➢ **Describe the key features of benign positional vertigo.**

Violent positional vertigo is usually provoked by certain head positions or movement. Nystagmus is also always positional, of brief duration with fatigability.

❏ ❏ ❏ ➢ **What are the key features of viral labyrinthitis or vestibular neuritis?**

Vertigo is severe, usually lasting three to five days, with nausea and vomiting. Symptoms usually regress over three to six weeks. Nystagmus may be spontaneous during the severe stage.

❏ ❏ ❏ ➢ **What is a major concern in a patient that presents with unilateral Parkinsonian features?**

Intracranial tumor.

❏ ❏ ❏ ➢ **Describe the key features of acoustic neuroma.**

Symptoms and signs may include unilateral high tone sensorineural hearing loss and tinnitus. Other signs and symptoms include decreased corneal sensitivity, diplopia, headache, facial weakness and positive radiographic findings. Vertigo usually appears late, more often presenting as a progressive feeling of imbalance. Vertigo may be provoked by changes in head movement. Nystagmus is frequently present and is usually spontaneous. The CSF may have elevated protein.

❏ ❏ ❏ ➢ **Describe the key features of vertebrobasilar insufficiency.**

Vertigo is nearly always positional, provoked by certain head positions. Nystagmus usually accompanies the vertigo. Other signs of arteriosclerosis may be found. Vertebrobasilar insufficiency is usually seen in older persons and may occur with other symptoms of brainstem ischemia, visual symptoms being the most common.

❏ ❏ ❏ ➢ **What's that little bone seen behind the tympanic membrane?**

The malleus..., the malleus.

❏ ❏ ❏ ➢ **What disease would you expect in a patient with a two week history of lower limb weakness?**

Guillain-Barré is usually an ascending weakness which begins in the lower extremity. With botulism poisoning, the weakness is descending.
Cranial nerves are typically affected first with myasthenia gravis.

❏ ❏ ❏ ➢ **What is the mortality rate of Wernicke's encephalopathy?**

10-20%. Treat with thiamine IV. Symptoms include ocular palsies, nystagmus, confusion, and ataxia.

❏ ❏ ❏ ➢ **Deep tendon reflexes are usually maintained in which of the following diseases: Myasthenia gravis, Guillain-Barré or Eaton-Lambert syndrome?**

Myasthenia gravis.
Reflexes are usually depressed in Eaton-Lambert syndrome and absent in Guillain-Barré.

❏ ❏ ❏ ➢ **On IVP, what is most indicative of severe urinary tract obstruction?**

A hyperdense nephrogram. Delayed filling may also be an indicator of obstruction.

❏ ❏ ❏ ➢ **How might a patient present with a hydatidiform mole?**

Hydatidiform mole presents with a larger than expected uterus and a positive pregnancy test.

❏ ❏ ❏ ➢ **Of the major tranquilizers, which one displays the most hypotensive tendency?**

Thorazine.

❏ ❏ ❏ ➢ **What is the most common cause for pain of odontogenic origin?**

Dental caries.

❏ ❏ ❏ ➢ **What factors and substances are known to decrease theophylline metabolism and increase theophylline levels?**

Age greater than 50, prematurity, liver and renal disease, pulmonary edema, CHF, pneumonia, obesity and viral illness in children. Drugs which increase theophylline levels include cimetidine, erythromycin, allopurinol, troleandomycin, BCP's, and quinolone antibiotics.

In smokers, however, theophylline half-life is decreased, causing decreased levels of serum theophylline. In addition to smoking, phenobarbital, phenytoin, rifampin, carbamazepine, marijuana smoking and exposure to environmental pollutants can decrease serum theophylline levels. Eating charcoal broiled foods may cause lowered theophylline levels.

❏ ❏ ❏ ➢ **What narcotic has the shortest half-life?**

Fentanyl has a half-life of about one half hour.

❏ ❏ ❏ ➢ **What therapy should be used for a patient with hemophilia A who suffers a head injury?**

Treat this patient with cryoprecipitate. Keep total volume as low as possible. Cryoprecipitate has an increased concentration of factor VIII complex and has less volume than fresh frozen plasma.

❏ ❏ ❏ ➢ **What is the most serious complication of abscessed anterior maxillary teeth?**

Septic cavernous sinus thrombosis. Results from extension of infection into the canine space and facial venous system.

❏ ❏ ❏ ➢ **What is the first therapy to initiate for a bleeding patient on warfarin with a high PT?**

D/C warfarin. Then administer a water soluble form of vitamin K. Give IM, consider test dose. If the bleeding is severe, fresh frozen plasma should be given containing active factors X, IX, VII and II (REMEMBER 1972).

❏ ❏ ❏ ➢ **What is a common electrolyte abnormality associated with transfusion of packed red blood cells?**

Hypocalcemia secondary to citrate toxicity. Citrate, when rapidly infused, binds ionized calcium and therefore decreases the calcium level. Hyperkalemia may also develop with rapid packed red blood cell transfusion, especially if the patient is in renal failure or if the blood products are old.

❏ ❏ ❏ ➢ **What invasive measurement should be performed to evaluate a patient with swelling of the face, neck and arms?**

CVP. Swelling of the face, neck and arms is suggestive of superior vena cava syndrome. To confirm superior vena cava syndrome, increased CVP pressure in the upper body and normal pressure in the lower extremities must be documented. Chest x-ray will detect only about 10 percent of the masses causing superior vena cava syndrome.

❏ ❏ ❏ ➢ **Describe Leriche's syndrome.**

Leriche's syndrome is characterized by buttock, calf, and back pain with impotence. It is usually seen with aortoiliac disease.

❏ ❏ ❏ ➢ **What diagnosis should be suspected for a patient who has suffered loss of vision and whose fundus is pale?**

Central retinal artery occlusion usually presents with acute, painless loss of vision.

❏ ❏ ❏ ➢ **What is the most common cause of otitis media in children?**

Strep pneumoniae and H. influenza.

❏ ❏ ❏ ➢ **Describe a patient with sigmoid volvulus.**

Patients with sigmoid volvulus are typically either psychiatric patients or elderly who suffer from severe chronic constipation. Symptoms include intermittent cramping, lower abdominal pain and progressive abdominal distention.

❏ ❏ ❏ ➢ **Describe a typical patient with intussusception.**

Intussusception typically occurs in children of ages 3 months to 2 years. The majority are in the 5 to 10 mo age group. It is <u>more</u> <u>common</u> in boys. The area of the ileocecal valve is usually the source of the problem.

❏ ❏ ❏ ➢ **What are the common symptoms and signs of hyperthyroidism?**

Symptoms include weight loss, palpitations, dyspnea, edema, chest pain, nervousness, weakness, tremor, psychosis, diarrhea, hyperdefecation, abdominal pain, myalgias and disorientation.
Signs include fever, tachycardia, wide pulse pressure, CHF, shock, thyromegaly, tremor, weakness, liver tenderness, jaundice, stare, and hyperkinesis. Mental status changes include somnolence, obtundation, coma, or psychosis. Pretibial myxedema may be found (a <u>true</u> misnomer!)

❏ ❏ ❏ ➢ **A patient suffers a rotational knee injury and hears a pop. Within 90 minutes hemarthrosis develops. What is the suspected location of the injury?**

The anterior cruciate.

❏ ❏ ❏ ➢ **What are radiological and laboratory findings of duodenal injury?**

Retroperitoneal air and increased serum amylase.

❏ ❏ ❏ ➢ **A patient has a fracture of the radial shaft. What associated injury should be ruled out?**

Distal radius-ulna joint dislocation, also known as a Galeazzi's fracture/dislocation. <u>G</u>reat <u>R</u>ays <u>D</u>own <u>D</u>eep! = GRDD

<u>GRDD</u> = <u>G</u>aleazzi, <u>R</u>adius fracture, <u>D</u>istal <u>D</u>islocation

182

❏ ❏ ❏ ➤ **G-6-PD is the first enzyme in the hexose monophoshate shunt pathway that generates NADPH. NADPH helps maintain reduced glutathione. In G-6-PD deficiency, which affects 11% of black American males, this enzyme deteriorates with age. So?**

Glutathione serves to protect hemoglobin from injury due to oxidants. If such injury occurs, denatured Hb or hemolysis may follow.

❏ ❏ ❏ ➤ **What drugs should be avoided in G-6-PD deficiency?**

ASA, phenacetin; primaquine, quinine and quinacrine; nitrofurans; sulfamethoxazole and sulfacetamide; and methylene blue are all associated with hemolysis. These are all oxidants.

❏ ❏ ❏ ➤ **What is the current therapeutic regimen for treatment of meningitis in a neonate?**

Initially, ampicillin and aminoglycoside were favored for treating the neonate with meningitis. However, today recommendations include <u>ampicillin</u> and <u>cefotaxime</u>. A combination used in infants up to 2 months of age will cover coliform, Group B streptococci, Listeria, and enterococcus. Over 2 months of age up to 6 years, cefotaxime alone is indicated.

❏ ❏ ❏ ➤ **What is the formula for calculating a change in potassium with changes in pH?**

For each pH increase of 0.1, expect the potassium to drop by 0.5 mmol/l.

❏ ❏ ❏ ➤ **A patient has alcoholic ketoacidosis (aka AKA); what is appropriate treatment?**

Alcoholic ketoacidosis usually presents with nausea, vomiting and abdominal pain occurring 24 to 72 h after cessation of drinking. No specific physical findings are typically evident, though abdominal pain is a common complaint/finding.
AKA is thought to be secondary to increased mobilization of free fatty acids with lipolysis to acetoacetate and ß-hydroxybutyrate.

Treatment usually includes <u>normal saline</u> and glucose. As acidosis is corrected, K^+ may drop. Sodium bicarbonate should not be given unless pH drops below 7.1.

❏ ❏ ❏ ➤ **A patient presents to the emergency department and is very sick. Your diagnosis is alcoholic ketoacidosis. Urine dip is *trace* positive for ketones. Now what do you think?**

God, I <u>LOVE</u> biochemistry!! I expect urine ketones to be few to none in some patients with AKA, as the nitroprusside test (Acetest®) is the common method used to test for ketones. I recall that this test measures positive for <u>Acetoacetate</u> and is less reactive to <u>Acetone</u> and is <u>not affected</u> by ß-hydroxybutyrate. *I know that ß-hydroxybutyrate is preferentially produced in AKA,* <u>thus it is both possible and likely to obtain a negative or weakly positive test for serum ketones in the presence of clinically significant AKA.</u>

2 Acetyl Co-A

$$O=CH3$$
$$SCo\text{-}A$$

H	H$^+$ +				
HO - C - CH3	NAD$^+$ NADH	$O=CH3$	H$^+$ CO$_2$	CH3	
C		CH2		$\alpha=$ C	
C		COO$^-$		CH3	

ß-Hydroxybutyrate   **Acetoacetate**   **Acetone**

❏ ❏ ❏ ➢ **Describe the symptoms of optic neuritis.**

The patient suffers a variable loss of central visual acuity with a central scotoma and change in color perception. The patient also has eye pain. The disk margins are blurred from hemorrhage and the blind spot is increased.

❏ ❏ ❏ ➢ **Compare and contrast primary and secondary myxedema.**

Primary:	Secondary :
Source: Thyroid	Pituitary
Frequency: Common, 95%	Ø common, 5%
+ Coarse voice	Ø Coarse voice
+ Goiter	Ø Goiter
Heart Big	heart small
+ Pubic hair	Ø Pubic hair
TSH elevated	TSH low
Iodine <2µg/dl	Iodine >2µg/dl

❏ ❏ ❏ ➢ **Which renal calculi are radiolucent and which renal calculi are radiopaque?**

Uric acid stones and blood clots are radiolUcent ureteral obstructions. 90 percent of all stones are radiopaque, composed of calcium oxalate, cysteine, calcium phosphate, or magnesium ammonium phosphate.

❏ ❏ ❏ ➢ **Antidote for arsenic?**

British Anti-Lewisite (BAL) 5 mg/kg IM.

❏ ❏ ❏ ➢ **Antidote for clonidine?**

Naloxone, tolazoline, and yohimbine may help. Care is primarily supportive.

❏ ❏ ❏ ➢ **Cyanide's harmful effects are due to its propensity to bind to metals and to disrupt the function of metal containing enzymes. Which is the most important of these?**

Cytochrome A$_3$, aka cytochrome oxidase, necessary for aerobic metabolism.

❏ ❏ ❏ ➢ **Antidote for cyanide?**

Amyl nitrite followed by sodium nitrite followed by sodium thiosulfate.

❏ ❏ ❏ ➢ **Why give nitrites for cyanide?**

Theory says nitrites form methemoglobin and methemoglobin strongly binds cyanide, decreasing binding to cytochrome A_3.

❏ ❏ ❏ ➢ **Why give sodium thiosulfate for cyanide?**

Rhodanase, an intrinsic enzyme, transfers cyanide from its attachment to methemoglobin to sulfur, forming thiocyanate. Thiocyanate is excreted. Sodium thiosulfate acts as a sulfur donor for this process.

❏ ❏ ❏ ➢ **Antidote for ethylene glycol?**

Ethanol and dialysis.

❏ ❏ ❏ ➢ **Antidote for gold?**

BAL.

❏ ❏ ❏ ➢ **Antidote for iron?**

Deferoxamine.

❏ ❏ ❏ ➢ **Antidote for lead?**

Dimercaptosuccinic acid (DMSA) or calcium EDTA.

❏ ❏ ❏ ➢ **Antidote for mercury?**

BAL.

❏ ❏ ❏ ➢ **Antidote for methanol?**

Ethanol and dialysis.

❏ ❏ ❏ ➢ **Antidote for nitrites?**

Methylene blue 1% 0.2 ml/kg IV over 5 minutes.
Severe methemoglobinemia requires exchange transfusion.

❏ ❏ ❏ ➢ **Antidote for organophosphates?**

Atropine with 2-PAM as indicated.

Great quotes series:

"Fools take to themselves the respect that is given to their office." Aesop

❑ ❑ ❑ ➤ **What are the common features of organic brain syndrome?**

Onset may be at any age.
Symptoms include visual hallucinations and perception of the unfamiliar as familiar.
Signs include mental status changes such as disorientation, clouded sensorium, asterixis or mild clonus and focal neurologic signs. Vital signs are most often within normal limits.

❑ ❑ ❑ ➤ **Describe the features of functional syndromes.**

Onset is usually at age less than 40.
Symptoms include auditory hallucination and perception of the familiar as unfamiliar.
Patients are usually oriented, cognitive function is usually normal and the sensorium is usually clear. Asterixis or myoclonus is not a feature of functional disease. Vital signs are usually normal without focal neurologic deficit.

❑ ❑ ❑ ➤ **Is the stomach more commonly injured with penetrating trauma or blunt trauma?**

The stomach is more commonly injured with penetrating trauma.

❑ ❑ ❑ ➤ **What is the most common body area affected in trauma that results in death?**

The head.

❑ ❑ ❑ ➤ **What is the most common cause of airway obstruction in trauma?**

CNS depression.

❑ ❑ ❑ ➤ **What is the most common wound associated with pericardial tamponade?**

Right ventricular injury.

❑ ❑ ❑ ➤ **What are the signs and symptoms of acute pericardial tamponade?**

Triad of hypotension, elevated CVP, and tachycardia is usually indicative of either acute pericardial tamponade or a tension pneumothorax in a traumatized patient. Muffled heart tones may be auscultated.

❑ ❑ ❑ ➤ **What EKG finding is pathognomonic of pericardial tamponade?**

Total electrical alternans. Pulsus paradoxus is nonspecific. Muffled heart tones are subjective findings and are difficult to appreciate.

❑ ❑ ❑ ➤ **What is the formula for correct infusion of peritoneal lavage fluid in a child?**

10 cc/kg of lactated Ringer's solution should be infused to allow accurate interpretation

of cell counts.

❐ ❐ ❐ ➤ **Name 2 retroperitoneal organs which may be injured without producing a positive DPL.**

Pancreas and duodenum.

❐ ❐ ❐ ➤ **Name 2 organs that do not tend to bleed enough to produce a positive DPL when injured.**

Bladder and small bowel.

❐ ❐ ❐ ➤ **What RBC count is considered positive in peritoneal lavage fluid analysis of a patient with blunt abdominal trauma?**

RBC counts of more than 100,000 per mm^3 are considered positive for both penetrating and blunt trauma to the abdomen.
5,000 RBCs per mm^3 is considered positive in a patient with low chest or high abdominal penetrating trauma where diaphragmatic perforation is a possibility.

❐ ❐ ❐ ➤ **Define sensitivity and specificity.**

Sensitivity is true positives divided by true positives plus false negatives. It represents how well a test identifies people who have a condition from among all the people who have the condition.

Specificity is true negatives divided by true negatives plus false positives. It is the percentage of people who do not have the disease correctly classified as negative by the test.

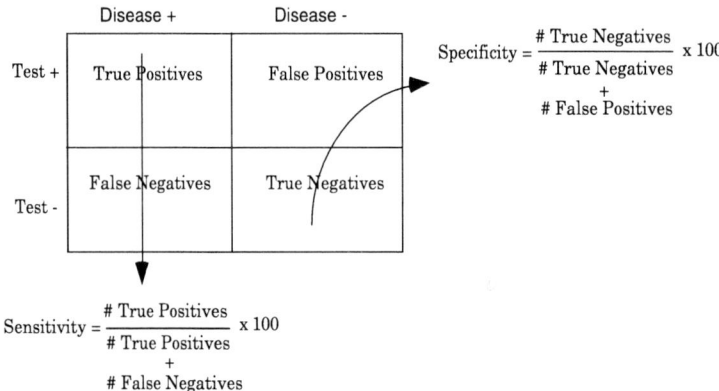

❐ ❐ ❐ ➤ **Describe the zones of the neck and the appropriate treatment for injuries to each zone.**

Zone 1 -- below the cricoid cartilage,
Zone 2 -- between the angle of the mandible and the cricoid cartilage,
Zone 3 -- above the angle of the mandible.

Treatment and evaluation:
Zones 1 and 3, angiography to evaluate major vessels.
Zone 2 requires surgical evaluation. ("2 surgery!!")

❏ ❏ ❏ ➤ **What is the cause of death secondary to untreated tension pneumothorax?**

Decreased cardiac output. The vena cava is compressed resulting in decreased right
heart blood return and concomitant severe compromise in stroke volume, blood pressure
and cardiac output.
[Editorial comment - 2° arrhythmias can also occur. V-tach in a young apparently
healthy person is 2° to a tension pneumothorax until proven otherwise. JNA]

❏ ❏ ❏ ➤ **How does a chronic pericardial effusion appear on chest x-ray?**

Gradual pericardial sac distention results in a "water bottle" appearance of the heart.

❏ ❏ ❏ ➤ **What are the symptoms and signs of adrenal insufficiency?**

Fatigue, nausea, anorexia, abdominal pain, change in bowel habits and syncope are
frequently reported symptoms.
Hyperpigmentation, hypertension, vitiligo and weight loss may be noted.
Laboratory abnormalities can include hypoglycemia, hyperkalemia, hyponatremia and
azotemia.

❏ ❏ ❏ ➤ **Treatment for myxedema coma may include:**

IV thyroid replacement with thyroxine, IV glucose, hydrocortisone and consideration of
water restriction.

❏ ❏ ❏ ➤ **What are the symptoms and signs of thyrotoxicosis?**

Weight loss and weakness may be reported.
Tachycardia and fever are common abnormal vital signs with hypotension and shock
occurring less frequently. Mental status changes of decreased consciousness or psychosis may be present. Signs of CHF, thyromegaly, tremor, eye signs including lid lag
and proptosis should also be sought.

❏ ❏ ❏ ➤ **How do patients present with central retinal artery occlusion?**

Patients present with a sudden, painless loss of vision in one eye.

❏ ❏ ❏ ➤ **Describe a patient with acute narrow angle closure glaucoma.**

Symptoms include nausea, vomiting and abdominal pain. Visual acuity is markedly
diminished.
The pupil is semi-dilated and nonreactive. There is usually a glassy haze over the
cornea and the eye is red and very painful. Intraocular pressure may be as high as 50
or 60 mmHg.

❏ ❏ ❏ ➤ **Describe the treatment of acute narrow angle glaucoma.**

Mannitol to decrease intraocular pressure.

Miotics, such as pilocarpine, to open the angle.

Carbonic anhydrase inhibitor to minimize aqueous humor production. Iridectomy is eventually performed to provide aqueous outflow.

❐ ❐ ❐ ➤ **What is the appropriate treatment for a hyphema?**

Elevate the head.

Other treatment is controversial, however, most ophthalmologists believe patients should be hospitalized. Treatment <u>may</u> include double eye patch, topical cortisone and cycloplegics. Visual acuity is often decreased.

❐ ❐ ❐ ➤ **Describe the classic symptoms and signs of retinal detachment.**

The patient is typically myopic and will complain of seeing a curtain coming down across his or her eye. This is usually accompanied by flashes of light but no discomfort. The patient may also see flashing lights, black dots, or sudden change in vision.

On funduscopic exam, the detached areas will appear gray in comparison to the normal pink retina.

Treatment includes bilateral eye patch, strict bedrest and consultation with an ophthalmologist for laser photocoagulation of the retinal detachment.

❐ ❐ ❐ ➤ **What type of streptococci cause acute post-streptococcal glomerulonephritis?**

Group A ß-hemolytic streptococci.

Physical exam may reveal facial edema and decreased urinary output that are the most common presenting findings. Urine may be dark. Laboratory findings include normochromic anemia due to hemodilution, increased sedimentation rate, numerous RBCs and WBCs in the urine with casts, and hyperkalemia. Hospitalization is advised.

❐ ❐ ❐ ➤ **Name the five major modified Jones criteria.**

Dr. Jones, the <u>EM</u> <u>P</u>hysician, is <u>SN</u>oring, she <u>C</u>an't <u>C</u>ome.

Dr. Jones, the <u>EM</u>	<u>E</u>rythema <u>M</u>arginatum
<u>P</u>hysician,	<u>P</u>olyarthritis
is <u>SN</u>oring,	<u>S</u>ubcutaneous <u>N</u>odules
she <u>C</u>an't	<u>C</u>arditis
<u>C</u>ome.	<u>C</u>h<u>o</u>rea

Other criteria include rheumatic fever or rheumatic heart disease, arthralgias, fever, prolonged PR interval on EKG, C reactive protein, elevated sedimentation rate, or antistreptolysin O titer.

❐ ❐ ❐ ➤ **What disorder is present when the five major modified Jones criteria are met?**

Rheumatic fever.

❐ ❐ ❐ ➤ **Describe the symptoms and signs of varicella (chickenpox).**

Varicella rash onset is one to two days after prodromal symptoms of slight malaise, anorexia and fever. The rash begins on the trunk and scalp. It first appears as faint macules, later becoming vesicles.

❏ ❏ ❏ ➢ **Describe the signs of roseola infantum.**

Roseola infantum usually affects children ages 6 months to 3 years. It is characterized by high fever that begins abruptly and lasts 3 to 5 days, possibly precipitating febrile seizures.   A rash appears as the temperature drops to normal.

❏ ❏ ❏ ➢ **Describe the symptoms and signs of rubella (German measles).**

Rubella begins after a mild 1 - 5 day prodrome of upper respiratory infection symptoms. A rash begins on the face and spreads quickly. Suboccipital and posterior auricular adenopathy are associated findings.

❏ ❏ ❏ ➢ **What is the standard dose of atropine in a child?**

0.02 mg/kg is the standard atropine dose.

❏ ❏ ❏ ➢ **What is the <u>most</u> <u>common</u> cause of bacterial meningitis in a child more than one month of age?**

Hemophilus influenzae.
S. pneumoniae is second most common.
N. meningitis is third most common.
This is treated with ampicillin and chloramphenicol. Single agent treatment with a third generation cephalosporin may also be used.

❏ ❏ ❏ ➢ **What is the initial dose of sodium bicarbonate in children during a cardiopulmonary arrest?**

1 mEq/kg.

❏ ❏ ❏ ➢ **How is the expected normal systolic blood pressure for a pediatric patient (toddlers and up) calculated?**

Multiply the age by 2 and add 90 to the result to determine expected systolic BP.

<u>Ave</u>rage SBP (mm Hg) = (Age x 2) + 90

<u>Low normal limit</u> SBP (mm Hg) = (Age x 2) + 70.

SBP for a term newborn is about 60 mm Hg.

❏ ❏ ❏ ➢ **How does sickle cell disease usually present in a patient older than 12 months?**

Initial symptoms are often pain in the joints, bones and abdomen. The child may have abdominal tenderness and even rigidity. Mild icterus and anemia may be present.

❏ ❏ ❏ ➢ **How does a child present with erythema infectiosum (fifth disease or slapcheek syndrome)?**

Fifth disease typically does not infect infants or adults. There are no prodromal symptoms. The illness usually begins with sudden appearance of erythema of the cheeks followed by a maculopapular rash on the trunk and extremities that evolve into a lacy pattern.

❒ ❒ ❒ ➢ **What is the correct dose of epinephrine and atropine during a pediatric code?**

Epinephrine 0.01 mg/kg/dose.
Atropine 0.02 mg/kg/dose.

❒ ❒ ❒ ➢ **What are the signs and symptoms of Kawasaki's disease?**

Kawasaki's initial presentation is with a high spiking fever, conjunctivitis, morbilliform rash, strawberry tongue, and erythema of the distal extremities with cervical adenopathy. It is a disease of the mucocutaneous lymph nodes. Patients should be hospitalized to rule out myocarditis, pericarditis and coronary aneurysms. Aspirin is therapeutic.

❒ ❒ ❒ ➢ **What is the initial antibiotic treatment for a child with epiglottitis?**

The most likely cause is H. influenzae; the child should be treated with a second or third generation cephalosporin.

❒ ❒ ❒ ➢ **What are the characteristics of a posterior hip dislocation?**

Posterior hip dislocations are typically caused by posteriorly directed force applied to the flexed knee. The extremity is shortened, internally rotated and adducted. Acetabular fractures are associated with this injury. 90% of hip dislocations are posterior.

❒ ❒ ❒ ➢ **Describe the key features of central cord syndrome.**

Central cord syndrome typically occurs with hyperextension injuries in older patients with spondylosis, degenerative changes or stenosis in the cervical spine. Symptoms include weakness that is more pronounced in the arms than the legs.

❒ ❒ ❒ ➢ **Key features of anterior spinal cord syndrome?**

The anterior cord syndrome involves compression of the anterior cord causing complete motor paralysis and loss of pain and temperature sensation distal to the lesion. Posterior columns are spared - light touch and proprioception are preserved.

❒ ❒ ❒ ➢ **What is the typical organism of a paronychia?**

Staphylococcus.

❒ ❒ ❒ ➢ **How does myasthenia gravis typically present?**

Weakness of voluntary muscles, usually the extraocular muscles.
Diagnostic confirmation relies on the edrophonium (Tensilon) test that we don't do.
Treatment includes neurologic consultation , anticholinesterases, steroids and thymectomy.

❑ ❑ ❑ ➤ **What visual deficit is typically associated with lesions at the optic chiasm?**

Optic chiasm lesions typically produce bitemporal hemianopsia.

❑ ❑ ❑ ➤ **On CT scan of the brain of an immunocompromised patient, a ring lesion is noted. The patient also has lymphadenopathy, fever, headache and confusion. What diagnosis is suspected?**

Toxoplasmosis secondary to Toxoplasma gondii cyst. The disease is typically treated with pyrimethamine and sulfadiazine.

❑ ❑ ❑ ➤ **What are the signs and symptoms of posterior inferior cerebellar artery syndrome?**

Cerebellar dysfunction such as vertigo, ataxia and dizziness.

❑ ❑ ❑ ➤ **Describe the signs and symptoms of neuroleptic malignant syndrome.**

Patients present with muscle rigidity, autonomic disturbances and acute organic brain syndrome.
Blood pressure and pulse fluctuate wildly and temperature may reach as high as 42 °C (108 °F).
Muscle necrosis may occur with resultant myoglobinuria.
Mortality ranges as high as 20%.

❑ ❑ ❑ ➤ **Describe the presentation of placenta previa.**

Placenta previa typically presents with painless bright red vaginal bleeding.

❑ ❑ ❑ ➤ **Describe the presentation of abruptio placentae.**

Dark red, painful, vaginal bleeding.

❑ ❑ ❑ ➤ **What is the <u>most</u> <u>common</u> growth plate (Salter class) injury?**

Salter II fracture.

❑ ❑ ❑ ➤ **Where is the most common site for esophageal foreign bodies to lodge?**

The cricopharyngeus muscle.

❑ ❑ ❑ ➤ **What is the <u>most</u> <u>common</u> organism causing a septic joint in a child?**

S. aureus.

❑ ❑ ❑ ➤ **What is the <u>most</u> <u>common</u> organism to cause a septic joint in an adolescent?**

Neisseria gonorrhoeae.

❑ ❑ ❑ ➤ **Signs of tension pneumothorax on physical exam include:**

Tachypnea, unilateral absent breath sounds, tachycardia, pallor, diaphoresis, cyanosis, tracheal deviation, hypotension and neck vein distention.

❏ ❏ ❏ ➢ **What is the most common cause of bacterial pneumonia, except for the first week of life?**

Streptococcus pneumoniae.

❏ ❏ ❏ ➢ **What is the most common cause of abdominal pain in children?**

Constipation.

❏ ❏ ❏ ➢ **What is the <u>most</u> <u>common</u> cause of an intestinal obstruction in a child under 2 years of age?**

Intussusception.

❏ ❏ ❏ ➢ **What is the most frequent carpal fracture.**

Navicular fracture.

❏ ❏ ❏ ➢ **What is the most frequently dislocated bone in the wrist?**

Lunate.
It is also the second most common fractured bone in the wrist.

❏ ❏ ❏ ➢ **What medications should be used to treat preeclampsia and eclampsia?**

Magnesium and hydralazine.

❏ ❏ ❏ ➢ **Do local anesthetics freely cross the blood brain barrier?**

Yes.
Most systemic toxic reactions to local anesthetics involve the CNS or cardiovascular system.

❏ ❏ ❏ ➢ **What is the <u>most</u> <u>common</u> cause of hemoptysis in the United States?**

Bronchitis and bronchiectasis.

❏ ❏ ❏ ➢ **What is the most common site of thrombophlebitis?**

The deep muscles of the calves, particularly the soleus muscle.

❏ ❏ ❏ ➢ **What is the <u>most</u> <u>common</u> cause of acute aortic regurgitation?**

Infectious endocarditis.

❐ ❐ ❐ ➣ **What are the most common causes of aortic stenosis (2)?**

Rheumatic fever and congenital bicuspid valve disease.

❐ ❐ ❐ ➣ **What is the <u>most</u> <u>common</u> cause of acute mitral regurgitation?**

Inferior wall infarcts.

❐ ❐ ❐ ➣ **What are the most common causes of pulsus paradoxus (2)?**

COPD and asthma.

❐ ❐ ❐ ➣ **What does Beck's triad consist of?**

Hypotension, elevated CVP (distended neck veins) and distant heart sounds.

❐ ❐ ❐ ➣ **What's it good for (Beck's triad that is)?**

A cute pericardial tamponade.

❐ ❐ ❐ ➣ **What is the <u>worst</u> way to confirm the diagnosis of a delayed pericardial injury after blunt trauma?**

Autopsy.

❐ ❐ ❐ ➣ **What is the <u>most</u> <u>common</u> conduction disturbance in acute myocardial infarction?**

First degree AV block.

❐ ❐ ❐ ➣ **How much fluid is needed in the pericardial sac to increase the cardiac silhouette on chest x-ray?**

About 250 ml.

❐ ❐ ❐ ➣ **What is the most common site of rupture in abdominal aortic aneurysms?**

Posterior lateral aorta.

❐ ❐ ❐ ➣ **What is the most common symptom in abdominal aortic aneurysm?**

Pain.

❐ ❐ ❐ ➣ **What is the most common dysrhythmia associated with Wolff-Parkinson-White syndrome?**

Paroxysmal atrial tachycardia.

❐ ❐ ❐ ➣ **What are the symptoms and signs of aortic stenosis?**

Exertional dyspnea, angina and syncope.
Narrowed pulse pressure with decreased SBP.
Slow carotid upstroke.
Prominent S_4.

❏ ❏ ❏ ➣ **What drugs are commonly associated with torsade de pointes?**

Type I-A antiarrhythmics - quinidine and procainamide.

These drugs lengthen the Q-T interval.

❏ ❏ ❏ ➣ **What common metabolic disorder is associated with hypercalcemia?**

Hypokalemia.

❏ ❏ ❏ ➣ **What does the urine dipstick show from a patient with myoglobinuria?**

The dipstick is "heme-positive" with few or no RBCs.

❏ ❏ ❏ ➣ **What is the <u>most</u> <u>common</u> cause of hepatitis transmitted through blood transfusions?**

Hepatitis C.

❏ ❏ ❏ ➣ **Are males or females more likely to get symptomatic gallstones?**

Females.

❏ ❏ ❏ ➣ **What is the <u>most</u> <u>common</u> type of ulcers?**

Duodenal ulcers are more commonly seen than gastric ulcers.

❏ ❏ ❏ ➣ **What is the differential diagnosis of a red eye with decreased visual acuity?**

Iritis, glaucoma and central corneal lesions.

❏ ❏ ❏ ➣ **A patient has a non-red, painful eye with decreased visual acuity. What diagnosis do you suspect?**

Optic neuritis.

❏ ❏ ❏ ➣ **What disease is associated with retrobulbar optic neuritis?**

MS.

❏ ❏ ❏ ➣ **How could mydriasis caused by third cranial nerve compression be distinguished from mydriasis caused by anticholinergic drugs or mydriatics?**

Mydriasis caused by third cranial nerve compression is reversible with pilocarpine, other causes are not.

❏ ❏ ❏ ➤ **What is the best method to open an airway while maintaining C-spine precautions?**

Jaw thrust.

❏ ❏ ❏ ➤ **What is the absolute contraindication to MAST?**

Pulmonary edema.

❏ ❏ ❏ ➤ **T/F: Increased blood pressure in hypovolemic patients associated with MAST application is primarily due to autotransfusion.**

NOT!
The primary mechanism of MAST appears to be due to increased peripheral vascular resistance. Autotransfusion of a few hundred ml of blood may occur but is not of great significance.

❏ ❏ ❏ ➤ **What is the <u>most</u> <u>common</u> complication of using an EOA?**

Tracheal intubation, 10%.

❏ ❏ ❏ ➤ **At what child's age is a cuffed ET tube preferred?**

6 y.

❏ ❏ ❏ ➤ **What is the formula for appropriate ET tube size in children greater than 1 y old?**

$$ET\ size = (Age + 16) / 4.$$

❏ ❏ ❏ ➤ **What is the correct ET tube size for a 1 - 2 y old?**

4.0 - 4.5 mm.

❏ ❏ ❏ ➤ **What is the correct ET tube size for a 6 mo old?**

3.5 - 4.5 mm.   Hey, we didn't *make up* these answers!...

❏ ❏ ❏ ➤ **What is the correct ET tube size for a newborn?**

3.0 - 3.5 mm.
Premature - 2.5 - 3.0 mm.

❏ ❏ ❏ ➤ **What is the distance from the mouth to 2 cm above the carina in men and women?**

Men 23 cm; women 21 cm.

❏ ❏ ❏ ➢ **What is an easy, if not precise, way to remember the times of HbCO half lives (based on the table shown previously)?**

> 6.0 h.
> 1.5 h.
> 0.5 h.

❏ ❏ ❏ ➢ **What is the treatment of hyperkalemia?**

Diurese with loop diuretic, e.g.., furosemide or ethacrynic acid.

Sodium polystyrene sulfonate ion exchange resin (Kayexalate) enema (associated Na load can cause failure). Hours before effect is seen.

1 ampule of D_{50}, insulin 5 to 10 units IV for redistribution (follow by 50 g glucose and 20 U insulin over 1 h). About 30 minutes for effect.

Sodium bicarbonate 50 - 100 mEq IV over 10 - 20 minutes. Five to ten minutes for effect.

Calcium. Calcium chloride has more Ca per ampule (13.4 mEq) than gluconate (4.6 mEq) and is faster acting. Give one ampule (10 ml of 10% solution) over 10 - 20 minutes. WATCH OUT if giving to a patient on digitalis, it will potentiate toxicity. Very rapid onset.

3% sodium chloride IV may serve as a temporary antagonist.

Peritoneal or hemodialysis.

Digoxin specific Fab (Digibind) if 2° to digitalis overdose.

❏ ❏ ❏ ➢ **Will you be asked a question on the above on the exam?**

Yes.

❏ ❏ ❏ ➢ **How should hypercalcemia be treated?**

Furosemide and normal saline. Mithramycin may be used, especially in hypercalcemia secondary to bone cancer. Other treatments include calcitonin, hydrocortisone, and indomethacin.

❏ ❏ ❏ ➢ **What is the <u>most</u> <u>common</u> cause of multifocal atrial tachycardia?**

COPD.

❏ ❏ ❏ ➢ **What is the treatment for multifocal atrial tachycardia?**

Treat underlying disorder.
Magnesium sulfate 2 grams over 60 seconds (with supplemental potassium to maintain serum K^+ above 4 mEq/l).
A second treatment is verapamil 10 mg IV.

❏ ❏ ❏ ➢ **What is the treatment of ectopic SVT due to digitalis toxicity?**

Stop digitalis, correct hypokalemia, consider digoxin specific Fab, magnesium IV, lidocaine IV or phenytoin IV.

❏ ❏ ❏ ➤ **What is the treatment of ectopic SVT not due to digitalis toxicity?**

Digitalis, verapamil or ß-blocker to slow rate.
Quinidine, procainamide or magnesium to decrease ectopy.

❏ ❏ ❏ ➤ **What is the treatment for verapamil-induced hypotension?**

Calcium gluconate 1 gram IV over several minutes.

❏ ❏ ❏ ➤ **What drugs are contraindicated for treatment of le torsade de pointes?**

A drug which prolongs repolarization (QT interval). For example, class Ia antiarrhythmics (quinidine, procainamide).
Other drugs that share this effect include TCAs, disopyramide, and phenothiazines.

❏ ❏ ❏ ➤ **What is the treatment of le torsade de pointes?**

Pacemaker cranked to 90 - 120 bpm to "overdrive" pace.
Isoproterenol.
Magnesium sulfate 2 grams IV.
The goal is to accelerate the heart rate and shorten ventricular repolarization. (If it's
me, start with the mag, SHP & JNA).

❏ ❏ ❏ ➤ **Discuss the treatment of digitalis toxicity.**

Charcoal.
Phenytoin (Dilantin) for ventricular arrhythmias (it increases AV node conduction) or
lidocaine.
Atropine or pace for bradyarrthymias.
Digoxin specific Fab (Digibind).

❏ ❏ ❏ ➤ **What hypos can lower the seizure threshold?**

Hypoglycemia, hyponatremia, and hypocarbia.

❏ ❏ ❏ ➤ **What are symptoms and signs of a vertebrobasilar artery lesion?**

Vertebral system supplies cerebellum and brain stem.
Vertigo, nausea, vomiting, ipsilateral 7th nerve deficit, contralateral hemiplegia.

Basilar artery occlusion leads to quadriplegia, coma or locked-in syndrome.

❏ ❏ ❏ ➤ **What motor function is spared in locked-in syndrome?**

Upward gaze.

❏ ❏ ❏ ➤ **What are signs and symptoms of a middle cerebral artery lesion?**

Hemiplegia or hemiparesthesias, homonymous hemianopsia and speech disturbance.

❏ ❏ ❏ ➤ **What is the most common cause of cerebral artery occlusion, embolic or thrombotic?**

Embolic.

❏ ❏ ❏ ➤ **What effects are likely to be present with an anterior cerebral artery lesion?**

Paralysis of contralateral leg with sensory loss in leg only and incontinence. No aphasia.

❏ ❏ ❏ ➤ **Discuss posterior cerebral artery syndrome.**

This vessel supplies occipital cortex and upper brainstem.
Hemianopsia or quadrantanopsia that patient may be unaware of, contralateral hemiparesis or hemiplegia possible but sensory loss is usually more prominent, recent memory loss (hippocampal), 3rd nerve palsy.

❏ ❏ ❏ ➤ **What deficits can result from ocular motor nerve paralysis?**

Ptosis as a result of levator palpebrae superioris/cranial nerve III injury. Lateral nerve gaze is controlled by cranial nerve VI, corneal reflex by cranial nerve V. The superior oblique muscle moves gaze downward and laterally; it is controlled by CN IV.

$$(LR_6 SO_4)_3$$

❏ ❏ ❏ ➤ **Describe the symptoms and signs of pressure on the first sacral root (S1).**

Symptoms of S1 injury include pain radiating to the mid-gluteal region, posterior thigh, posterior calf and down to the heel and sole of the foot.
Sensory signs are localized to the lateral toes. S1 root compression would typically involve the plantar flexor muscles of the foot and toes. The ankle reflex is decreased or absent.

❏ ❏ ❏ ➤ **In an infant, what is the most narrow segment of the airway?**

The cricoid cartilage ring. The glottic aperture is the most narrow part of the airway in the adult.

❏ ❏ ❏ ➤ **What is the ET tube size recommended for a term newborn infant?**

3 - 3.5 mm.
Premature infant requires a 2.5 mm tube.

❏ ❏ ❏ ➤ **What drug would you use to treat a patient in cardiac arrest secondary to hyperkalemia?**

Calcium chloride IV acts fastest.
Also provide NaHCO$_3$.

❏ ❏ ❏ ➤ **What are the potential complications of excess sodium bicarbonate?**

Cerebral acidosis, hypokalemia, hyperosmolality, and increased hemoglobin binding of oxygen.

❏ ❏ ❏ ➤ **What are the effects of dopamine at various doses?**

At 1 to 10 µg/kg, dopamine causes renal, mesenteric, coronary and cerebral vasodilation.
At 10 to 20 µg/kg, both α– and ß-adrenergic effects are present.
At 20 µg/kg, effects are primarily α–adrenergic.

❏ ❏ ❏ ➤ **What is the drug of choice for digitalis toxicity resulting in a ventricular arrhythmia?**

Phenytoin and digoxin specific Fab (Dilantin and Digibind).

❏ ❏ ❏ ➤ **What is the treatment for acute angle closure glaucoma?**

2% Pilocarpine drops every 15 minutes initially, acetazolamide (Diamox) 250 mg IV or 500 mg po, and po glycerol 1 g/kg with juice, or IV mannitol.

❏ ❏ ❏ ➤ **For each 100 increase in glucose, what is the effect on serum sodium?**

Each 100 increase in glucose decreases the serum sodium by 1.7 mEq/l.

❏ ❏ ❏ ➤ **What are common entities in the differential diagnosis of pinpoint pupils?**

Narcotic overdose, clonidine overdose, sedative hypnotic overdose including alcohol, cerebellar pontine angle infarct, and subarachnoid hemorrhage.

❏ ❏ ❏ ➤ **In a patient with tachycardia from cocaine abuse, what medications are appropriate?**

Sedation with benzodiazepines may calm the patient and decrease tachycardia.
Nitroprusside may be used to treat hypertension.
Caution must be used with ß-adrenergic antagonist agents alone as they may leave α–adrenergic stimulation unopposed, increasing the patient's risk for intracranial hemorrhage or aortic dissection.

❏ ❏ ❏ ➤ **What traditional anti-arrhythmic agents may be used to treat digitalis induced ventricular arrhythmias in addition to phenytoin?**

Lidocaine and bretylium. Procainamide and quinidine are contraindicated in digitalis toxicity.

❏ ❏ ❏ ➤ **In a trauma patient receiving multiple units of transfused blood, when should the blood products be supplemented with fresh frozen plasma?**

For each five units of transfused blood, fresh frozen plasma is usually given.

❏ ❏ ❏ ➤ **What is a complication due to citrate present in stored blood?**

Citrate may bind calcium and result in hypocalcemia.

❏ ❏ ❏ ➤ **What is an anaphylactoid reaction?**

Anaphylactoid reactions are very similar to anaphylaxis, however, they do not require prior exposure to the reaction product. Cases may result from radiopaque contrast media or medications such as NSAIDs.

❏ ❏ ❏ ➤ **A child has a mild anaphylactic reaction. What is the correct route and dose of epinephrine?**

The correct dose is 0.01 ml/kg of a 1:1,000 solution, up to 0.3 ml, SQ.

❏ ❏ ❏ ➤ **What is universal donor blood?**

Type Rh negative blood with anti-A and anti-B titers of less than 1:200 in saline.

❏ ❏ ❏ ➤ **When would orthostatic hypotension typically develop in a 70 kg adult?**

Loss of over 1000 cc of blood would probably result in orthostatic hypotension.
Class II hemorrhage (loss of 750-1500 ml) presents with tachycardia, normal BP and narrow pulse pressure.
Class III hemorrhage (loss of 1500 to 2000 ml) presents with tachycardia > 120, hypotension and decreased urine output.

❏ ❏ ❏ ➤ **What is a danger of rapid transfusion of whole blood?**

Citrate toxicity. This is more common in patients with liver failure. Signs and symptoms may include muscle tremors and prolonged QT segment which requires treatment with 10 grams of 10% calcium chloride. High citrate levels may lead to cardiac arrest if untreated.

❏ ❏ ❏ ➤ **What are the common presentations of a transfusion reaction?**

Myalgia, dyspnea, fever associated with hypocalcemia, hemolysis, allergic reactions, hyperkalemia, citrate toxicity, hypothermia, coagulopathies and altered hemoglobin function.

❏ ❏ ❏ ➤ **What are the signs of the Cushing reflex?**

Increased systolic blood pressure and bradycardia.

❏ ❏ ❏ ➤ **In the Glasgow Coma Scale a dead person gets a 3. What number of points are possible measuring eye-opening response?**

4.
(I've an eye 4 U).

❐ ❐ ❐ ➤ **What number of points is the best verbal response worth in the Glasgow Coma Scale?**

5.

❐ ❐ ❐ ➤ **What number of points is the best motor response worth in the Glasgow Coma Scale?**

6.

❐ ❐ ❐ ➤ **What are normal findings in the oculocephalic reflex?**

Conjugate eye movement is opposite to the direction of head rotation.

❐ ❐ ❐ ➤ **In testing a patient's oculovestibular reflex, what is the direction of nystagmus anticipated in response to cold-water irrigation; toward or away from the irrigated ear?**

Recall that nystagmus is <u>defined</u> as the direction of the fast component of saccadic eye movement.
Emergency physicians will commonly perform a crude but secure test of the oculovestibular reflex using ice water. After irrigation, nystagmus should be away from the irrigated ear.
Try the mnemonic COWS - <u>C</u>old <u>O</u>pposite, <u>W</u>arm <u>S</u>ame.

❐ ❐ ❐ ➤ **Signs and symptoms of an uncal herniation include:**

<u>Ipsilateral</u> <u>pupillary</u> <u>dilation</u> and either ipsilateral or contralateral hemiparesis.
Blunting of corneal reflex may occur.
Oculovestibular response may be lost.

❐ ❐ ❐ ➤ **Tonic eye movement toward irrigated ear in response to caloric testing in a comatose patient signifies.**

Life.

❐ ❐ ❐ ➤ **What effect do ß-blockers have on Prinzmetal's variant angina?**

ß-blockers typically worsen the syndrome by allowing unopposed α–adrenergic stimulation of the coronary arteries.

❐ ❐ ❐ ➤ **What are the symptoms and signs of an ophthalmoplegic migraine?**

Typical duration is 3 to 5 days. Patient may complain of diplopia.
Mydriasis and exotropia may be noted.
Palsies of the muscles served by cranial nerves III, IV and VI may occur.

❐ ❐ ❐ ➤ **Define strabismus.**

A lack of parallelism of the visual axis of the eyes.
Esotropia = medially deviated,
Exotropia = laterally deviated.

❐ ❐ ❐ ➤ **What common drugs cause bradycardia?**

Agents such as ß-blockers, cardiac glycosides, pilocarpine and cholinesterase inhibitors such as organophosphates are responsible for bradycardia.

Sympathomimetics such as amphetamines and cocaine, and anticholinergics, such as atropine and cyclic antidepressants, commonly cause tachycardia.

❐ ❐ ❐ ➤ **What drug commonly causes both horizontal and vertical nystagmus?**

Phencyclidine (PCP).

❐ ❐ ❐ ➤ **What life-threatening mnemonic may help recall of the signs of cholinergic poisoning?**

DUELS. These fighters are wet.

D   = diaphoresis,
U   = urination,
E   = eye changes (miosis),
L   = lacrimation,
S   = salivation.

❐ ❐ ❐ ➤ **What is the antidote for organophosphates?**

Atropine and pralidoxime (PAM).

❐ ❐ ❐ ➤ **How is an overdose of nitroprusside treated?**

Nitroprusside may induce methemoglobinemia. This is treated with 1% methylene blue solution.

❐ ❐ ❐ ➤ **For how long should sutures remain in the face, scalp or trunk, extremities and joints?**

Facial sutures	-3 to 5 days,
Scalp or Trunk	-7 to 10 days,
Extremities	-10 to 14 days,
Joints	-14 days.

❐ ❐ ❐ ➤ **What are the signs and symptoms of uncal herniation?**

Uncal herniation typically compresses the ipsilateral third cranial nerve resulting in ipsilateral pupil dilation. Contralateral weakness occurs because the pyramidal track decussates below this level. Occasionally, shift will be great enough to cause compression of both sides leading to a combination of ipsilateral or contralateral pupillary dilatation and weakness.

❏ ❏ ❏ ➢ **What is a common finding on sinus x-ray suggesting basilar skull fracture?**

Blood in the sphenoid sinus.

❏ ❏ ❏ ➢ **What bleeding sites are causes of subdural hemorrhages?**

Torn bridging veins.
Delayed hemorrhage from damaged parenchyma may also result in subdural hemorrhage.

❏ ❏ ❏ ➢ **In ordering x-rays of the face, what view gives the best view of the zygomatic arch?**

Modified basal view.
This is also called jug-handle, submentaloccipital or submental-vertical view.

❏ ❏ ❏ ➢ **What x-ray view should be ordered to evaluate the maxilla, maxillary sinus, orbital floor, inferior orbital rim or zygomatic bones?**

The Water's view.

❏ ❏ ❏ ➢ **How long can an extracted tooth survive?**

One percentage point of likely survivability is lost for each minute the tooth is out.
A tooth may survive 4 to 6 h longer in a commercial solution.
If no commercial solution is available place in milk or under patient's tongue.

❏ ❏ ❏ ➢ **Name five drugs or conditions that cause hypertension.**

S̲ympathomimetics
W̲ithdrawal
A̲nticholinergics
M̲AO Inhibitors
P̲hencyclidine (PCP).   Mnemonic for this is SWAMP.

❏ ❏ ❏ ➢ **Name five drugs or conditions that cause tachycardia.**

Sympathomimetics
Withdrawal
Anticholinergics
MAO Inhibitors
Phencyclidine (PCP).   SWAMP mnemonic.

❏ ❏ ❏ ➢ **Name six common drugs that can cause hyperthermia.**

S̲alicylates
A̲nticholinergics
N̲euroleptics
D̲initrophenols
S̲ympathomimetics and P̲CP.

A psychotic friend of mine (on Stelazine) with bad allergies was on the beach smoking some Jimson weed laced with PCP. She took some antihistamine for the allergies and ASA for the sunburn. She was then stung by a beach-bee and required epi, but right about then the drugs were kicking in and it took 12 beach security guards to hold her down for her shot. Boy was she HOT!
The mnemonic is SANDS-PCP.

❑ ❑ ❑ ➤ **What drugs/environmental exposures can induce bullous lesion formation?**

Sedative hypnotics, carbon monoxide, snake bite, spider bite, caustic agents, and hydro-carbons.

❑ ❑ ❑ ➤ **What drugs cause an odor of acetone on the breath?**

Ethanol, isopropanol and salicylates.
Ketosis often has the same odor.

❑ ❑ ❑ ➤ **What substances induce an odor of almonds on the breath?**

Cyanide, Laetrile, and apricot pits (latter two contain amygdalin).

❑ ❑ ❑ ➤ **What drugs induce an odor of garlic on the breath?**

DMSO, organophosphates, phosphorus, arsenic, arsine gas and thallium.

❑ ❑ ❑ ➤ **What drug induces an odor of peanuts on the breath?**

Vacor (RH-787).

❑ ❑ ❑ ➤ **What drugs induce a pear-like odor on the breath?**

Chloral hydrate and paraldehyde.

❑ ❑ ❑ ➤ **What compounds induce an odor of rotten eggs on the breath?**

Hydrogen sulfide, mercaptans and sewer-gas.

(Seen a lot of Sewer-Gas abusers in your practice?!@#?)

❑ ❑ ❑ ➤ **What is the mnemonic for remembering what drugs or conditions commonly cause seizures?**

SHAKE WITH eL SPOC!

S = salicylates,
H = hypoxia,
A = anticholinergics,
K = Karbon Monoxide (KO),
E = EtOH withdrawal,

W   = withdrawal,
I   = isoniazid,
T   = theophylline and tricyclics,
H   = hypoglycemia,

eL   = lead, lithium and local anesthetics,

S   = strychnine and sympathomimetics,
P   = PCP, phenothiazines and propoxyphene,
O   = organophosphates,
C   = camphor, cholinergics, carbon monoxide and cyanide.

❒ ❒ ❒ ➢ **What is a mnemonic for remembering the drugs that cause nystagmus?**

MALES TIP

M   = methanol,
A   = alcohol,
L   = lithium,
E   = ethylene glycol,
S   = sedative hypnotics and solvents,

T   = thiamine depletion and Tegretol (carbamazepine),
I   = isopropanol and
P   = PCP and phenytoin.

❒ ❒ ❒ ➢ **What is a mnemonic for remembering drugs that are radiopaque?**

BAT CHIPS!

B   = barium
A   = antihistamines,
T   = tricyclic antidepressants,

C   = chloral hydrate, calcium, cocaine condoms,
H   = heavy metals,
I   = iodine,
P   = phenothiazines, potassium,
S   = slow-release (enteric coated).

❒ ❒ ❒ ➢ **What is the antidote for Mercury, Arsenic and Gold (MAG) poisoning?**

BAL & Dimercaptosuccinic acid (DMSA).

Play BAL with a DMSAl named MAG!

❒ ❒ ❒ ➢ **What is the antidote for ß-blockers?**

Glucagon, likely drug of choice.

❒ ❒ ❒ ➢ **What is the antidote for ethylene glycol?**

Ethyl alcohol. Dialysis.

❏ ❏ ❏ ➢ **What three toxicologic emergencies may require immediate dialysis?**

Ethylene glycol, methyl alcohol and Amanita phalloides.

❏ ❏ ❏ ➢ **What is the antidote for iron?**

Deferoxamine.

❏ ❏ ❏ ➢ **What is the antidote for isoniazid?**

Pyridoxine.

❏ ❏ ❏ ➢ **Antidote for reversing benzodiazepine overdose?**

Flumazenil.

❏ ❏ ❏ ➢ **What is the antidote for lead?**

EDTA. EDTA is ONLY used for treating lead poisoning.
Penicillamine.
BAL.

❏ ❏ ❏ ➢ **What is the antidote for mercury?**

Penicillamine and BAL.

What is the antidote for organophosphates?

Atropine and PAM.

❏ ❏ ❏ ➢ **What is the antidote for tricyclic antidepressant overdose?**

Alkalinization.

❏ ❏ ❏ ➢ **Name some side effects of alkalization of the urine.**

Hypernatremia and hyperosmolality.

❏ ❏ ❏ ➢ **What drugs are commonly excreted using alkaline diuresis?**

BLIST

B = barbiturates (long-acting),
L = lithium (not so common),
I = INH,
T = TCAs,
S = salicylates.

❏ ❏ ❏ ➢ **What is the antidote for chronic bromide intoxication (bromism)?**

NaCl.

❏ ❏ ❏ ➢ **What drugs require immediate dialysis?**

Ethylene glycol and methyl alcohol.
Come on, you know it...yup, Amanita phalloides does too.

❏ ❏ ❏ ➢ **Can theophylline be dialyzed?**

Yes.

❏ ❏ ❏ ➢ **For what drugs may hemoperfusion be indicated?**

Salicylates, theophylline and long-acting barbiturates.

❏ ❏ ❏ ➢ **For what drugs may dialysis be indicated?**

Salicylates, theophylline and long-acting barbiturates.
Also - Methyl alcohol, ethylene glycol, amphetamine, lithium and thiocyanate.

❏ ❏ ❏ ➢ **What are the four mechanisms by which tricyclics induce toxicity?**

(1) Anticholinergic atropine-like effects 2° to competitive antagonism of acetylcholine.
(2) Block the reuptake of norepinephrine.
(3) A quinidine-like action on the myocardium.
(4) Alpha blocking action.

❏ ❏ ❏ ➢ **What are the symptoms and signs of anticholinergic effects?**

Peripheral effects include tachycardia, hyperpyrexia, mydriasis, vasodilatation, urinary retention, decreased GI motility, decreased secretions. Central effects include anxiety, disorientation, hallucinations, hyperactivity, delirium, seizures, coma and death. These patients are dry. In fact,
Dry as a bone,
Red as a beet,
Mad as a hatter,
Hot as a stone,
(Blind as a bat).

❏ ❏ ❏ ➢ **What are the four stages of acetaminophen toxicity?**

I (within h)   - anorexia, nausea, vomiting and diaphoresis.

II (24 - 48 h)   - liver function test abnormalities and right upper quadrant pain.

III (72-96 h)   - jaundice, return of GI symptoms, peak of liver function abnormalities, coagulation defects.

IV (4 d - 2 wk) - Get better or die.

❏ ❏ ❏ ➢ **When does acetaminophen become toxic?**

When there is no glutathione to detoxify its toxic intermediate.

❏ ❏ ❏ ➢ **How does N-acetylcysteine act to interrupt acetaminophen toxicity?**

Exact mechanism unknown, however, likely that NAC enters cells, and is metabolized to cysteine which is a precursor for glutathione. Thus it may increase glutathione stores.

❏ ❏ ❏ ➢ **Would you like to have FOUR <u>ACE</u>s.**

Of course! So check <u>ACE</u>tominophen level FOUR h after ingestion.

❏ ❏ ❏ ➢ **What is the early acid base disturbance seen in salicylate overdose?**

Respiratory alkalosis. Approximately 12 hours later, one might see an anion gap metabolic acidosis or mixed acid base picture.

❏ ❏ ❏ ➢ **In salicylate overdose, is hyperglycemia or hypoglycemia expected?**

This may present with either hyperglycemia or hypoglycemia.

❏ ❏ ❏ ➢ **What are common symptoms and signs of chronic salicylism?**

Fever, tachypnea, CNS alterations, acid base abnormalities, electrolyte abnormalities, chronic pain, ketonuria, and noncardiogenic pulmonary edema.

❏ ❏ ❏ ➢ **A patient presents with an acute salicylate ingestion. What symptoms are expected with a mild, a moderate and a severe overdose?**

Mild - Lethargy, vomiting, hyperventilation and hyperthermia.

Moderate - Severe hyperventilation and compensated metabolic acidosis.

Severe - Coma, seizures and uncompensated metabolic acidosis.

❏ ❏ ❏ ➢ **What is the treatment of salicylate overdose?**

Decontaminate, lavage and charcoal, fluid replacement, potassium supplementation, alkalize the urine with use of bicarbonate, cooling for hyperthermia, glucose for hypoglycemia, oxygen and PEEP for pulmonary edema, multiple dose activated charcoal, and dialysis.

❏ ❏ ❏ ➢ **A patient presents with vomiting, hematemesis, diarrhea, lethargy, coma and shock. What cause is suspected?**

Iron intoxication. Order a flat plate of the abdomen to look for concretions.

❏ ❏ ❏ ➢ **What iron level is considered toxic?**

Moderate overdose is considered to be 350 µg/dl, best measured 4 h after ingestion. The amount of <u>elemental</u> iron ingested is used in calculations. 20-40 mg elemental iron/kg is toxic.
Symptomatic patients receive treatment without waiting for lab tests.

❏ ❏ ❏ ➢ **Discuss the 4 stinking stages of iron toxicity.**

I (h) - Abdominal pain, vomiting, diarrhea, possible GI bleeding and 2° lethargy and metabolic acidosis. Due to direct corrosive effect of iron.

II (3-12 h) - GI symptoms resolve, M.D. falsely reassured.

III (>12 h) - Iron makes it into cells, blocks oxidative phosphorylation, catalyzes formation of free radicals. Cellular and organ disruption ensue with edema and venous pooling. Hepatic dysfunction, renal and cardiac failure can occur. Stage III occurs earlier in severe poisoning.

IV (days-wk) - Small bowel and gastric outlet obstruction.

❏ ❏ ❏ ➢ **What is the treatment of iron ingestion?**

If patient has ∅ symptoms ever for 6 h and is completely normal on exam, go home.

If patient has minimal symptoms and appears fine and has iron level close to maximum normal level (150 µg/dl) measured 4 h after ingestion, go home.

Cathartics for patients without diarrhea (controversial).
Hydration and treat GI hemorrhage.

Deferoxamine if:
    Moderate or severely symptomatic,
    Serum iron level > TIBC,
    Serum iron level > 350 µg/dl.

Deferoxamine is a specific agent for iron and will not chelate other metals. The IV dose of deferoxamine is 10 to 15 µg/kg/h.

❏ ❏ ❏ ➢ **What are the symptoms and signs of cyanide overdose?**

Dryness and burning in the throat, air hunger, and hyperventilation. If not removed from the toxic environment loss of consciousness, seizures, bradycardia and apnea follow prior to asystole.

❏ ❏ ❏ ➢ **What is the treatment for cyanide overdose?**

(0) Oxygen, CPR prn.
(1) Amyl nitrite perle inhaled.
(2) Sodium nitrite 10 cc of 3% solution in an adult which is 300 mg, or 0.2 - 0.33 ml/kg.
(3) Sodium thiosulfate 12.5 mg, in an adult which is 50 cc of a 25% solution or 1.0 - 1.5 ml/kg in a child (five times the volume of sodium nitrite).

Excess nitrites may require treatment with methylene blue for very, very rare case of dangerous methemoglobinemia.

❏ ❏ ❏ ➢ **What are the classic signs of PCP overdose?**

Hypertension, agitation, confusion, ataxia, vertical nystagmus, miosis, muscle rigidity, and catatonia.

❏ ❏ ❏ ➤ **What drugs can cause methemoglobinemia?**

Nitrites, local anesthetics, silver nitrate, amyl nitrite and nitrites, benzocaine, commercial marking crayons, aniline dyes, sulfonamides and phenacetin.

❏ ❏ ❏ ➤ **Atropine is used to treat:**

Organophosphate and carbamate overdose.

❏ ❏ ❏ ➤ **Pralidoxime (2-PAM) is used to treat:**

Organophosphate overdose.

❏ ❏ ❏ ➤ **Sodium chloride is used to treat:**

Chronic bromism.

❏ ❏ ❏ ➤ **Vitamin K is used to treat:**

Warfarin overdose.

❏ ❏ ❏ ➤ **Methylene blue is used to treat:**

Methemoglobinemia.

❏ ❏ ❏ ➤ **Pyridoxine is used to treat:**

Isoniazid and Gyromitra mushroom poisoning.

❏ ❏ ❏ ➤ **Name two selective cardioselective ß-blockers.**

Just remember the main cardioselective ß-blockers <u>M</u>etopralol and <u>A</u>tenolol from the mnemonic "Look <u>Ma</u>!, I'm cardioselective!"

❏ ❏ ❏ ➤ **Overdose of ß-blockers may result in:**

Nausea, vomiting, bradycardia, hypotension, respiratory depression, seizure, CHF, bronchospasm, hypoglycemia and hyperkalemia.

❏ ❏ ❏ ➤ **Evaluating a pediatric cervical spine film, what are the normal values?**

Predental space < 5 mm or < 3 mm in an adult.
The posterior cervical line attaching the base of the spinous process of C1 to C3 should be considered. If the base of C2 spinous process lies greater than 2 mm behind the posterior cervical line, a hangman's fracture should be suspected.
Anterior border of C2 to the posterior wall of the fornix distance < 7 mm.

Finally, anterior border of C6 to the posterior wall of the trachea distance would be 14 mm in children younger than 15 years of age, and less than 22 mm in an adult.

❏ ❏ ❏ ➢ **Describe a hangman's fracture.**

C2 bilateral pedicle fracture.

❏ ❏ ❏ ➢ **What are key features of a vertical compression fracture?**

Cervical and lumbar regions. Usually stable.

A Jefferson fracture of C1 may occur and is extremely unstable, although it is also very rare in occurrence.

❏ ❏ ❏ ➢ **Injury to what cervical area results in Horner's syndrome (ptosis, miosis, and anhidrosis)?**

Disruption of the cervical sympathetic chain at C7 to T2.

❏ ❏ ❏ ➢ **What spinal level corresponds with dermatomal innervation of:**
  a. Perianal region,
  b. Nipple line
  c. Index finger
  d. Knee
  e. Lateral foot.

a.	Perianal region	S2-S4
b.	Nipple line	T4
c.	Index finger	C7
d.	Knee	L4
e.	Lateral foot	S1

❏ ❏ ❏ ➢ **Describe a patient with a central cord syndrome.**

Injury to the ligamentum flavum and to the cord causing upper extremity neurologic deficit greater than lower extremity deficit.

❏ ❏ ❏ ➢ **Describe a patient with Brown-Séquard syndrome.**

Ipsilateral motor paralysis.
Ipsilateral loss of proprioception and vibratory sensation.
Contralateral loss of pain and temperature sensation.

❏ ❏ ❏ ➢ **Describe a patient with anterior cord syndrome.**

Complete motor paralysis and loss of pain and temperature sensation distal to the lesion.
Posterior column sparing results in intact proprioception and vibration sense.
Cause - occlusion of the anterior spinal artery or protrusion of fracture fragments into the anterior canal.

❏ ❏ ❏ ➤ **Under water conditions, oops. Under what conditions does trench foot or immersion foot develop?**

Trench foot occurs with exposure to wet or cold for days where the temperature is above freezing. The extremity develops superficial damage resembling partial thickness burns.

❏ ❏ ❏ ➤ **What is pernio (chilblain)?**

Chilblain refers to exposure of an extremity for a prolonged period of time to <u>dry</u> cold at temperatures above freezing. Patients develop superficial, small, painful ulcerations over chronically exposed areas. Sensitivity of the surrounding skin, erythema and pruritus may develop.

❏ ❏ ❏ ➤ **What is frost nip?**

Frost nip is the name for the condition preceding frostbite in which the skin becomes numb and blanched followed by cessation of discomfort. Sudden loss of cold sensation at the location of injury is a reliable sign of precipitant frostbite. Frost nip will proceed to frostbite if treatment is not initiated.

❏ ❏ ❏ ➤ **How is frostnip treated?**

Frostnip is the only form of frostbite which can be treated at the scene. It is treated by warming by hand, by breathing on the skin or by placing the frostnipped fingers or toes in the armpit (FUN!).
The affected part should not be rubbed. This may cause skin breakage, increases chances of infection, and does not thaw the tissues completely.

❏ ❏ ❏ ➤ **What is appropriate treatment for frostbite?**

The extremity in question should be rapidly rewarmed. Immerse in 42 °C circulating water for 20 min or until flushing is observed. <u>Dry heat should not be used</u>. Refreezing thawed tissue greatly increases damage. Remember tetanus prophylaxis.
Debride white or clear blisters as they contain toxic mediators (prostaglandin and thromboxanes). Hemorrhagic blisters should be left intact. Topical antibiotics such as silver sulfadiazine may be used. After admission, whirlpool treatments in warm antibiotic solution should be used twice per day.

Great quotes series:

“But facts are facts and flinch not.”

Robert Browning 1812-1889.

❏ ❏ ❏ ➤ **What are some common complications of frostbite?**

Rhabdomyolysis, permanent depigmentation of the extremity, and increased likelihood of subsequent cold injury.
X-ray approximately three to six months following frostbite injury reveals irregular, fine, punched out lytic lesions that may appear on the MTP, PIP and DIP joints, likely due to chronic subperiosteal inflammation.

❐ ❐ ❐ ➢ **Where do endoscopic perforations of the esophagus typically occur?**

They usually occur near the distal esophagus or at the site of pre-existing disease, such as a caustic burn.

❐ ❐ ❐ ➢ **What are the three most common sites of foreign body perforation of the esophagus?**

The levels of the cricopharyngeus muscle, the left mainstem bronchus, and the gastroesophageal junction.

❐ ❐ ❐ ➢ **What laboratory abnormalities may be anticipated in acute cyanide poisoning?**

An elevated anion gap - frequently 25 to 30 mEq/l, with lactic acidosis and decreased bicarbonate levels.

Venous PO_2 may be greater than 40 mm Hg due to decreased tissue oxygen extraction.

❐ ❐ ❐ ➢ **What is the <u>most</u> <u>common</u> site of penetrating ureteral injuries?**

Penetrating ureteral injuries typically occur in the upper one-third of the ureter.

In pelvic fractures the most common site of injury is where the ureter crosses the pelvic brim.

❐ ❐ ❐ ➢ **The most common cause of a coagulopathy in patients that require massive transfusions:**

Thrombocytopenia.

❐ ❐ ❐ ➢ **What percentage of ureteral injuries present without hematuria?**

One-third of ureteral injuries present without hematuria.

❐ ❐ ❐ ➢ **How may a posterior urethral tear be diagnosed in a male?**

High riding, boggy prostate suggests this injury.

❐ ❐ ❐ ➢ **Describe the mechanism of injury and signs & symptoms associated with an anterior urethral tear?**

Straddle or crush injury mechanism.
Severe perineal pain with blood usually found at the meatus.
Good urinary stream is maintained.

❐ ❐ ❐ ➢ **The best method of transporting an avulsed tooth?**

Under the patient's tongue. If unable, transport in milk, saline or a wet handkerchief.

❐ ❐ ❐ ➢ **What is the mechanism of a posterior urethral tear?**

Associated with pelvic fracture.
Urethral stricture, impotence and incontinence.

❏ ❏ ❏ ➤ **A patient has a pelvic fracture with suspected bladder or ureteral injury. What test should be performed first, a cystogram or an IVP?**

When a pelvic fracture is present or suspected, the cystogram is usually performed first so that distal ureteral dye from the IVP will not mimic extravasation from the bladder.

❏ ❏ ❏ ➤ **About what is the half-life of carboxyhemoglobin?**

6.0 h in 21% F_IO_2,
1.5 h in 100% F_IO_2 and
0.5 h in 3 atmospheres of hyperbaric 100% F_IO_2.

❏ ❏ ❏ ➤ **The most common cause of Ludwig's angina is:**

Odontogenic abscess of a lower molar. Most common pathogen is hemolytic strep.

❏ ❏ ❏ ➤ **The most common adverse effect of AZT:**

Granulocytopenia and anemia. Less commonly a myopathy.

❏ ❏ ❏ ➤ **Isopropyl alcohol, glycerol, or polyethylene glycol mixture is useful for treatment of what chemical burn?**

Phenol (carbolic acid).

❏ ❏ ❏ ➤ **The best means of transporting an amputated extremity:**

Wrapped in sterile gauze moistened with saline, placed in waterproof plastic bag, immersed in ice water.

❏ ❏ ❏ ➤ **What is the antidote for phosphorus poisoning?**

Copper sulfate 1% solution. Remove within 30 minutes.
Phosphorus may be identified by formation of insoluble black precipitate when swabbing with copper sulfate.

❏ ❏ ❏ ➤ **What is the dose of SQ/intradermal 10% calcium gluconate used to treat hydrofluoric acid skin burn.**

0.5 cc per cm^2 burned.

❏ ❏ ❏ ➤ **Explain the significant features of each "axis" in the DSM-III official diagnostic criteria and nomenclature for psychiatric illnesses.**

Axis I   - organic brain syndromes caused by intoxication or physical illness, and major psychiatric disorders including psychosis, affective disorders and disorders of substance use.

Axis II   - personality disorders including antisocial, schizoid and histrionic types.
Axis III   - medical problems such as heart disease and infections.
Axis IV   - life events that contribute to the patient's problems.
Axis V   - patient adaptation to these problems.

❏ ❏ ❏ ➤ **Which test is most reliable in predicting the severity of radiation exposure 48 h post exposure?**

Absolute lymphocyte count. Presence or absence of GI symptoms following near-lethal doses is a good indicator of mortality.

❏ ❏ ❏ ➤ **What local anesthetics may cause anaphylaxis?**

The ester derivatives containing para-aminobenzoic acid (PABA) are known to stimulate IgE antibody formation and cause anaphylaxis.

These include procaine and tetracaine.

❏ ❏ ❏ ➤ **What neighboring structures may be injured with a supracondylar distal humeral fracture?**

The median nerve and the brachial artery.

❏ ❏ ❏ ➤ **Which test best discriminates between functional and organic blindness?**

Optokinetic nystagmus.

❏ ❏ ❏ ➤ **What is the most common carpal fracture?**

Scaphoid (navicular); the more proximal the fracture, the more likely to develop avascular necrosis.

❏ ❏ ❏ ➤ **How may a lunate dislocation be diagnosed?**

Lateral view x-ray - the lunate appears dorsal or volar to its usual position within the radial fossa.

❏ ❏ ❏ ➤ **The most common ligament injured after an inversion ankle sprain?**

Anterior talo-fibular ligament.

❏ ❏ ❏ ➤ **How may a perilunate dislocation be diagnosed?**

AP and lateral x-ray - the lunate remains in alignment with the radial fossa and the other carpal bones appear displaced.

❏ ❏ ❏ ➤ **What is the cause of lymphogranuloma venereum?**

Chlamydia trachomatis.
Painful unilateral suppurative nodes may present with sinus tract.

216

Sx: Transient <u>ULCER</u> <u>IS</u> <u>PAINLESS.</u>
Dx: Compliment fixation.
Rx: Tetracycline, erythromycin, doxycycline.

❏ ❏ ❏ ➤ **What is the cause of granuloma inguinale?**

The bacterium Donovania granulomatis, recently renamed Calymmatobacterium granulomatis.

Dx: Bright, beefy-red, granulomatous lesions. Confirm diagnosis with finding of intracytoplasmic bacilli in macrophages (Donovan bodies).
Rx: Streptomycin, tetracycline, erythromycin, chloramphenicol, TMP/SMX.

❏ ❏ ❏ ➤ **The best diluent in solid lye ingestion is:**

Milk.

❏ ❏ ❏ ➤ **What is the cause of condylomata acuminata?**

Papova virus.

❏ ❏ ❏ ➤ **Incidence of trauma among elderly is less than, equal to, or greater than that of the general population?**

Equal.

❏ ❏ ❏ ➤ **What is the mechanism of injury responsible for the greatest portion of injuries in the elderly?**

Falls. Most falls are caused by tripping but other medical causes underlying the initial fall should always be sought.

❏ ❏ ❏ ➤ **The organ most severely affected in a blast injury:**

The lungs.

❏ ❏ ❏ ➤ **The organ most commonly affected in a blast injury:**

The ears.

❏ ❏ ❏ ➤ **A patient has previous focal deficits from CVA's. Is it true that such a patient may present with confusion when having suffered a new focal lesion.**

Yes. The presentation of a new focal lesion may be with generalized or non-focal symptoms in the context of previous insults.

❏ ❏ ❏ ➤ **A patient with a dementia gets a wound infection. Is it true that such a patient may present with a severe decrease in mental status.**

Yes. Normally minor insults may cause drastic changes in neurologic functioning in those with pre-existing deficits.

❏ ❏ ❏ ➢ **The most common cause of extrauterine surgical emergencies in pregnancy:**

Appendicitis.

❏ ❏ ❏ ➢ **A patient had right arm and hand paralysis from a previous CVA. That deficit is mostly compensated with only residual weakness remaining.   Should that patient subsequently have an episode of hyponatremia, can the presentation be with a right arm and hand paralysis?**

Sure. Formerly compensated deficits may return in response to a generalized neurological insult.

❏ ❏ ❏ ➢ **Red blood cell basophilic stippling is seen in what two disorders?**

Thalassemia and lead poisoning.

Zebe alert!

❏ ❏ ❏ ➢ **What triad is associated with Reiter's syndrome?**

Non-gonococcal urethritis, polyarthritis and conjunctivitis.
The conjunctivitis is the least common and is seen in only 30 percent of patients. Acute attacks respond well to NSAIDs.

❏ ❏ ❏ ➢ **What is the most common cause of immediate postpartum hemorrhage?**

Uterine atony followed by vaginal/cervical lacerations, and retained placenta or placental fragments.

❏ ❏ ❏ ➢ **What complications of rheumatoid arthritis require emergency treatment?**

Vasculitis. This should be promptly treated with systemic steroids, otherwise irreversible neuropathy may occur.

❏ ❏ ❏ ➢ **What is Felty's syndrome?**

Rheumatoid arthritis with splenomegaly and neutropenia. It is a late complication of rheumatoid arthritis.

❏ ❏ ❏ ➢ **What drugs are commonly known to induce a lupus reaction?**

Procainamide, hydralazine, isoniazid and phenytoin.

❏ ❏ ❏ ➢ **What is the most serious complication of dental infections, aside from possible respiratory compromise in Ludwig's angina?**

Septic cavernous sinus thrombosis.

❏ ❏ ❏ ➢ **What joint is <u>most</u> <u>common</u>ly affected with pseudogout?**

The knee. The causative agent is calcium pyrophosphate crystals.

❐ ❐ ❐ ➢ **What joint is <u>most</u> <u>commonly</u> affected with gout?**

The great toe MCP joint.

❐ ❐ ❐ ➢ **What are the complications of impetigo?**

Streptococcal induced impetigo can result in post-streptococcal glomerulonephritis.
<u>It has not been shown to be associated with rheumatic fever.</u>
Tx: erythromycin, dicloxacillin, cephalexin to help eliminate the skin lesions.
There is not clear proof that treatment prevents glomerulonephritis.

❐ ❐ ❐ ➢ **What are the clinical features of rubella (German measles)?**

Malaise, fever, headache, generalized lymphadenopathy, particularly the suboccipital
and the posterior auricular nodes, with a pinkish maculopapular rash that first appears
on the face.

❐ ❐ ❐ ➢ **How does measles (Rubeola) typically present?**

Fever, coryza and conjunctivitis. Pathognomonic Koplik's spots appear 2-4 d later on
the buccal mucosa followed by the spreading maculopapular rash starting on the forehead and upper neck radiating to truck and extremities.

❐ ❐ ❐ ➢ **The most common early manifestation of a significant radiation exposure is:**

Nausea and vomiting.

❐ ❐ ❐ ➢ **How does roseola infantum appear?**

Roseola is typified by a high fever for three to four days, followed by a macular or maculopapular rash that is profuse on the chest and abdomen and mild on face and extremities. Patient feels well with rash.

❐ ❐ ❐ ➢ **Describe the key features of the rash of Rocky Mountain Spotted Fever.**

Rocky Mountain Spotted Fever is caused by Rickettsia rickettsii and is transmitted by
Ixodidae ticks.
Patients get sick, with high fever, headache, chills and muscular pain. On about the 4th
d of fever, the rash begins on the wrists and ankles. The spread of rash is centripetal.

❐ ❐ ❐ ➢ **The most effective dermal decontaminate following radiation exposure:**

Wash with soap and water after removal of all clothes.

❐ ❐ ❐ ➢ **Describe the rash of scarlet fever.**

Sandpaper type texture rash beginning on the face, neck, chest, abdomen and spreads to
extremities. Patients may have strawberry tongue.

❏ ❏ ❏ ➢ **What is the most likely cause of unilateral transient loss of vision in a patient's eye (amaurosis fugax)?**

Carotid artery disease. This is usually the result of platelet emboli from plaques in the arterial system.

❏ ❏ ❏ ➢ **Syncope is a characteristic symptom of what valvular disease?**

Aortic stenosis.

❏ ❏ ❏ ➢ **What valvular lesion is most likely to cause syncope?**

Aortic stenosis.

❏ ❏ ❏ ➢ **The most common cause of a transudative pleural effusion?**

Congestive heart failure.

❏ ❏ ❏ ➢ **How does Landry-Guillain-Barré present?**

Presentation in the third to fourth decade of a rapidly progressive ascending transverse myelitis. Weakness begins in lower extremities. Bulbar musculature may eventually be involved.
Decrease or loss of DTRs is relatively specific for this disorder, though tick paralysis and Diphtheria neurotoxin can share this feature.

❏ ❏ ❏ ➢ **How does a patient present with Eaton-Lambert Syndrome?**

Proximal weakness with aching muscles especially in the lower extremities. Cranial nerve involvement is very rare.   Patients often have a dry mouth.
Unlike myasthenia gravis, which gets worse with activity, with E-L grip strength improves. There is no response to edrophonium test.

❏ ❏ ❏ ➢ **How is an acute hemorrhagic overdose of Coumadin best treated?**

Fresh frozen plasma, Vit K IM will help prevent subsequent hemorrhage.

❏ ❏ ❏ ➢ **Where does botulism toxin exert its effects?**

At the myoneural junction. It prevents the release of acetylcholine.

❏ ❏ ❏ ➢ **How does botulism present?**

Neurologic systems begin 24 - 48 hours after ingestion of contaminated foods. May start with nausea, vomiting or diarrhea.
Most common early neurologic complaints are related to the eye and bulbar musculature. Symptoms involve all muscles of the trunk and extremities. Intestinal and bladder involvement may include ileus and acute urinary retention.

❏ ❏ ❏ ➢ **Describe a patient with tick paralysis.**

A rapid progressive ascending paralysis that develops over one to two days. First systems occur in the extremities and trunk and move to bulbar musculature. It is almost identical to Guillain-Barré Syndrome.

❑ ❑ ❑ ➢ **Patient's with sickle cell trait most commonly present with:**

Hematuria and decreased urine concentrating ability.

❑ ❑ ❑ ➢ **Differentiate diphtheria with neurologic sequelae from toxicity due to botulism.**

Diphtheria vs. botulism - Diphtheria is an acute <u>febrile</u> illness with pseudomembranous oropharyngitis and cardiac involvement.

❑ ❑ ❑ ➢ **Differentiate neurologic sequela of botulism toxicity from neurologic deficits of Guillain-Barré syndrome.**

G-B is an ascending transverse myelitis. It does not begin with bulbar musculature.

❑ ❑ ❑ ➢ **How does infant botulism present?**

The usual source is raw honey. (Honey abusers, huh! We know your type...)
Presentation with lethargy, failure to thrive, progresses to paralysis and death.

❑ ❑ ❑ ➢ **What is the pathophysiology of myasthenia gravis?**

Circulatory antibody against ACh receptor which binds at the motor end plate. In myasthenics, ACh receptors are in short supply resulting in fatigable weakness.

❑ ❑ ❑ ➢ **What is the most serious transfusion reaction?**

Hemolytic. Treat with aggressive fluid replacement and Lasix.

❑ ❑ ❑ ➢ **What is the most common transfusion reaction?**

Febrile.

❑ ❑ ❑ ➢ **What diseases are associated with myasthenia gravis?**

Rheumatoid arthritis, pernicious anemia, SLE, sarcoidosis and thyroiditis. 10 - 25% have associated thymoma.

❑ ❑ ❑ ➢ **How does myasthenia gravis present?**

Muscular weakness with fatigability. Strength improves after resting. First muscles involved are usually the extraocular muscles (other bulbar muscles *may* present earlier). The first symptom is either diplopia or eyelid ptosis. Bright light may increase ptosis and diplopia and heat may increase muscle weakness. Proximal muscles are typically weakest. Respiratory muscle involvement can be life-threatening.

❏ ❏ ❏ ➢ **A patient presents with ocular, bulbar and limb weakness which gets worse during the day and decreases with resting - diagnosis?**

Myasthenia gravis.

❏ ❏ ❏ ➢ **The best emergent treatment of an Ellis III dental fracture in an adult:**

Cover tooth with moist cotton then dry aluminum foil, and refer immediately to an orthodontist.

❏ ❏ ❏ ➢ **What are some factors commonly associated with meningitis?**

Age less than 5 years or greater than 60 years, low socioeconomic status, male sex, crowding, black race, sickle cell disease, splenectomy, alcoholism, diabetes and cirrhosis, immunologic defects, dural defect from congenital, surgical or traumatic source, contiguous infections such as sinusitis, household contacts, malignancy, bacterial endocarditis, intravenous drug abuse and thalassemia major.

❏ ❏ ❏ ➢ **A patient has xanthochromic CSF with a low protein count. What is the most likely cause?**

Subarachnoid hemorrhage.

❏ ❏ ❏ ➢ **A patient has xanthochromic CSF with a high protein count (greater than 150 mg/dl). What is the most likely cause?**

Traumatic tap.

❏ ❏ ❏ ➢ **What disease is associated with periaqueductal petechial hemorrhages?**

Wernicke's disease.

❏ ❏ ❏ ➢ **What disorders are associated with cerebrocortical neuronal degeneration?**

Anoxic, hypoglycemic and hepatic encephalopathies.

❏ ❏ ❏ ➢ **What is the <u>most</u> <u>commonly</u> abused volatile substance?**

Toluene.

❏ ❏ ❏ ➢ **A patient presents with hypokalemia of 2.0, hyperchloremia and acidosis. What is the most likely toxicologic cause?**

Chronic toluene abuse.

❏ ❏ ❏ ➢ **A patient has been abusing nitrous oxide for a long time. What symptoms might be expected?**

Paresthesias and motor weakness may be present in chronic abusers. Such symptoms are often mistaken for symptoms of multiple sclerosis.

❏ ❏ ❏ ➤ **Describe the features of each of the three stages of PCP intoxication.**

Stage I - agitated or violent, normal vital signs.
Stage II - tachycardia, hypertension and unresponsive to pain.
Stage III - unresponsive, depressed respirations, seizures and death.

❏ ❏ ❏ ➤ **Should the urine be acidified in the treatment of PCP intoxication?**

Although acidification of the urine is theoretically advantageous, clinical experience has not shown this to be efficacious. Let's call that a "no."

❏ ❏ ❏ ➤ **Explain how methylene blue functions as an antidote for methemoglobinemia.**

A normal level of 3% methemoglobin is usually maintained by a NADPH - dependent enzyme. This enzyme capacity can be exceeded with oxidant poisoning.
Methylene blue enhances NADPH - dependent hemoglobin reduction by acting as a co-factor.
Methylene blue is usually only needed for MetHb levels > 30%; its dose is 1-2 mg/kg IV over 5 min.

❏ ❏ ❏ ➤ **A patient presents with belladonna alkaloid poisoning resulting in anticholinergic effects. Explain the dangers of treating this patient with physostigmine.**

Physostigmine acts to increase the acetylcholine levels. Doing so, it can precipitate a cholinergic crisis resulting in heart block and asystole. As a result, it is recommended to reserve physostigmine for life threatening anticholinergic complications.

Heart block and asystole.

❏ ❏ ❏ ➤ **Does botulism produce fever?**

No. This can be important in differentiating neurologic symptoms in a sick patient who could have diphtheria.

❏ ❏ ❏ ➤ **Describe a patient with Chlamydial pneumonia.**

Chlamydial pneumonia is usually seen in children 2 to 6 wk of age. The patient is afebrile. Patients do not appear toxic.

❏ ❏ ❏ ➤ **A patient has had three days of diarrhea which was abrupt in onset. The patient reports slimy green, malodorous stools that contain blood. In addition, the patient is febrile. What is the most likely cause?**

Salmonella.

❏ ❏ ❏ ➤ **Drug treatment for Campylobacter?**

Erythromycin or tetracycline.

❏ ❏ ❏ ➢ **In a child, does coarctation of the aorta typically cause cyanosis?**

No.

❏ ❏ ❏ ➢ **How much elemental iron will 100 mg of deferoxamine bind?**

About 8.5 mg of elemental iron is bound by 100 mg of deferoxamine.

❏ ❏ ❏ ➢ **Drug treatment for persistent Escherichia coli?**

Trimethoprim with sulfamethoxazole (TMP/SMX).

❏ ❏ ❏ ➢ **Drug treatment for Giardia lamblia?**

Quinacrine or metronidazole or furazolidone.

❏ ❏ ❏ ➢ **Drug treatment for persistent Salmonella?**

Ampicillin.
TMP/SMX.
Chloramphenicol.

❏ ❏ ❏ ➢ **Drug treatment for Shigella?**

TMP/SMX or Ciprofloxacin (if resistant).

❏ ❏ ❏ ➢ **Drug treatment for Yersinia?**

TMP/SMX.
Tetracycline.
3rd generation cephalosporin.

❏ ❏ ❏ ➢ **What are the 8 common clinical presentations of pediatric heart disease?**

Cyanosis, pathologic murmur, abnormal pulses, CHF, HTN, cardiogenic shock, syncope and tachyarrhythmias.

❏ ❏ ❏ ➢ **Complications of the use of sodium bicarbonate in severe metabolic acidosis include:**

Hypernatremia, paradoxical CSF acidosis, decreased oxygen unloading at the tissue level, hyperosmolality, dysrhythmias and hypokalemia.

❏ ❏ ❏ ➢ **What is the function of aldosterone?**

Aldosterone causes sodium conservation and K^+ excretion.
As a result, it causes increased resorption of sodium and fluid.

❏ ❏ ❏ ➢ **What drug will most rapidly decrease K^+?**

Calcium chloride IV (1 - 3 minutes).

❐ ❐ ❐ ➢ **What is a potential side effect of the use of Kayexalate?**

Kayexalate exchanges sodium for K⁺. As a result, sodium overload and CHF may occur.

❐ ❐ ❐ ➢ **What is Addison's disease?**

Deficiency or absence of mineralocorticoid (aldosterone). This results in increased sodium excretion. Potassium is retained. The urine cannot concentrate.

This can lead to severe dehydration, hypotension and circulatory collapse.

Deficiency of cortisol (also produced in the adrenal cortex) leads to metabolic disturbances, weakness, hypoglycemia and deceased resistance to infection.

❐ ❐ ❐ ➢ **What metabolic conditions will potentiate the toxic cardiac effects of digoxin?**

Hypokalemia and hypercalcemia.

❐ ❐ ❐ ➢ **What is the initial treatment for hypercalcemia?**

Saline and furosemide.
Then, if you've not yet sent the patient to the floor, calcitonin, mithramycin, hydrocortisone, and indomethacin.

❐ ❐ ❐ ➢ **What conditions lead to hypocalcemia?**

Shock, impaired production, pancreatitis, hypomagnesemia, alkalosis, decreased serum albumin, hypoparathyroidism, osteoblastic mets, and fat embolism syndrome.

❐ ❐ ❐ ➢ **What vital sign might be affected with hypermagnesemia?**

Hypermagnesemia causes hypotension because it relaxes vascular smooth muscle. Deep tendon reflexes may disappear.

❐ ❐ ❐ ➢ **What is the immediate treatment of thyroid storm?**

1st	-Draw blood for Free T4 index and free T3 and cortisol levels.
2nd	-Supportive care (avoid aspirin - it may increase free T3 and T4).
3rd	-IV glucocorticoids - 300 mg hydrocortisone per day.
4th	-Inhibit thyroid hormone synthesis - propylthiouracil 900-1200 mg or methimazole 90 - 120 mg.
5th	-Retard thyroid hormone release (iodine 1g q 8 hours IV).
6th	-Block peripheral thyroid hormone effects (propranolol 1 mg q 1 min. to total of 10 mg.

❐ ❐ ❐ ➢ **How is myxedema coma treated?**

IV thyroxine 400 - 500 mg infused slowly, then 50 - 100 mg every day. Caution, lower dose of thyroxine if cardiac ischemia or arrhythmias are present.

❏ ❏ ❏ ➤ **Common causes of hypercalcemia:**

PAM P SCHMIDT.

P   = Parathormone
A   = Addison's
M   = Multiple Myeloma

P   = Paget's

S   = Sarcoidosis
C   = Cancer
H   = Hyperthyroidism
M   = Milk - alkali Syndrome
I   = Immobilization
D   = Vitamin D Excess
T   = Thiazides

❏ ❏ ❏ ➤ **What is the treatment for adrenal crisis?**

100 mg hydrocortisone (Solu-cortef) IV bolus and 100 mg hydrocortisone added to IV solution. Then, 200 mg hydrocortisone q 6 h for 24 hours.

(Refer to your preferred text for discussion of simultaneous testing and treatment with dexamethasone and corticotropin instead).

❏ ❏ ❏ ➤ **What are the signs and symptoms of Wernicke's encephalopathy?**

Oculomotor disturbances are common, usually with nystagmus and ocular palsies. Abnormal mentation and ataxia may be present. Ophthalmoplegias and nystagmus usually respond to thiamine, however, mental changes are often irreversible.

❏ ❏ ❏ ➤ **When does alcoholic ketoacidosis commonly occur?**

It usually occurs in chronic alcoholics after an interval of binge drinking followed by one to three days of protracted vomiting, abstinence and decreased food intake.

❏ ❏ ❏ ➤ **ECG changes associated with tricyclic antidepressant overdose?**

Prolongation of the PR, QRS and QT interval, as well as conduction defects such as bundle branch block, typically on the right.

❏ ❏ ❏ ➤ **What is the treatment for TCA overdose?**

<u>Seizures</u>
    Alkalinization
    Diazepam
    Phenytoin
    Phenobarbital

<u>Tachycardia</u>
    Alkalinization by hyperventilation.

Blocks and Ventricular Arrhythmias
    Alkalinization by hyperventilation.
    Sodium bicarb
    Phenytoin (Unproven)
    Lidocaine (Unstudied)

Hypotension
    Alkalinization by hyperventilation.
    Fluids
    Sodium Bicarbonate
    Pressors: Epi, NE, Dopamine
    Digitalis (Unstudied)
    Physostigmine (in extremis)
    Charcoal hemoperfusion
    Cardiopulmonary bypass

❒ ❒ ❒ ➤ **What drugs should be avoided in treatment of TCA overdose?**

Absolute - Procainamide. Also quinidine, disopyramide, and ß-blockers.

Relative - Corticosteroids, dopamine, isoproterenol, low dose dobutamine, bretylium, amiodarone, encainide and flecainide.

❒ ❒ ❒ ➤ **What dose of ASA will cause mild to moderate toxicity?**

200 - 300 mg/kg. Greater than 500 mg/kg is potentially lethal.

❒ ❒ ❒ ➤ **What is the ferric chloride test and what toxic ingestion does it detect?**

Add a few drops of 10% ferric chloride solution to a few drops of urine. Violet purple color indicates presence of salicylic acid. Ketones or phenothiazines can lead to false positive results.

❒ ❒ ❒ ➤ **What is the treatment of lithium overdose?**

Saline diuresis and hemodialysis.

❒ ❒ ❒ ➤ **What is the treatment for chloral hydrate overdose?**

Hemodialysis and/or charcoal hemoperfusion will clear the active metabolite, trichloroethanol.

❒ ❒ ❒ ➤ **What are the common effects of barbiturate overdose?**

Hypothermia, hyperventilation, venodilation with hypotension and negative inotropic effect on the myocardium. Clear vesicles and bullae may also be seen.

❒ ❒ ❒ ➤ **What is the pediatric dose of naloxone?**

0.01 mg/kg to a dose of 0.8 mg, may repeat.

❐ ❐ ❐ ➢ **What electrolyte abnormality is commonly seen in salicylate toxicity?**

Hypokalemia.

❐ ❐ ❐ ➢ **What is the treatment for acetaminophen overdose?**

Charcoal, cathartics and N-acetylcysteine.

The other day I was playing poker with Tarot cards. I got a full house and 4 people died!

❐ ❐ ❐ ➢ **What electrolyte abnormality may mimic the signs and symptoms of hypocalcemia?**

Hypomagnesemia.

❐ ❐ ❐ ➢ **What are some key signs and symptoms of Thrombotic Thrombocytopenic Purpura (TTP).**

Thrombocytopenia, purpura, microangiopathic hemolytic anemia.
Presents with fever, fluctuating neurologic signs and renal complications. Untreated, the disease is almost uniformly fatal. Therapy includes steroids, splenectomy, plasmapheresis and exchange, and antiplatelet agents such as dipyridamole and aspirin.

❐ ❐ ❐ ➢ **How does a patient present with Boerhaave's syndrome?**

Boerhaave's syndrome is spontaneous esophageal perforation. It usually occurs after forceful vomiting. The patient suffers an acute collapse, chest and abdominal pain. A left pleural effusion is seen in 90 percent of patients on chest x-ray and most have mediastinal emphysema.

❐ ❐ ❐ ➢ **In what type of a patient is Staphylococcal pneumonia likely?**

Hospitalized, debilitated and drug abusing patients.

❐ ❐ ❐ ➢ **How low does the platelet count drop before spontaneous bleeding occurs .**

Below 50,000 per cubic millimeter spontaneous bleeding may occur.
CNS bleeds usually do not occur until counts drop below 10,000 per cubic millimeter.

❐ ❐ ❐ ➢ **What factors affect the prothrombin time (PT)? Which pathway is this?**

I, II, V, VII, and X. 125710.
Extrinsic.
PT is normal in hemophilia.
A normal PTT and increased PT suggests warfarin therapy, vitamin K deficiency, or liver disease.

❐ ❐ ❐ ➢ **What factors affect the partial thromboplastin time (PTT)? Which pathway is affected?**

VIII, IX, or XI. 8911.
Intrinsic.
Heparin increases PTT.

❏ ❏ ❏ ➤ **What affect will heparin or warfarin overdose have on the PT and PTT?**

Both cause increases in PT and PTT in excessive doses.

❏ ❏ ❏ ➤ **What are the five key lab findings in DIC?**

Increased PT, PTT, and fibrin degradation products.
Decreased fibrinogen and platelet levels.

❏ ❏ ❏ ➤ **In the thrombocytopenic patient, one unit of platelets will raise the platelet count by about how much?**

One unit raises the platelet count by $\approx$10,000 / mm^3.

❏ ❏ ❏ ➤ **What are the classic findings of shaken baby syndrome?**

Failure to thrive, lethargy.
Seizures.
Retinal hemorrhages.
CT may show subarachnoid hemorrhage or subdural hematoma from torn bridging veins.

❏ ❏ ❏ ➤ **Define spondylolysis.**

Spondylolysis is a defect in the pars interarticularis.

❏ ❏ ❏ ➤ **Define spondylolisthesis.**

Spondylolisthesis is forward movement of one vertebral body on the vertebra below it.

❏ ❏ ❏ ➤ **Define spondylosis.**

Spondylosis is degenerative change in the vertebrae which may also include osteophyte formation at the disk spaces.

❏ ❏ ❏ ➤ **T/F - High fever in neonates with bacterial pneumonia usually <u>follows</u> a period of general fussiness and decreased feeding.**

True.

❏ ❏ ❏ ➤ **Chlamydia pneumonia is more likely to occur in the neonate after how many weeks of age?**

Three weeks.

❏ ❏ ❏ ➤ **Conjunctivitis is an associated finding in about what percentage of neonates**

with Chlamydia pneumonia?

About 50%.

❑ ❑ ❑ ➢ **Neonates with Chlamydia pneumonia are usually tachypneic with a bad cough; are they febrile?**

Usually not.

❑ ❑ ❑ ➢ **What is the immediate treatment for cord prolapse?**

Displace the head cephalad.

❑ ❑ ❑ ➢ **What is the most common bacterium causing septic arthritis of the hip?**

Staphylococcus aureus.

❑ ❑ ❑ ➢ **What nerve may be injured in a distal femoral fracture?**

Peroneal nerve.

❑ ❑ ❑ ➢ **What is French Toast during the Renaissance?**

Something you can order at a place that advertises "Breakfast Anytime."

❑ ❑ ❑ ➢ **Newborns should stop losing weight by how many days after birth?**

About 6 days.

❑ ❑ ❑ ➢ **T/F - Stool color of neonates can be an important sign.**

False; with the exception of presence of blood, stool color is insignificant.

❑ ❑ ❑ ➢ **What is the difference between vomiting and regurgitation?**

Very little once it's on you!
Vomiting follows from forceful diaphragmatic and abdominal muscle contraction.
Regurgitation occurs without effort.

❑ ❑ ❑ ➢ **Is regurgitation dangerous in an otherwise thriving neonate?**

No.
It can be dangerous for newborns with failure to thrive or respiratory problems and it may be associated with chronic aspiration.

❑ ❑ ❑ ➢ **Projectile vomiting in the neonate is often associated with pyloric stenosis. When this is the case, such vomiting becomes a prominent sign after how many weeks of age?**

About two to three weeks.

❏ ❏ ❏ ➤ **What is the name for diarrhea associated with sepsis, otitis media, UTI or other systemic disease?**

Parenteral diarrhea.

❏ ❏ ❏ ➤ **Infectious diarrhea is most commonly viral. What are the two <u>most</u> <u>common</u> viruses?**

Rotavirus and Norwalkvirus.

❏ ❏ ❏ ➤ **T/F - Bacterial and parasitic etiologies of diarrhea in the neonate are rare.**

True.

❏ ❏ ❏ ➤ **What are some entities in the differential diagnosis of bloody diarrhea in the neonate?**

Necrotizing enterocolitis, bacterial enteritis, iatrogenic causes secondary to antibiotics, milk allergy.

❏ ❏ ❏ ➤ **Neonates with necrotizing enterocolitis are sick; what are some of the signs of sepsis to look for?**

Poor feeding, lethargy, fever, jaundice, abdominal distention, and poor color.

❏ ❏ ❏ ➤ **What should be considered in the case of a neonate who has never passed stool?**

Meconium ileus or plug, Hirschsprung's disease, intestinal stenosis or atresia.

❏ ❏ ❏ ➤ **Anal stenosis, hypothyroidism and Hirschsprung's disease can all present with what clinical sign?**

Constipation that was not initially present but which had onset prior to one month of age.

❏ ❏ ❏ ➤ **Describe the signs and symptoms, and x-ray tests, for diagnosing a slipped capital femoral epiphysis.**

Hip pain with restriction of internal rotation.
X-ray analysis should include anterior views of both hips and lateral views taken in a frogleg position.

❏ ❏ ❏ ➤ **Describe the signs and symptoms of a patient with chondromalacia patellae.**

Chondromalacia patellae typically occurs in young, active females.
The pain is localized to the knee. There is no effusion and no history of trauma.
Patella compression test is usually positive.

❏ ❏ ❏ ➤ **Describe the signs and symptoms of tarsal tunnel syndrome.**

Insidious onset of paresthesia, burning pain and numbness on the plantar surface of the foot. Pain radiates superiorly along the medial side of the calf. Rest decreases pain.

❏ ❏ ❏ ➢ **What is the cause of swimmer's itch (Schistosome dermatitis)?**

An invading cercariae.

❏ ❏ ❏ ➢ **Vector of malaria?**

Anopheles mosquito.

❏ ❏ ❏ ➢ **Insect vector of trypanosomiasis?**

Tsetse fly.

❏ ❏ ❏ ➢ **Infectious agent of elephantiasis?**

Nematode microfilaria.

❏ ❏ ❏ ➢ **What is the vector that transmits Chagas' disease (Trypanosoma Cruzi)?**

Reduviid (Assassin or kissing bug).

❏ ❏ ❏ ➢ **Cysticercosis is associated with:**

New onset seizure.

❏ ❏ ❏ ➢ **Hookworm is associated with what sort of anemia?**

Iron deficiency anemia.

❏ ❏ ❏ ➢ **Fish tapeworm (Diphyllobothrium latum) is associated with:**

Pernicious anemia.

❏ ❏ ❏ ➢ **Onchocerciasis (from Onchocerca volvalas) is associated with what visual deficit?**

Blindness.

❏ ❏ ❏ ➢ **Chagas' disease is associated with:**

Acute myocarditis. Trypanosoma Cruzi invades the myocardium resulting in myocarditis. Conduction defects may occur.

❏ ❏ ❏ ➢ **Roundworm is associated with:**

Small bowel obstruction.

❐ ❐ ❐ ➢ **Describe the presentation of a patient with post-extraction alveolitis:**

Pain of "dry socket" occurs on the 2nd or 3rd day after extraction.

❐ ❐ ❐ ➢ **Ludwig's angina typically involves what spaces in the head?**

The submental, the sublingual and submandibular spaces.

❐ ❐ ❐ ➢ **What are the signs and symptoms of a peritonsillar abscess?**

Sore throat, dysarthria (hot potato voice), odynophagia, ipsilateral otalgia, low grade fever, trismus, and uvular displacement.

❐ ❐ ❐ ➢ **What is the presentation of a patient with diphtheria?**

Sore throat, dysphagia, fever and tachycardia. A dirty tough gray fibrinous membrane that may be so firmly adherent that removal causes bleeding may be present in the oropharynx.
Corynebacterium diphtheriae exotoxin acts directly on cardiac, renal and nervous systems. Sure, it can cause ocular bulbar paralysis that may suggest botulism or, perhaps, myasthenia gravis.
The exotoxin may also cause flaccid limb weakness. Of note, such weakness may also include decreased or absent DTRs, a finding usually suggestive of Guillain-Barré or of tick paralysis (Dermacentor andersoni neurotoxin).

❐ ❐ ❐ ➢ **How does a patient present with a retropharyngeal abscess?**

Patients typically prefer a supine position. Retropharyngeal abscesses are common under 3 years of age. On examination, the uvula and tonsil are displaced away from the abscess. Soft tissue swelling and forward displacement of the larynx are present. Soft tissue x-ray films of the neck may assist in the diagnosis.

❐ ❐ ❐ ➢ **How does an adult with epiglottitis present?**

Pharyngitis and dysphagia are prominent symptoms. Adenopathy is uncommon. The patient may have a muffled voice and speak softly; hoarseness is rare. Pharyngitis is present and pain is out of proportion to objective findings.

❐ ❐ ❐ ➢ **What are the two most common pathogens in adult acute sinusitis?**

Streptococcus pneumoniae and Hemophilus influenzae.

❐ ❐ ❐ ➢ **What is rhinocerebral phycomycosis?**

Rhinocerebral phycomycosis, also known as mucormycosis, is a fungal infection typically seen in diabetic patients while in ketoacidosis, and in immunocompromised patients. The disease is rapidly fatal if not recognized and treated quickly. Treatment includes antifungal drugs and surgical debridement.

❐ ❐ ❐ ➢ **Where is the typical location of a Mallory-Weiss tear?**

The laceration typically occurs in the cardioesophageal region in the stomach, below the gastroesophageal junction. The bleeding usually stops spontaneously and does not typically require surgery. It can be diagnosed by endoscopy. It is associated with hiatal hernia.

❑ ❑ ❑ ➢ **Magnesium containing antacids may cause:**

Diarrhea.

❑ ❑ ❑ ➢ **Aluminum containing antacids may cause:**

Constipation.

❑ ❑ ❑ ➢ **What is the treatment for hepatic encephalopathy?**

Lactulose and poor per rectum neomycin.

❑ ❑ ❑ ➢ **When does an elevation of HBsAg occur in relation to symptoms of Hepatitis B?**

HBsAg always rises before clinical symptoms of hepatitis B.

❑ ❑ ❑ ➢ **Is hepatitis A associated with jaundice?**

Typically not, as more than 50 percent of the population have serologic evidence for hepatitis and do not recall being symptomatic.

❑ ❑ ❑ ➢ **Describe a patient with intussusception.**

Patients with intussusception are most likely very young. 70 percent occur within the first year of life. In children, the cause is thought to be secondary to lymphoid tissue at the ileocecal valve, whereas in adults, it is thought to be caused by local lesions, Meckel's diverticulum, or tumor. On exam, bowel sounds are usually normal. Intussusception typically involves the terminal ileum. Meckel's diverticulum is the single most common intrinsic bowel lesion involved.

❑ ❑ ❑ ➢ **Are adhesions a common cause of bowel obstruction in the large bowel?**

No. They are very common in the small bowel, but do not be fooled; they are extremely uncommon in large bowel obstructions.

❑ ❑ ❑ ➢ **Should salmonella be treated?**

Only if symptomatic infection persists. Treat with ampicillin, TMP/SMX, or chloramphenicol.

❑ ❑ ❑ ➢ **What is the most common cause of acute food-borne disease?**

Staph aureus and the enterotoxins it produces.

❏ ❏ ❏ ➤ **What are the common features of Vibrio parahaemolyticus?**

Organism associated with oysters, clams and crabs.
Symptoms include cramps, vomiting, dysentery and explosive diarrhea. Severe infections are treated with tetracycline and chloramphenicol.

❏ ❏ ❏ ➤ **What types of anorectal abscesses can be drained in the emergency department?**

Perianal, submucosal, and pilonidal abscesses can be drained in the emergency department.
Ischiorectal and supralevator abscesses need to be drained in the operating room.

❏ ❏ ❏ ➤ **Painful, bright red rectal bleeding is most often due to:**

Anal fissure.
External hemorrhoids present with acute painful thrombosis and are not typically associated with constant, bright red bleeding.
Internal hemorrhoids present with <u>painless</u> bright red bleeding, usually with defecation.

❏ ❏ ❏ ➤ **Where is the narrowest part of the ureter?**

The ureterovesicular junction.

❏ ❏ ❏ ➤ **What percentage of kidney stones are radiopaque?**

90 percent. Most are made of calcium oxalate.

❏ ❏ ❏ ➤ **In a patient with acute testicular pain, relief of pain with elevation of the scrotum (Prehn's sign) is classically associated with:**

Epididymitis.

❏ ❏ ❏ ➤ **Drug of choice for treating urinary tract infection due to Proteus mirabilis?**

Ampicillin. This is common in young boys.

❏ ❏ ❏ ➤ **Most common organism causing epididymitis in a 20 year old?**

Chlamydia trachomatis.

❏ ❏ ❏ ➤ **How should hydralazine be dosed for a preeclamptic patient?**

Hydralazine is given in 5 mg boluses every 20 minutes until adequate BP control is achieved or a total of 20 mg is reached.

❏ ❏ ❏ ➤ **What is the antidote of overdose of magnesium sulfate?**

Calcium gluconate infusion.

❐ ❐ ❐ ➢ **In an ectopic pregnancy, is an adnexal mass a common finding?**

No. An adnexal mass is actually found in less than 50 percent of cases. Abdominal pain is the most frequent sign. Amenorrhea is the second most common sign.

❐ ❐ ❐ ➢ **As pCO_2 increases, pH will decrease. By how much is the pH expected to decrease for every 10 mm Hg increase in pCO_2?**

pH decreases by 0.08 units for each increase of 10 mm of pCO_2.

❐ ❐ ❐ ➢ **How much protamine is required to neutralize 100 units of heparin?**

1 mg of protamine will neutralize ≈ 100 units of heparin. The maximum dose of protamine is 100 mg.

❐ ❐ ❐ ➢ **What is the <u>most common</u> symptom of a PE?**

Chest Pain (88%)
Dyspnea (84%)

❐ ❐ ❐ ➢ **What is the <u>most common</u> sign of a PE?**

Tachypnea (92%)
Rales (58%)

❐ ❐ ❐ ➢ **What is the <u>most common</u> radiographic finding of a PE?**

An elevated hemidiaphragm (41%).

❐ ❐ ❐ ➢ **What is the <u>most common</u> ECG finding of a PE?**

T-wave inversion (42%)

❐ ❐ ❐ ➢ **Of patients with a PE, what percentage have a normal ECG?**

Normal (13%).

❐ ❐ ❐ ➢ **Of patients with a PE, what percentage of ECG's show the classic $S_1 Q_3 T_3$ pattern?**

$S_1 Q_3 T_3$ (12%), incidence is 18% with massive PE

❐ ❐ ❐ ➢ **What test is most sensitive for evaluating a PE?**

Perfusion scan is the <u>most sensitive</u> test, even more so than a pulmonary angiogram. Unfortunately, it is not a specific test, as 5 percent of normal volunteers will have an abnormal scan, and virtually any pulmonary pathology will produce an abnormal scan.

❏ ❏ ❏ ➢ **What organisms are most commonly present in a pulmonary abscess?**

Mixed anaerobes.

❏ ❏ ❏ ➢ **What are some causes of thoracic outlet syndrome?**

Compression of the subclavian artery by an anomalous cervical rib, compression of the neurovascular bundle as it passes through the interscalene triangle, and compression of the neurovascular bundle in the retroclavicular space anterior to the first rib when the arms are hyperabducted. Symptoms are typically produced when the shoulders are moved backward and downward.

The <u>most</u> <u>common</u> cause is a cervical rib.

❏ ❏ ❏ ➢ **What is the <u>most</u> <u>common</u> cause of endocarditis in IV drug abusers?**

Staphylococcus aureus, most commonly involving the tricuspid valve.

❏ ❏ ❏ ➢ **What are the classic signs and symptoms of aortic stenosis?**

Left heart failure, angina and exertional syncope.

❏ ❏ ❏ ➢ **What patient position will enhance the murmur of mitral stenosis?**

Left lateral decubitus.

❏ ❏ ❏ ➢ **What is optimal patient position and maneuver for auscultation of aortic insufficiency?**

Have the patient sit up and lean forward with the hands tightly clasped. During exhalation, listen at the left sternal border.

❏ ❏ ❏ ➢ **What murmurs will the Valsalva maneuver increase?**

Only IHSS. All other murmurs are diminished.

❏ ❏ ❏ ➢ **What is the most common valvular disorder in the United States?**

Mitral valve prolapse.

❏ ❏ ❏ ➢ **What is the most common cause of endocarditis in late onset prosthetic valve endocarditis?**

Streptococcus viridans.

❏ ❏ ❏ ➢ **Symptoms of endocarditis?**

Fever, chills, malaise, anorexia, weight loss, back pain, myalgia, arthralgia, chest pain, dyspnea, edema, headache, stiff neck, mental status changes, focal neurologic complaints, extremity pain, paresthesia, hematuria and abdominal pain.

❏ ❏ ❏ ➢ **Key physical finding of "malignant" hypertension?**

Papilledema.

❏ ❏ ❏ ➢ **Key diagnostic features of coarctation of the aorta?**

Rib notching seen on x-ray. Significant differences in the blood pressure between the upper and lower extremities.

❏ ❏ ❏ ➢ **What is an interesting diagnostic feature of aortic regurgitation?**

Head bobbing.

❏ ❏ ❏ ➢ **What is the most common arrhythmia associated with digitalis?**

PVC (60%).
Ectopic SVT (25%).
AV Block (20%).

❏ ❏ ❏ ➢ **What effect does furosemide have on calcium excretion?**

Furosemide causes increased calcium excretion in the urine.

❏ ❏ ❏ ➢ **What is the <u>most</u> <u>common</u> arrhythmia in mitral stenosis?**

Atrial fibrillation.

❏ ❏ ❏ ➢ **The <u>most</u> <u>common</u> cause of CHF in an adult is:**

Hypertension.

❏ ❏ ❏ ➢ **What is the differential diagnosis of pulmonary edema with a normal size heart?**

Constrictive pericarditis, massive MI, non-cardiogenic pulmonary edema, and mitral stenosis (not mitral regurgitation).

❏ ❏ ❏ ➢ **How does dobutamine differ from dopamine?**

Dobutamine decreases afterload with less tendency to cause tachycardia.

❏ ❏ ❏ ➢ **Describe Kerley A and Kerley B lines.**

Kerley A lines are straight, non-branching lines in the upper lung fields.

Kerley B lines are horizontal, non-branching lines at the periphery of the lower lung fields.

❏ ❏ ❏ ➢ **Does nifedipine typically effect preload or afterload?**

Nifedipine is a vasodilator whose primary effects are on afterload reduction.

❏ ❏ ❏ ➢ **What effect does the Valsalva maneuver have on the heart?**

Valsalva decreases blood return to both the right and left ventricles. All murmurs decrease in intensity except IHSS.

❏ ❏ ❏ ➢ **Does prednisone cross the placenta?**

No. Prednisone is metabolized through prednisolone which does not cross the placenta.

❏ ❏ ❏ ➢ **You see a patient with a severe high concentration burn of hydrofluoric acid burn. How do you treat this patient?**

In addition to topical jelly and cutaneous injections of calcium gluconate, provide IV treatment with 10 cc. of 10% Calcium Gluconate (not calcium chloride) diluted in 50 cc. of D_5W. This is given via a pump over 4 h.

❏ ❏ ❏ ➢ **How should an ocular burn secondary to hydrofluoric acid be treated?**

Use calcium gluconate in a 1% solution mixed with saline and irrigate the eyes with this solution. The solution is made by diluting one part of standard 10% calcium gluconate solution with ten parts of saline which produces a 1% solution.

❏ ❏ ❏ ➢ **What electrolyte is depleted in a victim of a hydrofluoric acid burn?**

Hydrofluoric acid results in <u>hypocalcemia</u>. Patients may require calcium replacement. Keep in mind that normal signs and symptoms of hypocalcemia such as Chvostek's sign do not typically appear with hypocalcemia secondary to HF.

❏ ❏ ❏ ➢ **A 35 y old female presents with altered mental status and a temperature of 105 °F. The patient's muscles are rigid and she feels very hot in the trunk but her extremities are cool. What diagnosis is likely?**

Neuroleptic malignant syndrome. High fever and muscle rigidity should make you suspect a diagnosis of neuroleptic malignant syndrome. Check the CPK.

❏ ❏ ❏ ➢ **How should a patient with neuroleptic malignant syndrome be treated?**

1) Ice packs to the groin and axilla.
2) Cooling blankets.
3) Fan.
4) Alcohol evaporation.
5) Dantrolene at an IV rate of 0.8 to 3 mg/kg IV q 6 hours to a total of 10 mg/kg.

❏ ❏ ❏ ➢ **How should a patient with a black widow spider bite be treated?**

1) Antivenin.
2) IV calcium gluconate.
3) IV opiates plus IV benzodiazepines.

❐ ❐ ❐ ➢ **T/F - Centruroides scorpion antivenin should be considered for all Centruroides envenomations.**

NOT. False, false.
Scorpion antivenin is rarely necessary and is only typically used in children who have a severe (Grade IV) envenomation with peripheral motor and cranial nerve involvement. It is most important to use Centruroides antivenin only in severe cases as serum sickness or rash after administration is very common. In fact, as many as 60% of patients develop a rash or serum sickness secondary to this antivenin.

❐ ❐ ❐ ➢ **What is a significant complication of scorpion envenomation?**

Rhabdomyolysis.

❐ ❐ ❐ ➢ **In what states could a scorpion bite be deadly?**

Centruroides, which is the most toxic of scorpion stings, is only found in <u>Arizona</u>, California, Texas and New Mexico.

❐ ❐ ❐ ➢ **An elderly patient presents with the complaint of seeing halos around lights. What diagnosis is suspected?**

Glaucoma. Another presenting complaint of glaucoma is blurred vision. Also, consider digitalis toxicity.

❐ ❐ ❐ ➢ **A patient presents with back pain and complaints of incontinence. On exam, loss of anal reflex, and decreased sphincter tone is noted. What is your diagnosis?**

Cauda equina syndrome. The most consistent finding with cauda equina syndrome is <u>urinary retention</u>. On physical exam, expect saddle anesthesia, that is, numbness over the posterior superior thighs as well as numbness of the buttocks and perineum.

❐ ❐ ❐ ➢ **What is the most common site of lumbar disc herniations?**

98% of clinically important lumbar disc herniations are at the L4-5 or L5-S1 intervertebral levels.

Evaluate by checking for weakness of ankle and great toe dorsiflexors (L5). Also check pinprick sensation over the medial aspect of the foot (L5) and the lateral portion of the feet (S1).

❐ ❐ ❐ ➢ **What WBC count is expected during pregnancy?**

WBC counts of 15,000 to 20,000 are considered normal in pregnancy.

❐ ❐ ❐ ➢ **A trauma patient has a closed head injury with suspected elevated intracranial pressure. What treatments should be considered?**

1) Paralyze the patient and hyperventilate.
2) Maintain hypovolemia (fluid restrict).
3) Elevate the head of the bed to 30 degrees after the C-spine has been cleared.
4) Consider mannitol 500 ml. of a 20% solution over 20 minutes for a 70 kilogram adult.

Use of diuretics like furosemide is controversial. Steroids are no longer recommended. Barbiturate use is also not recommended. Mannitol use is also losing favor.

❏ ❏ ❏ ➢ **When monitoring a pregnant female trauma victim, which vital signs are more appropriate to follow - the mother's or those of the fetus?**

It is probably best to consider monitoring the fetal heart rate since it is more sensitive to inadequate resuscitation. Remember that the mother may lose 10 to 20% of her blood volume without change in vital signs whereas the baby's heart rate may increase or decrease above 160 or below 120 indicating significant fetal distress.

❏ ❏ ❏ ➢ **What two findings on physical exam are indicative of uterine rupture?**

Loss of uterine contour and palpable fetal part.

❏ ❏ ❏ ➢ **What physical exam findings may be discovered in abruptio placenta?**

Rapidly increasing fundal height secondary to bleeding into the uterus or a higher than expected fundal height.

❏ ❏ ❏ ➢ **What is the <u>number one</u> risk factor for uterine rupture?**

Previous cesarean section.

❏ ❏ ❏ ➢ **How should a diagnostic peritoneal lavage be performed for a pregnant patient?**

Use an open supraumbilical approach. Always make sure an NG tube and Foley are in place.

❏ ❏ ❏ ➢ **A gravid woman is sent to the OB floor for cardiotocographic monitoring after a motor vehicle accident. What findings will suggest problems with the fetus.**

On the OB floor, they will look for uterine contractions at a rate of greater than 8 per minute. They will also watch for late decelerations. Late deceleration are a slowing of the fetal heart rate near the end of a contraction.

❏ ❏ ❏ ➢ **An unconscious, 60 y old patient presents to the ED with a head injury. An ECG shows significant ST segment elevation. What is your concern?**

Although MI should be considered, don't forget the possibility of an intracerebral hemorrhage. This may also cause significant ST segment elevation.

❏ ❏ ❏ ➢ **Why should the use of atropine be considered in a pediatric patient prior to intubation?**

Many pediatric patients develop bradycardia associated with intubation. This can be prevented by pre-treatment with atropine (dose is 0.01 mg/kg).

❏ ❏ ❏ ➢ **What size tracheotomy tube is appropriate for an adult female and for an adult male?**

An adult female generally requires #4 tracheostomy tube and an adult male requires a #5.

❒ ❒ ❒ ➤ **After use of ketamine in a pediatric patient, what effects are expected?**

The child will have eyes wide open with a glassy stare, nystagmus, hyperemic flush and hypersalivation. There will also be a slight rise in the heart rate. A very rare complication of ketamine use is laryngospasm. Hallucinations are a common side-effect in children over the age of 10; as a consequence, ketamine should be restricted to use only in patients under the age of 10.

Ketamine may also cause sympathetic stimulation which increases intracranial pressure, and may cause random movements of the head and extremities. It is thus not a good sedative for children going to CT scan.

❒ ❒ ❒ ➤ **Contraindications to TAC?**

Mucus membranes, burns, and large abrasions. TAC used on the tongue and mucus membranes has led to status epilepticus and patient death.

❒ ❒ ❒ ➤ **Why are quinolones contraindicated in children?**

Quinolones impair cartilage growth.

❒ ❒ ❒ ➤ **A patient presents with a symmetric weakness which has been progressive over several days to weeks and has associated paresthesia. Diminished reflexes are noted. Diagnosis?**

Guillain-Barré syndrome. Other signs and symptoms are diminished reflexes, minimal loss of sensation, paresthesias, and leg weakness.

❒ ❒ ❒ ➤ **How is Guillain-Barré syndrome diagnosed in the ED?**

Suspect the diagnosis based on signs and symptoms, but confirmation requires nerve conduction studies performed as an inpatient.

❒ ❒ ❒ ➤ **What is the dose of acyclovir (Zovirax) used to treat herpes zoster infections in an immunocompetent adult?**

800 mg. po. five times per day for 7 to 10 days.
For herpes simplex genitalis, the dose is much lower, 200 mg. p.o. five times a day for ten days!

❒ ❒ ❒ ➤ **A patient is brought to the ED after exposure to ammonia gas. What are your chief concerns?**

Ammonia gas affects the upper respiratory tract and may cause significant laryngeal and tracheal edema. Administer warm humidified O_2 to soothe the bronchial tract. Bronchodilators may also be given by nebulization for bronchospasm. Be ready to intubate if severe upper airway edema occurs.

❑ ❑ ❑ ➢ **What signs and symptoms would lead to consideration of hyperbaric oxygen treatment for a patient with CO poisoning?**

History of, or current, unconsciousness, arrhythmia or ischemia, neurologic impairment greater than a mild headache, and/or a carboxyhemoglobin level over 40%.

6.0, 1.5, 0.5.

❑ ❑ ❑ ➢ **What are the indications for giving digitalis specific Fab?**

Ventricular arrhythmias.
$K^+ > 5.5$ mEq/L.
Unresponsive bradyarrhythmias.

Some authors refer to an ingestion of more than 0.3 mg/kg as requiring Fab (Digibind). The dose of Fab is:

    # vials required = 1.33 x mg ingested,

or use formula to determine dose based on serum digoxin level,
or give 10 vials (40 mg Fab each) if amount ingested is not known.

Adolescents and children have an even higher sensitivity to the serious complications of digoxin overdose and may need Fab therapy with ingestion of less than the recommended level of 0.3 mg. per kilogram.

Remember - in an acute overdose situation, the serum level of digitalis is unreliable in evaluating toxicity. Digitalis levels typically only become accurate after 4 to 6 hours; this is too long to wait for treatment.

❑ ❑ ❑ ➢ **You give digoxin specific antibody (Fab) to a digoxin-toxic patient with an elevated digoxin level. A repeat digoxin level is obtained after this treatment and it is much <u>higher</u> than the previous level! What gives? Didn't the Fab work?**

Digoxin assay measures free <u>and</u> bound digoxin, the latter increases ≈ 15 x via binding to Fab.

❑ ❑ ❑ ➢ **What electrolyte change is expected with a serious digoxin ingestion?**

Expect hyperkalemia. After Fab, potassium level may drop quickly and the patient may become hypokalemic. Monitor carefully.

❑ ❑ ❑ ➢ **A near drowning victim is comatose and intubated with a diagnosis of severe pulmonary edema. What specific pulmonary treatment should be provided in the Emergency Department?**

It is important to give these patients PEEP early. PEEP will decrease intrapulmonary shunting and prevent terminal airway closure.

Great quotes series:

"Victory at all costs, victory in spite of all terror, victory however long and hard the road may be; for without victory there is no survival."

Sir Winston Leonard Churchill, Speech, House of Commons, 13 May, 1940.

❐ ❐ ❐ ➣ **There are four types of hypersensitivity reactions. Name them in order:**

Hypersensitivity Reaction	Mediator	Example
Type 1 - Immediate	IgE binds allergen, includes mast cells and basophils	Food allergy. **Asthma in children.**
Type 2 - Cytotoxic	IgG & IgM antibody reactions to antigen on cell surface activates complement and killers	Blood transfusion rxn. ITP, hemolytic anemia. The least common rxn.
Type 3 - Immune complex, Arthrus	Complexes activate complement	Tetanus toxoid in sensitized persons. **Poststreptococcal glomerulonephritis.**
Type 4 - Cell mediated, delayed hypersensitivity	Activated T-lymphocytes	Skin tests

❐ ❐ ❐ ➣ **What distinguishes heat stroke from heat exhaustion?**

Heat exhaustion is progressive loss of electrolytes and body fluid depletion. Therapy is rehydration.

Heat stroke occurs when temperatures are above 42 °C and enzyme systems cease to function normally. As a result, there is necrosis, denaturing, and organ failure. Heat stroke requires much more aggressive treatment than simple fluid rehydration.

Remember - in patients with an altered sensorium and a core temperature above 42 °C, always suspect heat stroke. Half of patients will be diaphoretic.

❐ ❐ ❐ ➣ **What lab abnormalities may be found with heat stroke?**

High elevations in SGOT, SGPT and LDH.

❐ ❐ ❐ ➣ **How should a patient with heat stroke be treated?**

1) Cool the patient with lukewarm water and fans.
2) Pack the axillae, neck and groin with ice.
3) Give fluids cautiously as large boluses of fluids may precipitate pulmonary edema.
4) Treat shivering with chlorpromazine (Thorazine) 25 to 50 mg IV.

❐ ❐ ❐ ➣ **What complications can result from heat stroke?**

Renal failure, rhabdomyolysis, DIC, and seizures. Remember antipyretics will not help.

❐ ❐ ❐ ➢ **You are currently working locum tenens in <u>Arizona</u>, California, Texas and Mexico. As these states will have the deadly Centruroides scorpion, you are particularly concerned with scorpion sting treatment. How should a scorpion sting be treated?**

A scorpion sting should be treated with local ice compresses, analgesics, and perhaps antidote.

Patients who have extremity jerking, blurred vision, slurred speech, or hypersalivation probably will require antivenin as this represents a Grade IV envenomation with peripheral motor and cranial nerve involvement.

❐ ❐ ❐ ➢ **Describe the appearance of a black widow spider bite?**

Two tiny red marks with surrounding erythematous patch. The initial bite may be painless. If a "pinprick" type bite is followed by abdominal cramps, think of a black widow spider.

Exam reveals abdominal rigidity without true tenderness. Patients are restless and move about the gurney.

Antivenin should probably be given to patients who are pregnant, younger than 16 and older than 65, and symptomatic. It also should be given to patients with underlying cardiac disease.

Other treatments include calcium, diazepam (Valium), or methocarbamol (Robaxin). Traditional treatment also includes calcium gluconate.

❐ ❐ ❐ ➢ **What conditions may make the end tidal CO_2 monitor inaccurate?**

Monitor may be falsely yellow due to contamination from acid dilutants and drugs such as lidocaine-HCl and epinephrine-HCl. Contamination with vomitus or acid dilutants may produce false readings.

❐ ❐ ❐ ➢ **You are having a hard time remembering which anesthetics are amides and which anesthetics are esters. What is a fairly easy way of telling these two classifications of anesthetics apart?**

The word amide has an "i" in it and so do the am"i"des.

> Lidocaine (Xylocaine).
> Bupivacaine (Marcaine).
> Mepivacaine (Carbocaine).

> Esters on the other hand have no "i",
> Procaine (Novocain)
> Cocaine
> Tetracaine (Pontocaine)
> Benzocaine.

So remember - those with i's are amides. (In the first syllable only, the caines don't count! Thanks Pat!)

❐ ❐ ❐ ➢ **An elderly patient presents with sudden onset of severe abdominal pain followed by a forceful bowel movement. Diagnosis?**

Acute mesenteric ischemia. Keep in mind that abdominal series may be normal early in acute mesenteric ischemia. Possible late x-ray findings include:

Absent bowel gas, ileus, gas in the intestinal wall and thumb-printing of the intestinal

mucosa.
In most cases, films are normal or not specifically suggestive. Expect heme-positive stools. Patients especially prone to mesenteric ischemia include those with CHF and chronic heart disease.

❏ ❏ ❏ ➢ **Under what conditions does neurogenic pulmonary edema occur?**

Neurogenic pulmonary edema is commonly associated with increased intracranial pressure. It is commonly seen with head trauma, subarachnoid hemorrhage, and even with seizures.

❏ ❏ ❏ ➢ **A patient had a very severe headache two days ago. The headache is now subsiding and physical exam is normal. Should the possibility of a subarachnoid hemorrhage be evaluated, and if so, how?**

Yes. CT.
However, a significant percentage of scans will be negative 48 hours after intracranial hemorrhage.
LP done 2 to 3 days after a bleed should still be positive and xanthochromia typically persists for 7 to 10 days.

❏ ❏ ❏ ➢ **What are the classic signs and symptoms of adrenal insufficiency?**

Fatigue, weakness, GI symptoms, anorexia, hypotension, and dehydration. May also have the classic clue - history of chronic steroid use. Order plasma cortisol level. Remember - cortisol level should be drawn prior to giving steroid therapy.

❏ ❏ ❏ ➢ **What is the initial treatment for adrenal insufficiency (don't worry about Rx while Dx)?**

Fluids and hydrocortisone IV in a typical dose of 100 to 200 mg.

❏ ❏ ❏ ➢ **An elderly patient presents with altered mental status, a history of IDDM and is hypoglycemic. Core temperature is 32 °C. What endocrinologic condition is likely?**

Myxedema coma.
Other clues to look for are history of thyroid surgery, hypothyroidism, and use of anti-thyroid medications.

❏ ❏ ❏ ➢ **What three conditions may cause a falsely low sodium concentration?**

Pseudohyponatremia may be caused by:

Hyperglycemia.
Hyperlipidemia.
Hyperproteinemia.

❏ ❏ ❏ ➢ **A patient presents with very low sodium and you suspect SIADH. What lab findings would confirm the diagnosis?**

Serum osmolality should be low and urine sodium and osmolality should both be high. Remember - treatment of severe symptomatic hyponatremia includes a loop diuretic such as furosemide and simultaneous infusion of small boluses of 3% saline over 4 hours or 0.9 normal saline. Too rapid a correction of hyponatremia may result in neurologic sequelae.

❏ ❏ ❏ ➢ **A young competitive figure skater presents with a complaint of generalized weakness following practice. What might be the cause of this profound weakness?**

Hypokalemic "paralysis" is a cause of acute weakness.

❏ ❏ ❏ ➢ **How may hyperglycemic, hyperosmolar, non-ketotic coma be differentiated from DKA?**

Serum osmolality is higher in NKHC.
$NaHCO_3$ is normal in NKHC and depleted in DKA.
pH is usually maintained at >7.2 in NKHC.

❏ ❏ ❏ ➢ **How should non-ketotic hyperosmolar coma be treated?**

Fluids, fluids and more fluids. Such patients can be as much as 12 liters deficient. Give normal saline until adequate blood pressure and urinary output are established. Follow with half normal saline. When blood glucose falls to 250 to 300 mg, the solution should be changed to saline and glucose to avoid cerebral edema.
It is important to note that these patient's require very little insulin. Give as little as 5 to 10 units of insulin IV.
These patients are commonly deficient in potassium and will need 10 to 15 mEq per hour once urine flow has been established.
This disorder has a grave prognosis with up to a 50% mortality for severe cases.

❏ ❏ ❏ ➢ **T/F - Phenytoin is the drug of choice for a patient with non-ketotic hyperosmolar coma who experiences a seizure.**

False. Phenytoin is contraindicated in patients with hyperglycemic, hyperosmolar, non-ketotic coma.
Drugs of choice for treating this seizure disorder are lorazepam (Ativan) or diazepam (Valium). Phenobarbital use is also appropriate.

❏ ❏ ❏ ➢ **For what types of overdoses is activated charcoal _not_ indicated?**

Alcohol ingestion, electrolytes, heavy metals, lithium, hydrocarbons and caustic ingestions.

❏ ❏ ❏ ➢ **A young patient has a threatened abortion in the first trimester. Laboratory studies reveal she is Rh negative and her husband is Rh positive. Treatment?**

The patient will need 50 µg of Rh immunoglobulin (RhoGAM) IM. After the first trimester, the dose is increased to 300 µg IM.

❏ ❏ ❏ ➢ **What type of blood test is used to determine if a patient needs RhoGAM therapy?**

A Kleihauer-Betke checks for fetomaternal bleeding.

❏ ❏ ❏ ➢ **What are the signs and symptoms of preeclampsia?**

Upper abdominal pain, headache, visual complaints, cardiac decompensation, creatinine greater than 2, proteinuria greater than 100 mg per deciliter, and a blood pressure of greater than 160 mm Hg systolic or 110 mm Hg diastolic.

Preeclampsia is most common in nulliparous women late in pregnancy, typically after 20 weeks gestation. Look for edema, hypertension, and proteinuria to diagnose these patients.

The ED treatment for preeclampsia is IV hydralazine titrated to a blood pressure of 90 to 110 diastolic using 5 mg boluses q 20 to 30 minutes. Blood pressure must be lowered slowly to avoid compromising the uteroplacental blood flow. Patients with moderate to severe preeclampsia need IV magnesium (though its true utility is not well demonstrated).

❐ ❐ ❐ ➢ **What is the most commonly missed hip fracture?**

Femoral neck fracture.

❐ ❐ ❐ ➢ **Which is more common - a medial or a lateral tibial plateau fracture?**

The lateral tibial plateau is most commonly fractured. If AP and lateral films are negative, follow-up with oblique views if suspicious of a tibial plateau fracture.

❐ ❐ ❐ ➢ **What is the most commonly missed fracture in the elbow region?**

A radial head fracture. Like the navicular fracture, radiographic signs of a radial head fracture may not show up for days after the injury. A positive fat pad sign may be the only finding suggestive of this injury.

❐ ❐ ❐ ➢ **What are the two most common errors made in the intubation of a neonate?**

1) Placing the neck in hyperextension - this moves the cords even more anteriorly.
2) Inserting the laryngoscope too far.

❐ ❐ ❐ ➢ **What is the most common cause of food-borne <u>viral</u> gastroenteritis?**

Norwalk virus commonly found in shell fish.

❐ ❐ ❐ ➢ **What are the symptoms of "Chinese Restaurant" syndrome?**

Headache, dizziness, abdominal discomfort, facial flushing, and chest or facial burning. Symptoms typically start within an h of eating Chinese food.

❐ ❐ ❐ ➢ **A patient is in anaphylactic shock. She happens to be taking ß-blockers. She is not responding to epinephrine. What alternative agents might you consider?**

Norepinephrine, diphenhydramine, and glucagon.

❐ ❐ ❐ ➢ **A young boy is presented for evaluation after suffering a coral snake bite. He appears to be fine. What is appropriate management?**

Admit to the Intensive Care Unit and be ready for respiratory arrest. Coral snake bites appear minor at first. When symptoms begin, the patient may quickly progress to respiratory arrest. Coral snake venom is neurotoxic.

❑ ❑ ❑ ➢ **Describe the appearance of a coral snake.**

The snake is red, yellow and black. There is a black spot on the head. It is a round snake.

Coral snake bites typically do not cause immediate local pain whereas viper bites do. (Red on yellow, kill a fellow!)

❑ ❑ ❑ ➢ **What type of rattlesnake bite leads to most deaths?**

Diamond back rattlesnake is the cause of nearly all lethal snake bites in the United States. The Diamond Back accounts for only 3% of snake bites seen. Treat with 10 to 20 vials of antivenin.

❑ ❑ ❑ ➢ **How does a stupid idiot recognize a pit viper?**

If he gets close enough, he will observe an elliptical pupil that looks like a football stood on end.

❑ ❑ ❑ ➢ **What are some more common entities in the differential diagnosis of a limp or gait abnormality in a child?**

Legg-Calvé-Perthes disease, Osgood-Schlatter disease, infection, toxic transient tenosynovitis, patellofemoral subluxation, chondromalacia of patella, and slipped capital femoral epiphysis.

❑ ❑ ❑ ➢ **What are the treatment recommendations for a patient with cluster headache?**

Treat similarly to migraine except skip ß-blockers, add O_2, try lidocaine 4% in the ipsilateral nostril.

❑ ❑ ❑ ➢ **What is the treatment for trigeminal neuralgia?**

Carbamazepine (Tegretol) 100 to 200 mg. tid. Obtain baseline CBC and platelet count before starting carbamazepine.

❑ ❑ ❑ ➢ **What is the only absolute contraindication to IVP?**

Profound hypotension - the kidneys won't be perfused. Two relative contraindications are renal insufficiency with a creatinine greater than 1.6 and a history of allergic reactions.

❑ ❑ ❑ ➢ **What markers indicate that an HIV positive patient is at increased risk for opportunistic infections like PCP?**

An absolute CD-4 count of less than 200.

CD-4 lymphocytic percentage less than 20%.

❐ ❐ ❐ ➢ **What are the National Institutes of Health treatment recommendations for spinal cord injury?**

Give high dose methylprednisolone (Solu-medrol) 30 mg/kg bolus over 15 minutes followed by 45 minutes normal saline drip. Over the subsequent 23 hours the patient should receive an infusion of 5.4 mg/kg/h of methylprednisolone.

❐ ❐ ❐ ➢ **What is the <u>most</u> <u>common</u> cause of small bowel obstruction in the surgically virgin abdomen?**

Incarcerated hernia.

❐ ❐ ❐ ➢ **A patient with a temperature of 29 °C develops V-fib. Is defibrillation likely to be successful?**

Defibrillation should be attempted but is unlikely to be successful at temperatures less than 29 °C.

❐ ❐ ❐ ➢ **T/F - The presentation of infectious endocarditis in an IV drug abusing patient does <u>not</u> usually include a murmur.**

TRUE. Less than 1/2 present with a murmur.

❐ ❐ ❐ ➢ **How is a retropharyngeal abscess diagnosed on plain films of a one year old child?**

Look for prevertebral thickening of the soft tissues. More than 3 mm suggests the possibility of a retropharyngeal abscess. Air/fluid level may be present.

If still unsure, order a CT of the neck. On CT scan retropharyngeal abscesses are just anterior to the vertebral column, will appear in only a few cuts, and appear as a gray area of about the same density as the spinal canal on CT.

❐ ❐ ❐ ➢ **In what age child is use of an <u>uncuffed</u> tube most appropriate?**

Children under 6 should receive an uncuffed tube.

❐ ❐ ❐ ➢ **A straight (Miller) blade is preferred for intubating children of less than what age?**

4 y.

❐ ❐ ❐ ➢ **What is the Parkland formula for treating a pediatric burn victim?**

Ringer's lactate 4 ml/ %BSA/ kg over 24 h with 1/2 given in first 8 h.

❐ ❐ ❐ ➢ **Large burns in children less than 5 years of age may require:**

Colloid (5% Albumin or FFP) at 1 ml/ %BSA/ kg/ d

❏ ❏ ❏ ➣ **A burned pediatric patient is receiving fluids per the Parkland formula. How much *additional* fluid should be given for maintenance requirements?**

       100 ml/kg/d for each kg up to 10 kg
+   50 ml/kg/d for each kg from 10-20 kg
+   20 ml/kg/d for each kg thereafter.

❏ ❏ ❏ ➣ **When examining a lateral adult C-spine film, the predental space, that is the area between the dens and the anterior arch of C1, looks particularly wide. What width space is normal for an adult?**

Normal is 2.5 to 3 mm.

If this width is greater than 3 mm, consider that the transverse ligament has ruptured or is at least lax.

❏ ❏ ❏ ➣ **What is the upper limit of normal of prevertebral soft tissue at C3?**

Anything greater than 5 mm suggests hematoma or fracture.

❏ ❏ ❏ ➣ **What disease is commonly associated with central retinal vein occlusion?**

Hypertension.

❏ ❏ ❏ ➣ **What are common eye findings in patients with AIDS?**

Cotton wool spots and CMV retinitis.

❏ ❏ ❏ ➣ **What is Purtscher's retinopathy?**

Purtscher's retinopathy is associated with thoracic injuries and broken bones. Findings include retinal hemorrhage and cotton wool spots.

❏ ❏ ❏ ➣ **What are the common features of central vertigo?**

1) Symptoms are gradual and continuous.
2) Focal signs may be present.
3) Hearing loss is rare.
4) Nausea and vomiting.

❏ ❏ ❏ ➣ **What are the signs and symptoms of peripheral vertigo?**

1) Symptoms are usually <u>acute</u> and <u>intermittent</u>.
2) Hearing loss is <u>common</u>, nausea and vomiting are severe.

❏ ❏ ❏ ➣ **In the evaluation of retropharyngeal abscess, what is the most common age of the patient, how do they present, what diagnostic tests are used in the evaluation, and what treatment modalities are recommended?**

Retropharyngeal abscess is most commonly seen in children less than 4 years of age.

Usual presentation is with dysphagia, muffled voice, stridor, sensation of a lump in the throat.
Patients usually prefer to lie supine.

Diagnosis is made with a soft tissue lateral neck film which may demonstrate edema and air/fluid levels. CT may be useful.

Treatment includes airway, IV antibiotics and admission to the ICU. Intubation may rupture the abscess.

❐ ❐ ❐ ➢ **The causes of epiglottitis include:**

Hemophilus influenzae is by far <u>most</u> <u>common.</u>
Pneumococcus, staphylococcus, and Branhamella may also be causes.
Presentation is most common among children within a few years of age 5.
Dogma to <u>never</u> attempt direct visualization of epiglottis is being questioned.

❐ ❐ ❐ ➢ **What is the most common cause of Ludwig's angina?**

Ludwig's angina is often associated with dental infections. Hemolytic streptococcus or mixed anaerobic infections are most common.

It is commonly seen in elderly and debilitated patients. It often presents with sublingual pain, protruding tongue, dysphonia, brawny induration, and stridor.

❐ ❐ ❐ ➢ **A set of perennial favorites from our friend, René Le Fort! What is a Le Fort I fracture?**

A maxilla fracture extending to the nasal aperture often missed on x-ray.

❐ ❐ ❐ ➢ **What is a Le Fort II fracture?**

A "pyramidal" fracture extends vertically through the maxilla, through maxillary sinuses and infraorbital rims and across nasal bridge. Usually confirmed with Waters' view.

❐ ❐ ❐ ➢ **What is a Le Fort III fracture?**

Craniofacial dysfunction includes fracture through the frontozygomatic suture lines, across the orbits and through the base of the nose. Le Fort I or II may also be present.

❐ ❐ ❐ ➢ **What is the usual cause of facial cellulitis in children less than 3 years of age?**

H. influenzae.
In adults- Staph or Strep.

❐ ❐ ❐ ➢ **A trauma patient presents with a complaint of severe burning pain in the upper extremities and associated neck pain. On physical exam, the patient has good strength in his upper extremities and no obvious neurologic deficits in the lower extremities. Although the C-spine series is negative, what problem is still suspected?**

Central cord syndrome. This injury is due to hyperextension of the spinal cord.

Diagnostic findings include upper extremity neurologic symptoms and minimal or no lower extremity symptoms.
Tingling, paresthesias, burning pain, and severe weakness or paralysis in the upper extremities with little or no symptoms in the lower extremities.

❑ ❑ ❑ ➤ **An asthmatic patient suddenly develops a supraventricular tachycardia. Blood pressure is normal and the QRS complex is also narrow. What therapy is most appropriate?**

Verapamil.

Avoid the use of adenosine as it is relatively contraindicated and may exacerbate bronchospasm in asthmatic patients. Also avoid ß-blockers.

❑ ❑ ❑ ➤ **How is a laryngeal fracture diagnosed on plain films?**

On a lateral soft tissue x-ray of the C-spine, check for retropharyngeal air, and elevation of the hyoid bone.
The hyoid bone is usually at the level of C3 if there is no evidence of a laryngeal fracture.

Elevation of the hyoid bone above C3 suggests a laryngeal fracture.

❑ ❑ ❑ ➤ **Differentiate between a hypertensive emergency and a hypertensive urgency.**

Elevated BP + end organ damage = hypertensive emergency.
Elevated BP + no symptoms or signs of end organ damage = hypertensive urgency; usually DBP > 115 mm Hg. Requires acute treatment.

❑ ❑ ❑ ➤ **A patient presents with a history of forehead contusion. She cannot move her arms; lower extremity strength is intact. X-rays of the neck are normal. What is the suspected diagnosis?**

Central cord syndrome. We just did this!
Management includes maintaining C-spine precautions, CT or MRI of the C-spine and neurosurgical consultation.

❑ ❑ ❑ ➤ **What are the antibiotics of choice in a wound resulting from a skin diving incident?**

Ciprofloxacin or TMP/SMX.

❑ ❑ ❑ ➤ **How should a jelly fish sting be treated?**

Rinse with saline.
Apply 5% acetic acid (vinegar) locally to the wound for approximately 30 minutes. In addition, corticosteroid agents may be applied topically. No antibiotics are necessary.
Tetanus prophylaxis.
Chironex flexeri antivenin only for this coelenterate.

❑ ❑ ❑ ➤ **A young man was found on the street by police and is brought to the ED. He has a temperature of 105 °F, altered mental status and muscle rigidity. You find a bottle**

of thioridazine (Mellaril) in his pocket. What conditions should be considered?

Meningitis , encephalitis, hyperthyroidism, anticholinergic or strychnine poisoning and heat stroke come to mind. Another disease that should be considered is <u>neuroleptic malignant syndrome</u> .

Patients may also have hypotension, hypertension, and tachycardia.

❏ ❏ ❏ ➤ **When does dysbaric air embolism typically occur?**

DAE always develops within minutes of surfacing after a dive. Symptoms are sudden and dramatic and include loss of consciousness, focal neurologic symptoms such as monoplegia, convulsions, blindness, confusion, and sensory disturbances.

Sudden loss of consciousness or other acute neurologic deficits immediately after surfacing is due to DAE unless proven otherwise. Treatment includes high flow oxygen and rapid transport for hyperbaric oxygen treatment.

❏ ❏ ❏ ➤ **A patient's blood gases reflect a mixed metabolic acidosis and respiratory alkalosis; what cause immediately comes to mind?**

Salicylate intoxication.

❏ ❏ ❏ ➤ **A two y old has jammed a pencil into her lateral soft palate. What complication might develop?**

Ischemic stroke is a complication of soft palate pencil injuries that results in contralateral hemiparesis.

❏ ❏ ❏ ➤ **What is the appropriate paralyzing agent to use when intubation is required in a seizing patient?**

Use pancuronium (Pavulon) as succinylcholine has greater tendency to increase serum potassium and to increase ICP.

❏ ❏ ❏ ➤ **Distinguish the key differences between strychnine and tetanus poisoning:**

Tetanus poisoning produces constant muscle tension whereas strychnine produces tetany and convulsions with episodes of relaxation between muscle contractions.

❏ ❏ ❏ ➤ **What is the common name for Dermacentor andersoni?**

Wood tick.

❏ ❏ ❏ ➤ **What neurologic disorder presents similarly to symptoms caused by Dermacentor andersoni (Wood Tick) bite?**

Guillain-Barré. Recall that tick paralysis may have decreased or absent DTRs as a clinical finding. Such DTRs may also be found associated with diphtheria exotoxin.

❏ ❏ ❏ ➤ **What nerve supplies taste to the anterior two thirds of the tongue, the lacrimal and salivary glands?**

Cranial nerve VII.

❏ ❏ ❏ ➤ **What disease is associated with anti-acetylcholine receptor antibodies that affect the post-synaptic neuromuscular site and is seen more commonly in females with a peak incidence in the third decade of life?**

Myasthenia gravis. 50% of myasthenia gravis patients have thymomas and 75% have lymphoid hyperplasia.

❏ ❏ ❏ ➤ **What antibiotics should be avoided in myasthenia gravis patients?**

Polymyxin and aminoglycosides have curare-like properties and may cause paralysis in these patients.

❏ ❏ ❏ ➤ **A baby presents to your emergency department with no facial movement, the lids sag and the child has a poor suck. She does not seem to move much and seems very weak. What causes do you consider?**

Myasthenia gravis or baby botulism.

❏ ❏ ❏ ➤ **A patient complains of pronounced weakness when attempting to climb stairs and even becomes tired when they do such simple tasks as brushing their teeth. Diagnosis?**

Myasthenia gravis.

❏ ❏ ❏ ➤ **What is the treatment for myasthenia gravis?**

Steroids, thymectomy, immunosuppressive drugs, plasmapheresis, and cholinergic agents such as pyridostigmine.

❏ ❏ ❏ ➤ **What disease is tick paralysis very similar to?**

It is very Guillain-Barré like.

❏ ❏ ❏ ➤ **Eaton-Lambert syndrome is associated with what class of diseases?**

Malignancies, particularly oat-cell carcinoma.
Symptoms include aching muscle pain and weakness (the latter usually less than associated with MG); cranial nerves are not usually involved.
Muscle strength may increase with repeated action in contradistinction to greater weakness with use encountered in MG.

❏ ❏ ❏ ➤ **What is a chalazion?**

This is a Meibomian gland granuloma.

❏ ❏ ❏ ➤ **How should a chalazion be treated?**

Surgical curettage.

❏ ❏ ❏ ➤ **Patient presents with eye pain. She has a constricted pupil, ciliary flush, and red injected sclera at the limbus. Diagnosis?**

Acute iritis.

❏ ❏ ❏ ➤ **A patient presents with loss of central vision. Likely diagnosis?**

A retrobulbar neuritis is likely. MS is associated with about 25% of cases of retrobulbar neuritis.

Macular degeneration and central retinal vein occlusion can also lead to loss of central vision.

❏ ❏ ❏ ➤ **I am used to treat acute angle closure glaucoma (and occasionally in vain attempts to treat retinal artery occlusion). I also play a role in treatment and prevention of acute mountain sickness. I decrease aqueous humor production via my mechanism of being a carbonic anhydrase inhibitor. What is my name?**

Acetazolamide (Diamox).

❏ ❏ ❏ ➤ **A patient presents with fever, neck pain or neck stiffness and trismus. Exam reveals pharyngeal edema with tonsil displacement and edema of the parotid area. Diagnosis?**

PARAPHARYNGEAL Abscess.

❏ ❏ ❏ ➤ **A patient presents with hearing loss, nystagmus, complaint of facial weakness, and diplopia. Vertigo is provoked with sudden movement. A lumbar puncture reveals elevated CNS protein. What diagnosis is suspected?**

An acoustic neuroma.

❏ ❏ ❏ ➤ **Can a parapharyngeal abscess present with an associated finding of edema in the area of the parotid gland?**

Yes.

❏ ❏ ❏ ➤ **In a trauma patient, facial dimpling of the cheek is associated with:**

Zygomatic arch fracture.

❏ ❏ ❏ ➤ **What x-rays should be ordered to diagnose a fracture of the zygoma?**

A jug handle, Water's view or submental view.

❏ ❏ ❏ ➤ **What are the key features of Stevens-Johnson Syndrome?**

It is a bullous form of erythema multiforme with involvement of mucous membranes. It may cause corneal ulcerations, anterior uveitis and blindness.

❏ ❏ ❏ ➢ **Blood is originating from a tooth after trauma. What Ellis classification?**

3.

❏ ❏ ❏ ➢ **What are the most common drugs causing TEN?**

Phenylbutazone, barbiturates, sulfa drugs, anti-epileptics and antibiotics.

❏ ❏ ❏ ➢ **Rhomboid shaped crystals from a joint aspiration are associated with:**

Pseudogout.

❏ ❏ ❏ ➢ **Needle shaped crystals are associated with:**

Gout.

❏ ❏ ❏ ➢ **What is the most common site of aseptic necrosis?**

The hip.

❏ ❏ ❏ ➢ **Acute treatment for gout?**

Colchicine, indomethacin and other NSAIDs.

❏ ❏ ❏ ➢ **Most common presentation of a Charcot's joint?**

A swollen ankle and a" bag of bones" appearance on x-ray.

❏ ❏ ❏ ➢ **On x-ray you see Charcot's joints. Diagnosis?**

Diabetes.

❏ ❏ ❏ ➢ **What is the most common cause of Charcot's joint?**

Diabetic peripheral neuropathy.

❏ ❏ ❏ ➢ **What is the most common tendon affected in calcified tendonitis?**

The supraspinatus.

❏ ❏ ❏ ➢ **Which epicondyle is involved in tennis elbow?**

The lateral epicondyle.

❏ ❏ ❏ ➢ **What is the <u>most</u> <u>common</u> and second most common site of infectious arthritis?**

The knee is the most common and the hip is the second most common.

Staphylococcus is the <u>most</u> <u>common</u> cause.

❏ ❏ ❏ ➣ **At what cervical level is the hyoid bone normally found?**

The third cervical vertebra.
If the hyoid is above this level a laryngeal fracture should be suspected.

❏ ❏ ❏ ➣ **At what cervical level is the thyroid located?**

Level of the fourth cervical vertebra.

❏ ❏ ❏ ➣ **What is the most common site of cervical disc herniation?**

C5-C6. Patient will complain of bilateral shoulder pain.

❏ ❏ ❏ ➣ **What nerve is located in the tarsal tunnel?**

The tibial nerve.

❏ ❏ ❏ ➣ **A patient has difficulty squatting and arising. Likely spinal pathology?**

L4 root compression with involvement of quadriceps.
(Don't even *think about* X-linked Duchenne's muscular dystrophy!)

❏ ❏ ❏ ➣ **What STD pathogens cause *painful* ulcers?**

Type II Genital Herpes and chancroid.

STD	Ulcer	Node
Genital Herpes	**Painful**	Painful
Chancroid	**Painful**	Painful
Syphilis	Painless	Less Painful
Lymphogranuloma Venereum	Painless	Moderately

❏ ❏ ❏ ➣ **A patient presents with a complaint of pain at the site of the deltoid insertion with radiation into the back of the arm (C5 distribution). On exam, there is increased pain with active abduction from 70° - 120°. X-rays reveal calcification at the tendinous insertion of the greater tuberosity. Diagnosis?**

Supraspinatus tendonitis.

❏ ❏ ❏ ➣ **Absent knee jerk. What level?**

L4.

❏ ❏ ❏ ➣ **Absent Achilles reflex. What level?**

S1.

❏ ❏ ❏ ➤ **Paresthesia of the great toe. Level?**

L5.

❏ ❏ ❏ ➤ **Paresthesia of the little toe. Level?**

S1.

❏ ❏ ❏ ➤ **What is the most common site of compartment syndrome?**

Anterior compartment of the leg.

❏ ❏ ❏ ➤ **Describe the leg position associated with an anterosuperior hip dislocation.**

Anterosuperior - External rotation and slight abduction. In the pubic type, the hip is extended and in the iliac type, it is slightly flexed.

❏ ❏ ❏ ➤ **Describe the leg position associated with an obturator hip dislocation.**

In an obturator dislocation there is external rotation, flexion and abduction.

❏ ❏ ❏ ➤ **Posterior hip dislocation - leg position?**

Internal rotation, flexion and abduction. Most common type.

❏ ❏ ❏ ➤ **A patient in the ED cannot recall ever having a tetanus shot. The nurse gives him a tetanus shot. Later, he develops a hypersensitivity reaction and recalls that he recently had a tetanus shot. What type of reaction does he have?**

Type 3 - arthrus reaction.
Type 3 reactions are caused by immune complexes or antigen-antibody complexes that activate complement and platelets forming aggregates and complexes with IgE.

❏ ❏ ❏ ➤ **A positive TB test is what type of reaction?**

Type 4 - cell mediated, delayed hypersensitivity.
Type 4 reactions do not involve complement or antibodies.

❏ ❏ ❏ ➤ **What drugs commonly cause erythema multiforme?**

Carbamazepine, penicillin, sulfa, pyrazolone, phenytoin, barbiturates.

❏ ❏ ❏ ➤ **What <u>aerobe</u> is <u>most</u> <u>commonly</u> found in cutaneous abscesses?**

Staphylococcus aureus.

❏ ❏ ❏ ➤ **What is the most common gram negative aerobe found in cutaneous abscesses?**

Proteus mirabilis.

❏ ❏ ❏ ➢ **Describe the Gram stain appearance of Staphylococcus aureus.**

Gram positive cocci in grape-like clusters.

❏ ❏ ❏ ➢ **What is the <u>most</u> <u>common</u> cause of cellulitis in children less than 3 years of age?**

Hemophilus influenzae.

❏ ❏ ❏ ➢ **What is the <u>most</u> <u>common</u> cause of cellulitis in the adult?**

Staphylococcus aureus.

❏ ❏ ❏ ➢ **What is the cause of erysipelas?**

Group A , ß-hemolytic streptococci.

❏ ❏ ❏ ➢ **How is erysipelas treated?**

Penicillin.

Erythromycin for penicillin allergic patients.

❏ ❏ ❏ ➢ **What is the most common cause of toxic shock syndrome?**

Staphylococci. Toxins C and F are the proteins that mediate toxic shock syndrome.

❏ ❏ ❏ ➢ **A child presents to the ED with a history of fever, conjunctival hyperemia, and erythema of the mucus membranes with desquamation. Diagnosis?**

Kawasaki's Disease. Remember - Kawasaki's Disease may have lesions resembling erythema multiforme.

❏ ❏ ❏ ➢ **Clostridium tetanus, a Gram and anaerobe, produces a neurotoxin. Is it an endotoxin or an exotoxin?**

Tetanospasmin is an exotoxin. Its major effect is prevention of transmission of inhibitory neurons in anterior horn cells resulting in motor system disinhibition.

❏ ❏ ❏ ➢ **What are some of the common causes of prerenal acute renal failure?**

Volume depletion and decreased effective volume (CHF, sepsis, cirrhosis).

❏ ❏ ❏ ➢ **What are the causes of acute renal failure which are renal in nature?**

Acute Tubular Necrosis, acute interstitial nephritis, acute glomerulonephritis and vascular disease.

❏ ❏ ❏ ➢ **What are the causes of post-renal failure?**

Ureteral and urethral obstruction.

❏ ❏ ❏ ➢ **What findings mark the presentation of a patient with rapidly progressive glomerulonephritis?**

Most common - hematuria.
Also edema (periorbital), HTN, ascites, pleural effusion, rales, and anuria.

❏ ❏ ❏ ➢ **What arrhythmia is frequently encountered during renal dialysis.**

Hypokalemia induced ventricular fibrillation.

❏ ❏ ❏ ➢ **In which trimester of pregnancy is UTI and pyelonephritis most common?**

Third.

❏ ❏ ❏ ➢ **What is inflammation of the foreskin called?**

Balanitis or balanoposthitis.

❏ ❏ ❏ ➢ **What is phimosis?**

A condition in which the foreskin cannot be retracted posterior to the glans.   The preliminary treatment is a dorsal slit.

❏ ❏ ❏ ➢ **What is paraphimosis?**

A condition in which the foreskin is retracted posterior to the glands and cannot be advanced over the glans.

❏ ❏ ❏ ➢ **What are causes of priapism?**

Prolonged sex (I *hate* it when...), leukemia, sickle cell trait and disease, blood dyscrasias, pelvic hematoma or neoplasm, syphilis, and urethritis.
Drugs - Phenothiazines, prazosin, tolbutamide, anticoagulants, corticosteroids.

❏ ❏ ❏ ➢ **What causes a green to gray frothy vaginal discharge with mild itching.**

Trichomonas vaginitis. On physical exam, the cervix may have a strawberry appearance (20%).

❏ ❏ ❏ ➢ **Describe the presentation of a patient with Gardnerella vaginitis?**

On physical exam, note a frothy, gray-white, fishy smelling vaginal discharge. Wet mount may show clue cells (clusters of bacilli on the surface of epithelial cells).

Sherlock Holmes always uses his magnifying lens to look for *Clues* in the *Garden*.

❐ ❐ ❐ ➢ **Do you know why I *hate* it when my foot falls asleep during the day?**

It'll be up <u>all</u> <u>night</u>!

❐ ❐ ❐ ➢ **Sulfamethoxasole may lead to hemolysis in a patient with:**

G6PD deficiency.

❐ ❐ ❐ ➢ **What disease is associated with <u>painless</u> bright red bleeding per vagina in the third trimester?**

Placenta previa.

❐ ❐ ❐ ➢ **<u>Painful</u> third trimester vaginal bleeding likely represents?**

Abruptio placenta.

❐ ❐ ❐ ➢ **What affect does pregnancy have on BUN and creatinine?**

Both the creatinine and BUN are decreased. This is as the result of increased renal blood flow and increased glomerular filtration rate.

❐ ❐ ❐ ➢ **When can one auscultate the fetal heart?**

Ultrasound-   6 weeks.

Doppler-   10 - 12 weeks.

Stethoscope-   18 - 20 weeks.

❐ ❐ ❐ ➢ **Describe a Brudzinski sign:**

Flexion of the neck produces flexion of the knees.

❐ ❐ ❐ ➢ **Describe Kernig's sign:**

Extension of the knees from the flexed thigh position results in strong passive resistance.

❐ ❐ ❐ ➢ **What is the normal opening pressure in a spinal tap?**

15 cm H_2O.

❐ ❐ ❐ ➢ **What is the normal CSF protein level?**

40 mg/dl

❐ ❐ ❐ ➢ **What opening pressure and protein level are expected in bacterial meningitis?**

Opening pressure of near 30 cm H_2O and protein level of greater than 150 mg/dl.

Glucose level will drop with bacterial meningitis, with TB and with fungal infections.

❐ ❐ ❐ ➤ **What does the India ink test show?**

Cryptococcus neoformans.

❐ ❐ ❐ ➤ **What is the most significant pathophysiologic mechanism of death from cyclic antidepressants?**

Myocardial depression, including hypotension and conduction blocks.

❐ ❐ ❐ ➤ **Of patients who die from CA overdose, what percentage are awake and alert at the time of first prehospital contact?**

25%.

❐ ❐ ❐ ➤ **What are some common side effects of phenothiazine use?**

Malaise, hyperthermia, tachycardia, anticholinergic effects, and quinidine-like membrane stabilization. The most dangerous side effect is neuroleptic malignant syndrome.

❐ ❐ ❐ ➤ **How should stable ventricular tachyarrhythmias associated with phenothiazine overdose be treated?**

Lidocaine and phenytoin.

❐ ❐ ❐ ➤ **Which antibiotic may either increase or decrease lithium secretion?**

Tetracycline.

❐ ❐ ❐ ➤ **How is lithium overdose treated?**

Lavage, saline diuresis, furosemide, and hemodialysis.
Alkalinization *may* be appropriate.

❐ ❐ ❐ ➤ **Is phenobarbital more quickly metabolized by children or by adults?**

Adults. Neonates are especially slow at metabolizing phenobarbital.

❐ ❐ ❐ ➤ **How should barbiturate poisoning be treated?**

Supportive, charcoal, alkalinization of the urine, charcoal hemoperfusion or hemodialysis.

❐ ❐ ❐ ➤ **What drugs increase the half-life of phenytoin?**

Sulfonamides, isoniazid, dicumarol, and chloramphenicol.

❐ ❐ ❐ ➤ **What hypersensitivity skin rashes are noted with phenytoin use?**

Lupus-like and Stevens-Johnson syndrome.

❏ ❏ ❏ ➢ **What are the cardiac effects of phenytoin?**

Inhibits sodium channels, decreases the effective refractory period and automaticity in the Purkinje fibers. Little effect on QRS width or action potential duration.

❏ ❏ ❏ ➢ **What is the lethal dose of phenytoin?**

20 mg/kg.

❏ ❏ ❏ ➢ **What symptoms are expected with a phenytoin level of > 20, of > 30, and of > 40 μg/ml?**

> 20 - lateral gaze nystagmus.
> 30 - lateral gaze nystagmus plus increased vertical nystagmus with upward gaze.
> 40 - lethargy, confusion, dysarthrias, and psychosis.

❏ ❏ ❏ ➢ **In endocarditis (all comers), what is the most commonly involved cardiac valve?**

Mitral > Aortic > Tricuspid > Pulmonic.

❏ ❏ ❏ ➢ **Infectious endocarditis in an IV drug abuser most commonly affects which valve?**

#1 - Tricuspid.
#2 - Pulmonary.

❏ ❏ ❏ ➢ **What is the <u>most</u> <u>common</u> causative bacterium associated with right-sided endocarditis in IV drug abusers?**

S. aureus.
<u>Left- sided</u> endocarditis in IV drug abusers is likely due to E. coli, streptococcus, Klebsiella, Pseudomonas and Candida.

❏ ❏ ❏ ➢ **A heroin addict presents with pulmonary edema. What is the best treatment?**

Naloxone, O_2 and ventilatory support.
Don't bother using diuretics. This seems like a good test question.

❏ ❏ ❏ ➢ **What is the <u>most</u> <u>common</u> neurologic complication of IV drug abuse?**

Nontraumatic mononeuritis - painless weakness 2 -3 h after injection.

❏ ❏ ❏ ➢ **Name two frequently observed organisms causing septic arthritis in drug addicts.**

Serratiae and Pseudomonas.
These are rare causes in non-addicts.

❑ ❑ ❑ ➢ **An alcoholic patient presents with complaints of abdominal pain and blurred vision. The patient is very photophobic and blood gases reveal a metabolic acidosis. Diagnosis?**

Methanol poisoning. These patients may describe seeing something resembling a snow-storm.

❑ ❑ ❑ ➢ **What is the mechanism of action of clonidine?**

Clonidine is a central acting α–agonist. It leads to decreased sympathetic outflow and lowers catecholamine levels.

❑ ❑ ❑ ➢ **What is the lethal dose of methanol?**

30 ml.
Formate levels in methanol poisoning are greatest in vitreous humor.

❑ ❑ ❑ ➢ **What alcohol poisoning is suggested by a plasma bicarbonate level of zero (cipher, null, empty set, zip, Ø)?**

Methanol.

It also produces a large osmolar gap and large anion gap. Methanol poisoning is treated with IV ethanol and hemodialysis.

❑ ❑ ❑ ➢ **Positive birefringent calcium oxalate crystals are pathognomonic for poisoning with what substance?**

Ethylene glycol.
The lethal dose of ethylene glycol is 100 ml.

❑ ❑ ❑ ➢ **What are the signs and symptoms of ethylene glycol poisoning?**

Hallucinations, nystagmus, ataxia, papilledema, and a large anion gap.

❑ ❑ ❑ ➢ **How should ethylene glycol poisoning be treated?**

Gastric lavage, sodium bicarbonate, thiamine and pyridoxine, IV ethanol and hemodialysis.

❑ ❑ ❑ ➢ **What are the major lab findings in a patient with isopropanol poisoning?**

Elevated osmolal gap.
Acetonemia and acetonuria. Acetone.
Ø acidosis.

❑ ❑ ❑ ➢ **A patient presents to the ER with ataxia, altered mental status, and sixth nerve palsy. What is your diagnosis?**

Wernicke's encephalopathy.

❐ ❐ ❐ ➢ **What are the signs and symptoms of isopropanol poisoning?**

Sweet odor of breath (acetone), hypotension and hemorrhagic gastritis, CNS depression from isopropanol and from its metabolite, acetone.

❐ ❐ ❐ ➢ **What is the treatment of cocaine toxicity?**

Sedate with benzodiazepine.
Treat unresponsive hypertension with nitroprusside or phentolamine.
Return to text book to re-read discussion of <u>worsening</u> symptoms with ß-adrenergic antagonists.

❐ ❐ ❐ ➢ **Vertical nystagmus?**

<u>PCP</u>.
(O.K., there *are* some other causes...brainstem disease, vestibular disease.)

❐ ❐ ❐ ➢ **X-ray finding in a patient with salicylate toxicity:**

Noncardiogenic pulmonary edema.

❐ ❐ ❐ ➢ **Describe central nervous system affects of salicylate poisoning:**

Lethargy, confusion, seizures, and respiratory arrest.

❐ ❐ ❐ ➢ **Salicylate levels should ideally be checked how long after an ingestion?**

6 h.

❐ ❐ ❐ ➢ **What is the minimum likely toxic dose of salicylates?**

150 mg/kg.

❐ ❐ ❐ ➢ **Salicylate <u>level</u>, measured at 6 h after ingestion, greater than _____ is associated with toxicity.**

45 mg/dl.

❐ ❐ ❐ ➢ **ACEtominophen <u>level</u>, measured 4 ACEs after ingestion, greater than _____ is associated with toxicity.**

150 µg/ml.

❐ ❐ ❐ ➢ **For what drugs will alkalinization of the urine increase excretion?**

CA's, salicylates, and long-acting barbiturates.
May be of some use to enhance lithium excretion.

❏ ❏ ❏ ➤ **What are the signs of salicylate poisoning?**

Hyperventilation, hyperthermia, mental status changes, nausea, vomiting, abdominal pain, dehydration, diaphoresis, ketonuria, metabolic acidosis, and respiratory alkalosis.

❏ ❏ ❏ ➤ **A child presents with lethargy, seizures, and hypoglycemia. A history of several days of preceding viral syndrome symptoms is elicited. Name two disorders that should be considered.**

Reye's syndrome and salicylate intoxication.

❏ ❏ ❏ ➤ **What laboratory test can aid in evaluation of a possible toxic iron ingestion?**

Total iron binding capacity measured 3 to 5 hours after ingestion.
If serum iron level is significantly less than the total iron binding capacity, a toxic iron ingestion is less likely.

❏ ❏ ❏ ➤ **What is the antidote for a toxic ingestion of iron?**

Deferoxamine chelates only free iron.

❏ ❏ ❏ ➤ **Deferoxamine should be given for a serum iron level greater than:**

350 µg/dl.

❏ ❏ ❏ ➤ **Deferoxamine should be given for what ratio of serum iron to total iron binding capacity?**

Give deferoxamine if serum iron is > total iron binding capacity.

❏ ❏ ❏ ➤ **How many hours after an iron ingestion should total iron binding capacity be measured. Feel the Force, Luke; we just did this.**

3-5 h.

❏ ❏ ❏ ➤ **What type of hydrocarbons are most toxic?**

"Oh no...not that reverse viscosity stuff!"

Kinematic viscosity (u), shear rates unrelated to apparent viscosity (∂) neglecting Fähraeus-Lindqvist effect.

O.K. - Thus, substances with <u>low</u> viscosities (measured in Saybolt Seconds Universal (SSU)) are <u>more</u> toxic than higher viscosity compounds. Your gasoline, kerosene and paint thinner (all aliphatic hydrocarbons with SSU's of < 60), are all more toxic than your motor oil, your tar and your petroleum jelly, which all have SSUs > 100.

Of the compounds with SSUs < 60, the most toxic are those that are not aliphatic, including your benzene, toluene, xylene and tetrachloroethylene.

❏ ❏ ❏ ➤ **What is the most reliable site for detecting central cyanosis?**

The tongue.

❐ ❐ ❐ ➢ **You are taking boards and are presented with a patient with a history of placement of an aortic graft or of abdominal aortic aneurysm. The patient has been vomiting up some coffee ground emesis. What infrequent entity needs to be considered?**

The dreaded aortoenteric fistula. These patients may present with a limited herald bleed before massive bleeding develops.
A CT showing air in the periaortic area is indicative of need for immediate surgery.

❐ ❐ ❐ ➢ **What is a common complication of pancuronium?**

Tachycardia from its vagolytic action.
Pancuronium tachycardia can give you an ulcer; that is Pantac can give you an ulcer!

❐ ❐ ❐ ➢ **What is the most common cause of hypermagnesemia in a patient with renal failure?**

Patient use of compounds high in magnesium, such as antacids.
This can result in neuromuscular paralysis.
Consider IV calcium.
Saline and furosemide assisted diuresis may not help this patient with renal failure, so consider dialysis.

❐ ❐ ❐ ➢ **What is the treatment for torsade de pointes?**

Untwisting.

❐ ❐ ❐ ➢ **How much energy should be used in cardioversion of an unstable infant with a wide complex tachycardia?**

0.5 to 1.0 J/kg.

❐ ❐ ❐ ➢ **How much energy should be used to cardiovert unstable VF in an infant?**

2 J/kg.

❐ ❐ ❐ ➢ **What is the most common malposition of the nasotracheal tube?**

Into the piriform sinus. The second most common malposition is the esophagus.

❐ ❐ ❐ ➢ **What is the <u>most</u> <u>common</u> physical sign of a PE?**

Tachypnea.

❐ ❐ ❐ ➢ **What are the three most common presenting signs of aortic stenosis?**

Syncope, angina, and heart failure.

268

❏ ❏ ❏ ➤ **When do CK levels first begin to rise and when do they peak in an MI?**

CK - MB earliest rise 6-8 h.
Peak 24-30 h.
Normalizes 48 h.

❏ ❏ ❏ ➤ **When does LDH first begin to rise and when does it peak in an MI?**

LDH-I (from heart) earliest rise 12 to 24 h.
Peak 48 to 96 h.

❏ ❏ ❏ ➤ **What is the effect of nitrates on preload and afterload?**

Nitrates mostly dilate veins and venules to decrease preload.

❏ ❏ ❏ ➤ **Inferior wall MIs commonly lead to what two types of heart block (via mechanism of damage to autonomic fibers in the atrial septum giving increased vagal tone impairing AV node conduction)?**

First degree AV block.
Mobitz Type I (Wenckebach) second-degree AV block.
Sinus bradycardia can also occur.

Progression to complete AV block is not common.

❏ ❏ ❏ ➤ **Anterior wall MIs may directly damage intracardiac conduction. This may lead to what type of arrhythmias?**

The dangerous type! Mobitz II second-degree AV block that can suddenly progress to complete AV block.

❏ ❏ ❏ ➤ **What are some of the potential, sometimes rare, complications of Mycoplasma pneumonia?**

Non-pulmonary: Hemolytic anemia, aseptic meningitis, encephalitis, Guillain-Barré syndrome, pericarditis, and myocarditis.

Pulmonary: ARDS, atelectasis, mediastinal adenopathy, pneumothorax, pleural effusion and abscess.

❏ ❏ ❏ ➤ **Under what conditions should Staphylococcal pneumonia be considered as a possible diagnosis?**

Although it only accounts for 1% of bacterial pneumonias, it should be considered in patients with sudden chills, hectic fever, pleurisy and cough, especially following a viral illness such as measles or influenza.

❏ ❏ ❏ ➤ **Of the following anesthetics, which has the shortest duration of action - lidocaine, procaine, bupivacaine or mepivacaine?**

Procaine.

❏ ❏ ❏ ➤ **Differential diagnosis of a ring lesion on CT scan:**

Toxoplasmosis, lymphoma, fungal infection, TB, CMV, Kaposi's, and hemorrhage.

❐ ❐ ❐ ➢ **Does erythema multiforme itch?**

Not typically. It may be tender.

❐ ❐ ❐ ➢ **A patient presents with granuloma inguinale. What does it look like?**

Papular, nodular or vesicular painless lesions. These can progress to extensive destruction of local tissues.
Cause is Calymmatobacterium granulomatis.

❐ ❐ ❐ ➢ **What causes chancroid?**

Hemophilus ducreyi.
Painful necrotic ulcerative lesions and painful nodes.

❐ ❐ ❐ ➢ **Describe lesions associated with Chlamydia.**

Painless shallow ulcerations, papular or nodular lesions or herpetiform vesicles wax and wane.

❐ ❐ ❐ ➢ **What type of diarrhea causing disease may be transmitted by pets?**

Yersinia.

❐ ❐ ❐ ➢ **What state is associated with akinetic mutism?**

N. Dakota is a bucolic state.
Akinetic mutism is an abulic state (which is like a coma vigil). Patients seem awake and may have eyes open. They respond to questions very slowly.
The cause is typically due to depressed frontal lobe function.

❐ ❐ ❐ ➢ **What is normal blood pressure in a newborn?**

60 mmHg.

❐ ❐ ❐ ➢ **What is the initial drug of choice to treat SVT in a pediatric patient.**

Adenosine 0.1 mg/kg is drug of choice.
Digoxin 0.02 mg/kg may take ≈ 4 h for conversion.
Verapamil may be used in children > 2 years of age. It is contraindicated in younger children due to several deaths.
Synchronized cardioversion at 0.5-1.0 J/kg.

❐ ❐ ❐ ➢ <u>After</u> **the first mo of life, what is the number one cause of meningitis and of pneumonia in children?**

Most common cause of meningitis after the first mo of life is H. influenza.

Most common cause of pneumonia after the first mo of life is S. pneumoniae; H. influenza is the second most common cause.

For bacteremia in children greater than one mo, the <u>most</u> <u>common</u> causes are S. pneumoniae (70%) and H. influenza (20%) of the time.

❐ ❐ ❐ ➢ **Discuss infantile spasms.**

Onset is by 3 to 9 months of age, typically lasts seconds, and may occur in single episodes or bursts.   The EEG is most often abnormal.
85% of these patients go on to be mentally handicapped.

❐ ❐ ❐ ➢ **Erythema multiforme can be associated with which anticonvulsants?**

Phenobarbital, phenytoin and carbamazepine.

❐ ❐ ❐ ➢ **Hepatic failure is commonly associated with what anticonvulsant?**

Valproic acid.

❐ ❐ ❐ ➢ **A patient presents with fever, neck pain and trismus.   Exam reveals pharyngeal edema with tonsil displacement and edema of the *parotid* area.   Diagnosis?**

PARAPHARYNGEAL abscess.

❐ ❐ ❐ ➢ **Does H. influenza typically cause abscesses?**

No.

❐ ❐ ❐ ➢ **What drugs, activities and cooking habits are associated with increasing clearance of theophylline (decreasing the theophylline level)?**

Phenytoin, phenobarbital, cigarette smoking and charcoal Bar-B-Queing.

❐ ❐ ❐ ➢ **Anaphylaxis is a common cause of what type of renal failure?**

Prerenal.

❐ ❐ ❐ ➢ **What are the end products of methanol, of ethylene glycol and of isopropyl alcohol metabolism?**

Methanol   - formate.
Ethylene glycol   - oxalate and formate.
Isopropyl alcohol - acetone.

❐ ❐ ❐ ➢ **What type of alcohol ingestion is associated with hypocalcemia?**

Ethylene glycol.

❐ ❐ ❐ ➢ **What type of alcohol ingestion is associated with hemorrhagic pancreatitis?**

Methanol.

❏ ❏ ❏ ➢ **Arsenic produces an odor on the breath similar to what?**

Garlic.

❏ ❏ ❏ ➢ **When does ECM show up in Lyme disease?**

Stage I - 3 to 32 days after the bite.

❏ ❏ ❏ ➢ **For what disorder is vigorous digital massage of the orbit indicated?**

Central retinal artery occlusion.
DO NOT do this in central vein occlusion!

❏ ❏ ❏ ➢ **What pathogen is suggested by a pneumonia with a single rigor?**

Pneumococcus.

❏ ❏ ❏ ➢ **What pathogen does a strawberry cervix suggest?**

Trichomonas.

❏ ❏ ❏ ➢ **What are the key features of Ellis Type I, II, and III?**

Enamel, dentin, pulp.
Enamel, dentin, pulp. Pulp bleeds.

❏ ❏ ❏ ➢ **What is the vector and causative organism of Lyme disease?**

The vector is Ixodes dammini and the organism is Borrelia burgdorferi. It is the most frequently transmitted tick-borne disease.

❏ ❏ ❏ ➢ **Q fever cause:**

Coxiella burnetii, aka Rickettsia burnetii.
First found in Dermacentor andersonii tick.
Fever, headache, malaise, chest pain.

❏ ❏ ❏ ➢ **A hordeolum is:**

A Meibomian gland infection, usually of upper lid.

❏ ❏ ❏ ➢ **Ludwig's angina pathology:**

Hemolytic streptococci, staphylococcus, mixed aerobes and anaerobes.

❏ ❏ ❏ ➢ **The three most common locations of malignant melanoma:**

1) Skin.
2) Eye.
3) Anal canal.

❏ ❏ ❏ ➢ **What is the initial dose of blood to be given in children?**

10 ml/kg of packed RBCs.

❏ ❏ ❏ ➢ **What is achalasia?**

Disorder of esophageal motility and incomplete relaxation of the lower esophagus.

❏ ❏ ❏ ➢ **Suspected mesenteric ischemia may be virtually confirmed by what invasive exam other than laparotomy?**

Angiography.

❏ ❏ ❏ ➢ **Enterotoxin producing organisms that can cause food poisoning:**

Clostridium.
Staph aureus.
Vibrio cholerae.
E. coli.

❏ ❏ ❏ ➢ **Antibiotics should be avoided in what infectious diarrhea?**

Salmonella. Clear exceptions are in severe cases of diarrhea in immunocompromised patients and in children less than 6 months of age.

❏ ❏ ❏ ➢ **Anal fissures:**

Crohn's.

❏ ❏ ❏ ➢ **Diphtheria - growth medium:**

Loffler's medium or tellurite.
O.K.

❏ ❏ ❏ ➢ **Three disorders that are associated with decreased DTRs:**

Guillain-Barré.
Tic paralysis due to Dermacentor andersoni (Wood Tick) bite.
Diphtheria exotoxin.

❏ ❏ ❏ ➢ **What is the most common cause of bacterial pneumonia in children greater than 4 weeks of age?**

S. pneumoniae is the most common.
H. influenza is the second most common.

❏ ❏ ❏ ➢ **Likely cause of CHF in a premature infant?**

Premature infants = PDA.

❏ ❏ ❏ ➢ **Likely cause of CHF presenting in the first 3 d of life?**

First 3 d = transposition of the great vessels which will cause cyanosis and failure.

❏ ❏ ❏ ➢ **Likely cause of CHF presenting in the first week of life?**

First week = hypoplastic left ventricle.

❏ ❏ ❏ ➢ **Likely cause of CHF presenting in the second week of life?**

Second week = coarctation.

❏ ❏ ❏ ➢ **Do you treat Shigella with antibiotics?**

In general, yes.

❏ ❏ ❏ ➢ **What is a pinguecula?**

It is a yellowish nodule, particularly on the nasal aspect of the eye, but it may be lateral. Often caused by wind and dust.

❏ ❏ ❏ ➢ **What is a pterygium?**

It is a chronic growth over the medial or lateral aspect of the cornea approaching the pupil. It is much thicker than pingueculae.

❏ ❏ ❏ ➢ **What is the most common cause of painless upper GI bleeding in an infant or child?**

Varices from portal hypertension.

❏ ❏ ❏ ➢ **What is the <u>most</u> <u>common</u> cause of major painless lower GI bleeding in an infant or child?**

Meckel's diverticulum.

❏ ❏ ❏ ➢ **Common cause of orbital cellulitis:**

Staph aureus.

❏ ❏ ❏ ➢ **Who should receive prophylaxis after exposure to Neisseria meningitidis?**

People living with the patient or having close intimate contact.

❏ ❏ ❏ ➢ **Name some common hydrocarbons that are considered to be most toxic and**

have SSU's of less than 60.

Aromatic hydrocarbons, halogenated hydrocarbons, mineral seal oil, kerosene, naphtha, turpentine, gasoline and lighter fluid.

Others considered less toxic have SSU's greater than 100, such as grease, diesel oil, mineral oil, petroleum jelly, paraffin wax, and tar.

❐ ❐ ❐ ➢ **What drug is absolutely contraindicated in the treatment of hydrocarbon poisoning?**

Epinephrine as it sensitizes the myocardium, potentially leading to arrest.

❐ ❐ ❐ ➢ **What drug is contraindicated in a glue sniffing patient?**

Epinephrine. Like solvent abusers, these patients may be scared to death.

❐ ❐ ❐ ➢ **What is a delayed complication of acid ingestion?**

Pyloric stricture.

❐ ❐ ❐ ➢ **What is the difference between carbamates and organophosphates?**

Carbamates produce similar symptoms as organophosphates, however, the bonds in carbamate toxicity are reversible.

❐ ❐ ❐ ➢ **What are key signs and symptoms of organophosphate poisoning?**

Ataxia, abdominal pain and cramping, blurred vision, seizures, ataxia and miosis.

❐ ❐ ❐ ➢ **A patient presents with miotic pupils, muscle fasciculations, diaphoresis and diffuse oral and bronchial secretions. The patient has an odor of garlic on his breath. What is your diagnosis?**

Organophosphate poisoning.

❐ ❐ ❐ ➢ **What ECG changes may be associated with organophosphate poisoning?**

Prolongation of the QT interval, and ST and T wave abnormalities.

❐ ❐ ❐ ➢ **What is the key laboratory finding in the diagnosis of organophosphate poisoning?**

An elevated red blood cell cholinesterase level.

❐ ❐ ❐ ➢ **Treatment of organophosphate poisoning?**

Decontaminate, charcoal, atropine and pralidoxime prn.

❐ ❐ ❐ ➢ **What are the key features in the diagnosis of Trench foot?**

Exposure must be for one to two days of wet, cold temperatures above freezing.
Trench foot represents a superficial partial burn with no deep tissue damage.

❏ ❏ ❏ ➤ **What is chilblain?**

Chilblain is prolonged exposure to dry cold.

❏ ❏ ❏ ➤ **At about what core body temperature does shivering cease?**

30 to 32 °C.

❏ ❏ ❏ ➤ **What is the sequence of arrhythmia development in a patient with hypothermia?**

Bradycardia → Atrial fibrillation → Ventricular fibrillation → Asystole.

❏ ❏ ❏ ➤ **What is the common pathogen in a cat bite?**

Pasteurella multocida.

❏ ❏ ❏ ➤ **What would you expect to find in the hippocampus of a patient with rabies?**

Negri bodies. Incubation for rabies is 30 to 60 days. Treatment includes cleaning of the wound, rabies immune globulin, and Human Diploid Cell Vaccine. Remember, 1/2 the rabies immune globulin goes around the wound and the other half goes IM.

❏ ❏ ❏ ➤ **How do you treat the bite of a megalopyge opercularis caterpillar?**

Calcium gluconate, 10 ml of a 10% solution IV.
Stings cause immediate rhythmic pain.

❏ ❏ ❏ ➤ **What is the rumpel-leede phenomenon found in Rocky Mountain Spotted Fever?**

Don't know and don't care.

❏ ❏ ❏ ➤ **What kind of tick transmits Rocky Mountain Spotted Fever?**

The female andersoni tick. It transmits rickettsia rickettsii.

❏ ❏ ❏ ➤ **What is the most common symptom in Rocky Mountain Spotted Fever?**

Headache occurs in 90% of patients.

❏ ❏ ❏ ➤ **Describe the rash of Rocky Mountain Spotted Fever.**

It is a macular rash, 2 to 6 mm in diameter, and located on the wrists and palms, spreading to the soles and trunk.

❏ ❏ ❏ ➤ **What tick transmits Lyme disease?**

The Ixodes dammini tick.
Sphirochete Borrelia burgdorfi is diagnosed by culture on Kelly's medium.

❏ ❏ ❏ ➤ **Describe skin lesion seen in Lyme disease.**

A large distinct circular skin lesion called erythema chronicum migrans. It is an annular erythematous lesion with central clearing.

❏ ❏ ❏ ➤ **Describe a patient with tick paralysis.**

Bulbar paralysis, ascending flaccid paralysis, paresthesias of hands and feet, symmetric loss of deep tendon reflexes and respiratory paralysis.

❏ ❏ ❏ ➤ **What drug is contraindicated in a Gila monster bite?**

Meperidine (Demerol).
(May be synergistic with venom!)

What is the causative organism of otitis externa?

Pseudomonas.

❏ ❏ ❏ ➤ **Signs and symptoms of Lyme Disease, stages I-III:**

I   Erythema Chronicum Migricans.
    Malaise, fatigue, headache, arthralgias, fever, chills.

II Neurologic, cardiac.
    Headache, meningoencephalitis, facial nerve palsy,
    radiculoneuropathy, ophthalmitis and 1°, 2° and 3° AV blocks.

III Arthritis.
    Knee > shoulder > elbow > TMJ > ankle > wrist > hip >hands > feet.

❏ ❏ ❏ ➤ **A diver levels off at 33 feet. How many atmospheres of pressure is he experiencing?**

Two. Sea level is one, 33 feet is two, 66 feet is three, etc.

❏ ❏ ❏ ➤ **After a diver surfaces, she immediately experiences aphasia, paralysis and blindness. Diagnosis?**

Dysbaric air embolism.

❏ ❏ ❏ ➤ **After a blast injury, the most life threatening injury is likely to have occurred where?**

In the lungs.

❒ ❒ ❒ ➢ **Describe the wound resulting from AC .**

AC produces an entrance and exit wound of similar size.
The damage from AC is usually worse than that from DC.

❒ ❒ ❒ ➢ **Describe a DC wound.**

Small entrance wound, large exit wound.

❒ ❒ ❒ ➢ **What type of arrhythmia does lightning produce?**

It is a DC and produces asystole.

❒ ❒ ❒ ➢ **What type of arrhythmia does AC tend to produce?**

Ventricular fibrillation.

❒ ❒ ❒ ➢ **A patient, who works in a plant that makes chemical deodorizers presents after exposure to phenol. Treatment?**

Clean the patient with olive oil and water.

❒ ❒ ❒ ➢ **What are the <u>most</u> <u>common</u> complaints in a patient with carbon monoxide poisoning?**

The <u>most</u> <u>common</u> is headache. Also dizziness, weakness, and nausea.

❒ ❒ ❒ ➢ **What signs and symptoms are expected after radiation exposures of 100 REM, 300 REM, 400 REM and 2000 REM, less than two hours post exposure?**

100 REM produces nausea and vomiting.
300 REM produces erythema.
400 REM produces diarrhea.
2000 REM produces seizures.

❒ ❒ ❒ ➢ **What drug blocks the uptake of radioactive iodine?**

Potassium iodine.

❒ ❒ ❒ ➢ **Psilocybin mushroom is associated with:**

Hallucinations.

❒ ❒ ❒ ➢ **In brain stem herniation is decorticate or decerebrate posturing expected?**

Decerebrate posturing (hyperextension)
Decorticate posturing is flexion of the upper extremities and extension of the lower extremities.

❏ ❏ ❏ ➤ A patient presents after experiencing trauma to the head. The patient has an elevated systolic blood pressure and bradycardia. Diagnosis?

Cushing reflex.

❏ ❏ ❏ ➤ What are the three components to the Glasgow coma scale, and how many points is each worth?

Eye opening (4).
Verbal response (5).
Motor response (6).

❏ ❏ ❏ ➤ What is the name for a flexion mechanism fracture through the anterior aspect of a vertebral body that is associated with ligamentous damage and an anterior cord syndrome?

A teardrop fracture.

❏ ❏ ❏ ➤ Describe the corneal reflex.

Conducted by the ophthalmic branch of the 5th nerve and the afferent branch of the facial (7th) nerve.

❏ ❏ ❏ ➤ What is the most unstable cervical spine injury?

Rupture of transverse atlantal ligament > dens fracture > burst fracture (flexion teardrop) > bilateral facet dislocation.

❏ ❏ ❏ ➤ What is the eponym for a C1 burst fracture from vertical compression?

Jefferson fracture.

❏ ❏ ❏ ➤ A patient in a motor vehicle accident sustains a hyperextension injury of the neck. Plain films reveal a C2 bilateral facet fracture through the pedicles. You describe this fracture in consultation with the neurosurgeon. What type of fracture have you described?

A Hangman's fracture.

❏ ❏ ❏ ➤ A patient has an avulsion fracture of the spinous process of C7 with a history of a hyperflexion mechanism. Diagnosis?

Clay shoveller's fracture - fracture involving the spinous process of C6, C7, or T1. The mechanism is usually flexion or a direct blow.

❏ ❏ ❏ ➤ A patient suffers a bilateral interfacetal dislocation. What is your concern?

Injury occurs as a result of flexion and is very unstable with ligament disruption.

❏ ❏ ❏ ➤ What is the most unstable <u>fracture</u> of the cervical spine?

A dens fracture with rupture of the atlantal ligament.

❐ ❐ ❐ ➢ **Stable or unstable: a Clay shoveller's fracture?**

Stable.

❐ ❐ ❐ ➢ **Stable or unstable: fracture of the posterior arch of C1?**

Stable.

❐ ❐ ❐ ➢ **Name the four stable cervical spine fractures.**

Simple wedge.
Clay shovelers.
Pillar.
C1 posterior neural arch.
The rest are unstable or potentially unstable!

❐ ❐ ❐ ➢ **A patient presents with a history of a blow to the forehead. Her neck was hyperextended. Patient complains of weakness in the arms with minimal weakness in the lower extremities. Diagnosis?**

Central cord syndrome.

❐ ❐ ❐ ➢ **You see a patient with an obvious traumatic spinal cord lesion. On physical exam, he has motor paralysis, loss of gross proprioception and loss of vibratory sensation on one side, and loss of pain and temperature sensation on the opposite side. Diagnosis?**

Brown-Séquard's syndrome.

❐ ❐ ❐ ➢ **What is the most common cause of shock in patients with blunt chest trauma?**

Pelvic (or extremity) fracture.

❐ ❐ ❐ ➢ **What is a frequent complication of ethmoid sinusitis?**

Orbital cellulitis.

❐ ❐ ❐ ➢ **What is the most common site of aspiration pneumonitis?**

Right lower lobe.

❐ ❐ ❐ ➢ **What is the most common ECG finding associated with a myocardial contusion?**

ST-T wave abnormalities.

❐ ❐ ❐ ➢ **What is the most common valvular injury associated with blunt cardiac injury?**

A ruptured aortic valve.

❏ ❏ ❏ ➤ **What is the most common site of a traumatic aortic laceration?**

The vast majority occur just distal to the left subclavian artery.

❏ ❏ ❏ ➤ **What is the most common x-ray finding in traumatic rupture of the aorta?**

Widening of the superior mediastinum.

❏ ❏ ❏ ➤ **What is the most accurate x-ray finding in traumatic rupture of the aorta?**

Rightward deviation of the esophagus more than 1 - 2 cm.

❏ ❏ ❏ ➤ **A patient presents with a history of high speed traumatic injury to the chest. On physical exam, a systolic murmur over the precordium is auscultated The patient has a slightly hoarse voice. The nurse tells you the pulse is also stronger in the upper extremities. Diagnosis?**

Traumatic rupture of the aorta.

❏ ❏ ❏ ➤ **A patient presents with a history of chest trauma, a systolic murmur and an infarct pattern on ECG. Diagnosis?**

Traumatic ventricular septal defect.

❏ ❏ ❏ ➤ **A person with a history of a motor vehicle accident has x-ray findings of retroperitoneal air seen on a flat plate of the abdomen. What is a likely diagnosis?**

Duodenal injury. Tentative test is a contrast study. Extravasation confirms a duodenal injury.

❏ ❏ ❏ ➤ **On an x-ray of the hand, the AP view shows a triangular shaped lunate. Diagnosis?**

Lunate dislocation.
Lateral films will show a cup spilling out water.

❏ ❏ ❏ ➤ **What x-ray view is required to diagnose a perilunate dislocation?**

Lateral view.

❏ ❏ ❏ ➤ **A patient presents describing a snapping sensation in the wrist and a click. Diagnosis:**

Scaphoid dislocation.

❏ ❏ ❏ ➤ **X-ray of the hand reveals a 3 mm space between the scaphoid and the lunate. Diagnosis?**

Scaphoid dislocation.

❏ ❏ ❏ ➤ **In a boxer's fracture, how much angulation of the 5th metacarpal neck is acceptable.**

45 degrees.

❏ ❏ ❏ ➤ **What ligament in the hand is commonly injured in a fall while skiing?**

Thumb MCP joint ulnar collateral ligament rupture.

❏ ❏ ❏ ➤ **Posterior dislocation of the shoulder is often missed with a standard issue radiographic shoulder series. What x-ray view aids in diagnosis?**

The "Y" view.

❏ ❏ ❏ ➤ **Name the four muscles of the rotator cuff.**

Supraspinatus, infraspinatus, teres minor and the subscapularis. Patients with a rotator cuff tear will not be able to fully abduct or to internally or externally rotate the arm normally.

❏ ❏ ❏ ➤ **What is the usual mechanism of injury in a supracondylar fracture?**

A fall on the outstretched arm.

❏ ❏ ❏ ➤ **What artery is commonly injured with a supracondylar fracture?**

Brachial artery.

❏ ❏ ❏ ➤ **What nerve is commonly injured with a supracondylar fracture?**

The median nerve.

❏ ❏ ❏ ➤ **Elbow. X-ray. Anterior fat pad sign! Diagnosis?**

Radial head fracture.

❏ ❏ ❏ ➤ **What nerve injury is associated with a medial epicondyle fracture?**

Ulnar nerve.

❏ ❏ ❏ ➤ **Type I pelvic fracture?**

Fracture of individual pelvic bone without a break in the pelvic ring.

❏ ❏ ❏ ➤ **Type II pelvic fracture?**

Single fracture of the pelvic ring.

❏ ❏ ❏ ➢ **Type III pelvic fracture?**

Double break in the pelvic ring. This is an unstable fracture.

❏ ❏ ❏ ➢ **What is the characteristic x-ray finding of a Type IV fracture of the pelvis?**

Fracture of the acetabulum.

❏ ❏ ❏ ➢ **About how many liters of blood can a patient lose in the retroperitoneal space?**

About 4 liters.

❏ ❏ ❏ ➢ **Which type of pelvic fracture has the greatest amount of bleeding?**

Type III. There is a double break in the pelvic ring.

❏ ❏ ❏ ➢ **A patient presents to the emergency department with a history of a limp. Physical exam reveals pain with extension and abduction of the hip. Diagnosis?**

Greater trochanteric fracture, the result of an avulsion at the insertion site of the gluteus medius.

❏ ❏ ❏ ➢ **A patient presents with a history of hearing an audible pop in the knee and ankle as he fell. Diagnosis?**

Tear of the anterior cruciate and Achilles tendon rupture.

❏ ❏ ❏ ➢ **What nerve may be injured with a knee dislocation?**

The peroneal nerve.

❏ ❏ ❏ ➢ **What is the most common site of a stress fracture in the foot?**

Second and third metatarsal.

❏ ❏ ❏ ➢ **What is the most frequent cause of superior vena cava obstruction?**

Bronchogenic carcinoma.

❏ ❏ ❏ ➢ **What is the most common level of malignant spinal cord compression?**

Thoracic.

❏ ❏ ❏ ➢ **What is the most common site of bursitis?**

Olecranon.

❏ ❏ ❏ ➢ **What is the most common cause of subarachnoid hemorrhage in teenagers?**

AV malformations.

❏ ❏ ❏ ➢ **A patient presents with a painful, red eye and a decrease in visual acuity. What is the differential?**

Central corneal lesions, glaucoma, and iritis.

❏ ❏ ❏ ➢ **What is the most common symptom of acute mesenteric ischemia?**

Abdominal pain.

❏ ❏ ❏ ➢ **Where does pulmonary embolism rank in terms of lethality in the United States?**

It is the third most common cause of death in the United States.
About 650,000 cases occur annually with overall mortality of 8%.

❏ ❏ ❏ ➢ **What are the most common findings of osteomyelitis on x-ray?**

Periosteal elevation and demineralization.

❏ ❏ ❏ ➢ **For what conditions is hydralazine commonly used?**

Treatment of preeclampsia and eclampsia.

❏ ❏ ❏ ➢ **What is the most common cause of acute aortic regurgitation?**

Infectious endocarditis.

❏ ❏ ❏ ➢ **What is the most common congenital valvular disease?**

Bicuspid aortic valve.

❏ ❏ ❏ ➢ **What infarct is most commonly associated with acute mitral regurgitation?**

Inferior wall.

❏ ❏ ❏ ➢ **What metabolic abnormality is commonly associated with hypercalcemia?**

Up to 1/3 will have hypokalemia.

❏ ❏ ❏ ➢ **What form of hepatitis is most commonly transmitted through blood transfusions?**

Hepatitis C.

❏ ❏ ❏ ➢ **On funduscopic exam, microaneurysms and soft exudates are typical of:**

Hypertension.

❏ ❏ ❏ ➤ **On funduscopic exam, macular microaneurysms and hard exudates are typical of:**

Diabetes.

❏ ❏ ❏ ➤ **In a patient with retrobulbar optic neuritis, what is the most likely cause?**

Multiple sclerosis.

❏ ❏ ❏ ➤ **How is pancuronium reversed?**

Atropine and neostigmine.

❏ ❏ ❏ ➤ **What paralyzing drug typically causes transient hyperkalemia?**

Succinylcholine.

❏ ❏ ❏ ➤ **What are the contraindications to succinylcholine use?**

Rhabdomyolysis, narrow angle glaucoma, neurologic disorders, renal failure, myopathies, muscle trauma and burns.

❏ ❏ ❏ ➤ **What are the initial symptoms of a patient with hypocalcemia?**

Paresthesias around the mouth and fingertips, irritability, hyperactive deep tendon reflexes and seizures.

❏ ❏ ❏ ➤ **What ECG change is associated with hypocalcemia?**

Prolonged T waves.

❏ ❏ ❏ ➤ **A patient is digitalis toxic. What electrolytes will need to be replaced?**

It is important to replace potassium and magnesium.

❏ ❏ ❏ ➤ **What EKG changes are expected in hypokalemia?**

Low voltage QRS.
Flattening of T waves.
Depressed ST segment.
Prominent P and U waves.
Prolonged QT and PR intervals

❏ ❏ ❏ ➤ **What ECG changes may be seen in hyperkalemia?**

Tall or peaked T waves.
Prolonged QT and PR intervals.
Diminished P wave amplitude.

Depressed ST segments.
QRS widening.

❒ ❒ ❒ ➢ **What ECG findings are anticipated with hypercalcemia?**

Depressed ST segments.
Widened T waves.
Decreased QT intervals.
Bradycardia.
BBBs leading to 2° and 3° heart blocks.

❒ ❒ ❒ ➢ **What ECG findings suggest hypomagnesemia?**

Prolonged QT and PR intervals.
Widened QRS.
Depressed ST segments.
Inverted T waves.

❒ ❒ ❒ ➢ **What is the most common complication of verapamil and how should it be treated?**

Hypotension, treated with calcium gluconate IV over several minutes.

❒ ❒ ❒ ➢ **Third degree heart block is often seen in what type of myocardial infarction?**

Acute anterior wall myocardial infarction.

❒ ❒ ❒ ➢ **What is the most common arrhythmia associated with Wolff-Parkinson-White syndrome?**

PAT. The patient presents with angina, syncope, and shortness of breath.

❒ ❒ ❒ ➢ **How may mydriasis caused by mydriatics and anticholinergic drugs be distinguished from those caused third cranial nerve compression?**

Pilocarpine. Pilocarpine will reverse cranial nerve compression but will have no effect on anticholinergic drugs or mydriatics.

❒ ❒ ❒ ➢ **During CPR, the mean cardiac index is what percentage of normal?**

25%.

❒ ❒ ❒ ➢ **Outline treatment of atrial flutter.**

Cardioversion 25 to 50 joules, verapamil, digoxin, propranolol, procainamide, and quinidine.

❒ ❒ ❒ ➢ **How should atrial fibrillation be treated?**

Procainamide, digoxin, verapamil, and propranolol.
Cardioversion with 100 to 200 joules.

❏ ❏ ❏ ➢ **Why is verapamil a bad choice to treat ventricular tachycardia?**

Verapamil could increase heart rate and decrease blood pressure, without converting the rhythm.

❏ ❏ ❏ ➢ **What drugs should never be used in atrial fibrillation with Wolff-Parkinson-White?**

Digitalis, verapamil, and phenytoin.
Atrial fibrillation with Wolff-Parkinson-White should be treated with cardioversion or procainamide.

SVT with Wolff-Parkinson-White should be treated with verapamil or adenosine.

❏ ❏ ❏ ➢ **What does VVI mean?**

Ventricular pace, ventricular sense, and inhibited.

❏ ❏ ❏ ➢ **What complications can result from excessive lidocaine administration?**

Seizures and methemoglobinemia.

❏ ❏ ❏ ➢ **Name the drug of choice for Wolff-Parkinson-White with atrial flutter or fibrillation?**

Procainamide.

❏ ❏ ❏ ➢ **What makes the first heart sound?**

Closure of the mitral valve and left ventricular contraction.

❏ ❏ ❏ ➢ **What makes the second heart sound?**

Closure of the pulmonary and aortic valves.

❏ ❏ ❏ ➢ **What is the cause of the third heart sound.**

This is caused by the deceleration of blood flowing into the ventricle when the ventricle reaches its final stages of filling.

❏ ❏ ❏ ➢ **What is the cause of the fourth heart sound?**

It is caused by vibrations of the left ventricular muscle, the mitral valve and the left ventricular flow tract.

❏ ❏ ❏ ➢ **What is a common pathologic cause of an S_3?**

Congestive heart failure.

❒ ❒ ❒ ➤ **What is the pathologic cause of an S₄?**

Often decreased left ventricular compliance due to acute ischemia.
Other causes include: aortic stenosis, subaortic stenosis, HTN, coronary artery disease, myocardiopathy, anemia and hyperthyroidism.

❒ ❒ ❒ ➤ **What is the chief effect of dopamine and what is the chief complication of dopamine?**

The chief effect is prompt elevation of blood pressure with ß-adrenergic effects at low doses and α–adrenergic effects at high doses.
The primary complication is tachycardia which unfortunately, increases myocardial oxygen demand.

❒ ❒ ❒ ➤ **What is the chief effect of dobutamine?**

Dobutamine increases the cardiac contractility. It has only minor effects on peripheral α–receptors.
It can increase cardiac output without increasing blood pressure.

❒ ❒ ❒ ➤ **What effect does morphine have on preload and afterload?**

Morphine decreases both preload and afterload.

❒ ❒ ❒ ➤ **Does furosemide affect preload or afterload?**

Furosemide decreases preload.

❒ ❒ ❒ ➤ **What is the most common cause of post splenectomy sepsis?**

Streptococcus pneumonia.

❒ ❒ ❒ ➤ **What laboratory findings are expected in a child with pyloric stenosis?**

Hypokalemia, hypochloremia, and metabolic alkalosis.

❒ ❒ ❒ ➤ **What is the most common cause of tricuspid regurgitation?**

Right heart failure secondary to left heart failure, typically caused by mitral stenosis.

❒ ❒ ❒ ➤ **What drug is preferred to treat hypertension in a patient with renal failure?**

Labetalol (metabolized in the liver).

❒ ❒ ❒ ➤ **Treatment for a propranolol overdose?**

Glucagon.

❒ ❒ ❒ ➤ **Preferred treatment for a patient with hypertensive encephalopathy?**

Nitroprusside and labetalol.

❑ ❑ ❑ ➢ **What x-ray findings may occassionally be seen in ischemic bowel disease?**

"Thumb" printing on the plain film and a ground glass appearance with absence of bowel gas.

❑ ❑ ❑ ➢ **A patient with currant jelly sputum is likely to have what type of pneumonia?**

Klebsiella or type 3 Pneumococcus.

❑ ❑ ❑ ➢ **What two diseases does the deer tick, Ixodes dammini, transmit?**

Lyme disease and Babesia.

❑ ❑ ❑ ➢ **How do patients present with Babesia infection?**

Intermittent fever, splenomegaly, jaundice, and hemolysis. The disease may be fatal in patients without spleens. The disease can simulate rickettsial diseases like Rocky Mountain spotted fever. Treatment is with clindamycin and quinine.

❑ ❑ ❑ ➢ **Time for a food question! There are 9 questions in this book that deal with either strawberry tongue, strawberry cervix, currant jelly sputum or currant jelly stool. Describe the pathology associated with each of these.**

Strawberry tongue - Scarlet fever, Kawasaki's disease.
Strawberry cervix - Trichomonas.
Currant jelly sputum - Klebsiella, less commonly type 3 Pneumococcus.
Currant jelly stool - Intussusception.

❑ ❑ ❑ ➢ **What is the most frequently transmitted tick-borne disease?**

Lyme disease.
Causative agent - spirochete Borrelia burgdorferi.
Vector - Ixodes dammini (deer tick) also I. pacificus, Amblyomma americanum, and Dermacentor variabilis.

❑ ❑ ❑ ➢ **What is the second most common tick borne disease?**

Rocky Mountain spotted fever.
Causative agent - Rickettsia rickettsii.
Vector - Female Ixodid ticks Dermacentor andersonii (wood tick) and D. variabilis (American dog tick).

❑ ❑ ❑ ➢ **If you melt enough dry ice, can you swim without getting wet?**

Probably not!

BIBLIOGRAPHY

BOOKS:

Adler, J.N. & Plantz, S.H. Emergency Medicine Pearls of Wisdom (1st Ed.). 1993.

Advanced Cardiac Life Support. Dallas: American Heart Association, 1987.

Advanced Trauma Life Support. Chicago: American College of Surgeons, 1990.

Anderson, J.E. Grant's Atlas of Anatomy (8th Ed.). Baltimore: Williams & Wilkins, 1983.

Auerbach, P.S. Management of Wilderness and Environmental Emergencies (2nd Ed.). St. Louis: C.V. Mosby Company, 1989.

Bakerman, S. A B C'S of Interpretive Laboratory Data (2nd Ed.). Greenville: Interpretive Laboratory Data, Inc., 1984.

Barkin, R.M. Emergency Pediatrics (3rd Ed.). St. Louis: C.V. Mosby Company, 1990.

Berkow, R. The Merck Manual (15th Ed.). Rahway: Merck Sharp & Dohme Research Laboratories, 1987.

Bork, K. Diagnosis and Treatment of Common Skin Diseases. Philadelphia: W.B. Saunders Company, 1988.

Bryson, P.D. Comprehensive Review in Toxicology (2nd Ed.) Aspen Publishers, Inc., 1989

DeGowin, E.L. Bedside Diagnostic Examination (4th Ed.). New York: Macmillan Publishing Co. Inc., 1981.

Fitzpatrick, T.B. Color Atlas and Synopsis of Clinical Dermatology. New York: McGraw-Hill Publishing Company, 1990.

Harris, J.H. The Radiology of Emergency Medicine (2nd Ed.). Baltimore: Williams and Wilkins, 1981.

Harrison, T.R. Principles of Internal Medicine (11th Ed.). New York: McGraw-Hill Book Company, 1987.

Harwood-Nuss, A. The Clinical Practice of Emergency Medicine. Philadelphia: J.B. Lippincott Company, 1991.

Hoppenfeld, S. Physical Examination of the Spine and Extremities. Norwalk: Appleton-Century-Crofts, 1976.

Leaverton, P.E. A Review of Biostatistics (3rd Ed.). Boston: Little Brown and Company, 1986.

Marriott, H.J.L. Practical Electrocardiography (7th Ed.). Baltimore: Williams and Wilkins, 1983.

Moore, K.L. Clinically Oriented Anatomy. Baltimore: Williams & Wilkins, 1982.

Perkins, E.S. An Atlas nf Diseases of the Eye (3rd Ed.). London: Churchill Livingstone, 1986.

Physicians' Desk Reference (44th Ed.). Oradell: Medical Economics Company Inc., 1990.

Plantz, SH. Emergency Medicine PreTest, Self-Assessment and Review, McGraw- Hill, 1990.

Plantz, S.H. & Adler, J.N. Emergency Medicine Pearls of Wisdom, Second Edition. Boston: Harvard Medical School and Watertown: Mount Auburn Press, 1993.

Rivers, C.S. Preparing for the Written Board Exam in Emergency Medicine. Milford: Emergency Medicine Educational Enterprises, Inc. 1992.

Robbins, S.L. Pathologic Basis of Disease (3rd Ed.). Philadelphia: W.B. Saunders Company, 1984.

Rosen, P. Emergency Medicine Concepts and Clinical Practice (3rd Ed.). St. Louis: Mosby Year Book, 1992.

Rowe, R.C. The Harriet Lane Handbook (11th Ed.). Chicago: Year Book Medical Publishers, Inc., 1987.

Simon, R.R. Emergency Orthopedics The Extremities (2nd Ed.). Norwalk: Appleton & Lange, 1987.

Simon, R.R. Emergency Procedures and Techniques (2nd Ed.). Baltimore: Williams and Wilkins, 1987.

Slaby, F. Radiographic Anatomy. New York: John Wiley & Sons, 1990.

Squire, L.F. Fundamentals of Radiology (3rd Ed.). Cambridge: Harvard University Press, 1982.

Stedman, T.L. Illustrated Stedman's Medical Dictionary (24th Ed.). Baltimore: Williams & Wilkins, 1982.

Stewart, C.E. Environmental Emergencies. Baltimore: Williams and Wilkins, 1990.

Textbook of Pediatric Advanced Life Support. Dallas: American Heart Association, 1988.

The Hand Examination and Diagnosis (2nd Ed.). London: Churchill Livingstone, 1983.

The Hand Primary Care of Common Problems (2nd Ed.). London: Churchill Livingstone, 1990.

Tintinalli, J.E. Emergency Medicine A Comprehensive Study Guide (3rd Ed.). New York: McGraw-Hill, Inc., 1992.

Weinberg, S. Color Atlas of Pediatric Dermatology (2nd Ed.). New York: McGraw-Hill, 1990.

Weiner, H.L. Neurology for the House Officer (4th Ed.). Baltimore: Williams & Wilkins, 1989.

Wilkins, E. W. Emergency Medicine (3rd Ed.). Baltimore: Williams & Wilkins, 1989.

COURSES:

Eye Emergencies, Chicago, IL 1991.

ENT Emergencies, Chicago, IL 1991.

CRIT Course, Springfield, MA 1992.

Emergency Medicine Board Review, Chicago, IL 1991.

Emergency Medicine Specialty Review, Chicago, IL 1991.

Emergency Medicine Interactive Review, Boca Raton, FL 1992.

Emergency Medicine Board Review, Columbus, OH 1992.